Phlebotomy
Principles and Practice

Jahangir Moini, MD, MPH
Professor of Allied Health Sciences
Everest University
Melbourne, FL

Reviewers

Deyal Riley, CHI, CPT
Instructor of Phlebotomy
Washtenaw Community College
Phlebotomy Education Inc.

Michael Paulson
Critical Care Flight Paramedic
Director of Education/Owner
Allied Healthcare Educator
Subject Matter Expert
Trinity Medical Academy, Inc.
New Port Richey, FL

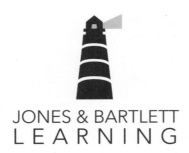

JONES & BARTLETT
LEARNING

World Headquarters
Jones & Bartlett Learning
5 Wall Street
Burlington, MA 01803
978-443-5000
info@jblearning.com
www.jblearning.com

Jones & Bartlett Learning books and products are available through most bookstores and online booksellers. To contact Jones & Bartlett Learning directly, call 800-832-0034, fax 978-443-8000, or visit our website, www.jblearning.com.

Substantial discounts on bulk quantities of Jones & Bartlett Learning publications are available to corporations, professional associations, and other qualified organizations. For details and specific discount information, contact the special sales department at Jones & Bartlett Learning via the above contact information or send an email to specialsales@jblearning.com.

Phlebotomy: Principles and Practice is an independent publication and has not been authorized, sponsored, or otherwise approved by the owners of the trademarks or service marks referenced in this product.

Some images in this book feature models. These models do not necessarily endorse, represent, or participate in the activities represented in the images.

This publication is designed to provide accurate and authoritative information in regard to the Subject Matter covered. It is sold with the understanding that the publisher is not engaged in rendering legal, accounting, or other professional service. If legal advice or other expert assistance is required, the service of a competent professional person should be sought.

Production Credits

Publisher: William Brottmiller
Executive Editor: Cathy L. Esperti
Senior Acquisitions Editor: Joseph Morita
Managing Editor: Maro Gartside
Production Manager: Tracey McCrea
Marketing Manager: Grace Richards
Manufacturing and Inventory Control Supervisor: Amy Bacus

Composition: Publishers' Design and Production Services, Inc.
Cover Design: Kristin E. Parker
Rights & Photo Researcher: Sarah Cebulski
Cover Image: Blood cells: © Sashkin/ShutterStock, Inc.; Test tubes: © Rob Bouwman/ShutterStock, Inc.
Printing and Binding: Manufactured in the Unites States by RR Donnell
Cover Printing: Manufactured in the United States by RR Donnelley

To order this product, use ISBN: 1-978-1-7637-5260-9

Library of Congress Cataloging-in-Publication Data
Moini, Jahangir, 1942–
    Phlebotomy : principles and practice / Jahangir Moini.
        p. ; cm.
    Includes bibliographical references and index.
    ISBN 978-0-7637-9906-9 (pbk.)
    I. Title.
    [DNLM: 1. Phlebotomy—methods. 2. Hematologic Tests. 3. Specimen Handling—methods. QY 25]
    616.07'561—dc23
                                                                2011052779

6048

Printed in the United States of America
17 16 15   10 9 8 7 6 5 4 3

Brief Table of Contents

Chapter 1 Introduction to Phlebotomy 1

Chapter 2 Fundamentals of the Medical Laboratory 9

Chapter 3 Communication Skills for Phlebotomists 15

Chapter 4 Terminology and Abbreviations 23

Chapter 5 Anatomy and Physiology of the Cardiovascular System 35

Chapter 6 Common Disorders and Conditions Related to Phlebotomy 53

Chapter 7 Hematology, Hemostasis, Blood Types, and Transfusions 63

Chapter 8 Clinical Chemistry and Serology Tests 77

Chapter 9 Microbiology 83

Chapter 10 Safety, Infection Control, and Standard Precautions 93

Chapter 11 Phlebotomy Equipment 109

Chapter 12 Phlebotomy Procedures 123

Chapter 13 Specimen Collections and Special Procedures 141

Chapter 14 Specialized Phlebotomy 153

Chapter 15 Complications of Phlebotomy 161

Chapter 16 Urinalysis and Non-blood Specimens 167

Chapter 17 Specimen Handling and Transport 179

Chapter 18 Compliance 187

Chapter 19 Computer Technology 193

Appendix A Units of Measurement and Conversion Tables 201

Appendix B Common Laboratory Tests 203

Appendix C NAACLS Phlebotomy Competencies   207

Appendix D Reference Laboratory Values   211

Appendix E ABC Laboratories Blood Transfusion Consent Form   213

Appendix F Military Time   215

Answer Key   217

Glossary   221

Index   233

Credits   249

Table of Contents

Reviewers   xi

About the Author   xiii

Dedication   xv

Acknowledgments   xvii

Preface   xix

Chapter 1   Introduction to Phlebotomy   1
Outline   **1**
Objectives   **1**
Key Terms   **1**
Introduction   **2**
The History of Phlebotomy   **2**
Becoming a Successful Phlebotomist   **2**
Roles and Responsibilities of
   Phlebotomists   **3**
Phlebotomy Education and Certification   **3**
Legal and Ethical Issues   **3**
Rules and Regulations   **4**
   Clinical and Laboratory Standards
      Institute   **4**
   Clinical Laboratory Improvement Act   **4**
   National Accrediting Agency for Clinical
      Laboratory Sciences   **4**
   Joint Commission   **4**
   College of American Pathologists   **4**
   State Board of Health   **4**
Classifications of Law   **4**
   Civil Law   **4**
   Criminal Law   **5**
   Preventive Law   **5**
   Ethics   **5**
Patient Self-Determination Act   **5**
Patient's Bill of Rights   **6**
Quality Assurance and Quality Control   **6**
   Quality Assurance Guidelines   **6**

   Quality Control Guidelines   **6**
Summary   **7**
Critical Thinking   **7**
Websites   **8**
Review Questions   **8**

Chapter 2   Fundamentals of the Medical
Laboratory   9
Outline   **9**
Objectives   **9**
Key Terms   **9**
Introduction   **9**
The Medical Laboratory   **9**
   Laboratory Divisions   **10**
   Laboratory Staff   **11**
   Laboratory Hazards   **12**
Professionalism   **12**
Record Keeping   **12**
Summary   **12**
Critical Thinking   **12**
Websites   **12**
Review Questions   **12**

Chapter 3   Communication Skills for
Phlebotomists   15
Outline   **15**
Objectives   **15**
Key Terms   **15**
Introduction   **15**
The Communication Cycle   **15**
Types of Communication   **16**
   Verbal Communication   **16**
   Nonverbal Communication   **17**
   Written Communication   **18**
   Telephone and Computer
      Communication   **18**
Improving Your Communication Skills   **19**

Interactions with Other
    Individuals   **19**
Barriers to Communication   **20**
Defense Mechanisms   **20**
Summary   **20**
Critical Thinking   **20**
Websites   **21**
Review Questions   **21**

Chapter 4   Terminology and
              Abbreviations   23
Outline   **23**
Objectives   **23**
Introduction   **23**
The Language of Medicine   **23**
    Word Roots   **23**
    Prefixes   **23**
    Suffixes   **23**
    Combining Forms   **26**
Common Medical Terminology Related
    to the Cardiovascular System   **26**
    Common Terms Related to the
        Cardiovascular System   **26**
    Common Terms Related to
        Anatomy and Physiology   **29**
    Cardiovascular
        System—Abbreviations   **29**
    Laboratory and
        Phlebotomy—Abbreviations   **30**
Summary   **32**
Critical Thinking   **32**
Websites   **32**
Review Questions   **33**

Chapter 5   Anatomy and Physiology of the
              Cardiovascular System   35
Outline   **35**
Objectives   **35**
Key Terms   **35**
Introduction   **36**
The Heart   **37**
    Structures of the Heart   **38**
    Conduction System   **40**
    Functions of the Heart   **41**
The Blood Vessels and
    Circulation   **41**
    Blood Vessels   **41**
    Blood Pressure   **43**
    Blood Circulation   **44**
Summary   **48**

Critical Thinking   **51**
Websites   **51**
Review Questions   **51**

Chapter 6   Common Disorders and
              Conditions Related to
              Phlebotomy   53
Outline   **53**
Objectives   **53**
Key Terms   **53**
Introduction   **54**
Cardiovascular Disorders   **54**
    Coronary Artery Disease   **54**
    Angina Pectoris   **54**
    Myocardial Infarction   **55**
    Cardiac Arrhythmias   **55**
    Hypertension   **55**
    Cardiomyopathy   **56**
    Carditis   **56**
    Heart Failure   **56**
    Cardiac Arrest   **56**
    Pulmonary Edema   **56**
    Rheumatic Fever   **56**
    Valvular Heart Disease   **56**
    Mitral Valve Prolapse   **56**
    Shock   **56**
Blood Vessel Disorders   **57**
    Atherosclerosis   **57**
    Arteriosclerosis   **57**
    Emboli   **57**
    Aneurysms   **57**
    Phlebitis   **57**
    Thrombophlebitis   **57**
    Varicose Veins   **58**
Blood Disorders   **58**
    Anemias   **58**
    Polycythemia   **59**
    Hemochromatosis   **59**
    Leukemias   **59**
    Lymphatic Diseases   **60**
    Transfusion Incompatibility
        Reaction   **60**
    Clotting Disorders   **60**
Summary   **61**
Critical Thinking   **61**
Websites   **61**
Review Questions   **61**

Chapter 7   Hematology   63
  Outline   63
  Objectives   63
  Key Terms   63
  Introduction   64
  Hematology   64
    Red Blood Cells   65
    White Blood Cells   66
    Platelets   69
    Plasma   69
  Hemostasis   70
    Serum   71
    Plasma   71
  Appearance of Serum and
    Plasma   72
    Blood Clotting   72
  Blood Types and Transfusions   73
  Summary   75
  Critical Thinking   76
  Websites   76
  Review Questions   76

Chapter 8   Clinical Chemistry and Serology
    Tests   77
  Outline   77
  Objectives   77
  Key Terms   77
  Introduction   78
  Specimen Requirements   78
  Chemistry Panels or Profiles   78
    Hepatic Profile   78
    Renal Profile   78
    Lipid Profile   78
    Cardiac Profile   80
    Thyroid Profile   80
  Glucose Testing   80
  Serology and Immunology Tests   80
    Rapid Tests   80
    Common Serology Tests   80
  Drug Testing   80
  Summary   81
  Critical Thinking   81
  Websites   81
  Review Questions   81

Chapter 9   Microbiology   83
  Outline   83
  Objectives   83
  Key Terms   83

  Introduction   84
  Microorganisms   84
  Classifications of
    Microorganisms   84
    Bacteria   84
    Viruses   87
    Fungi   87
    Protozoa   87
  Microbial Growth   87
  Microbes and the Human Body   88
  Microscope   88
    Structure   88
    Protection   89
  Summary   89
  Critical Thinking   90
  Websites   90
  Review Questions   90

Chapter 10   Safety, Infection Control, and
    Standard Precautions   93
  Outline   93
  Objectives   93
  Key Terms   93
  Introduction   94
  Physical Hazards   94
    Fire Hazards   95
    Electrical Hazards   96
    Mechanical Hazards   96
    Chemical Hazards   96
    Disposal of Chemicals   98
    Chemical Spill Cleanup   98
  Patient Safety Related to Latex
    Products   99
  Infection Control   100
    Pathogens and Infections   100
    Nosocomial Infections   100
  Chain of Infection   101
    Infectious Agent   101
    Reservoir Host   101
    Portal of Exit   101
    Mode of Transmission   101
    Portal of Entry   102
    Susceptible Host   102
  Standard Precautions   102
    Biologic Hazards   102
    Blood-borne Pathogens
      Standard   102
    Disposal of Hazardous
      Wastes   103

Safety Showers and the Eyewash Station **103**

Sharps/Needlestick Injury Prevention **104**

Exposure Control **104**

Prevention of Disease Transmission **104**

Hand Washing **104**

Sanitization **105**

Disinfection **106**

Sterilization **106**

Decontamination **106**

Cardiopulmonary Resuscitation **106**

Summary **106**

Critical Thinking **107**

Websites **107**

Review Questions **107**

Chapter 11 Phlebotomy Equipment 109

Outline **109**

Objectives **109**

Key Terms **109**

Introduction **110**

Types of Equipment **110**

Gloves **110**

Other Personal Protective Equipment **110**

Tourniquets **111**

Venoscopes **111**

Antiseptics **111**

Evacuated Tubes **111**

Needle Holders **112**

Additive and Nonadditive Tubes **112**

Anticoagulants **113**

Syringes **114**

Needles **115**

Butterfly Collection Systems **116**

Lancets **117**

Micropipettes **117**

Microcollection Tubes **117**

Gauze Pads **117**

Bandages **118**

Centrifuge **118**

Blood-Drawing Chair **118**

Infant Phlebotomy Station **119**

Specimen Collection Trays **119**

Sharps Containers **120**

Needle Safety **120**

Summary **121**

Critical Thinking **121**

Websites **121**

Review Questions **122**

Chapter 12 Phlebotomy Procedures 123

Outline **123**

Objectives **123**

Key Terms **123**

Introduction **124**

Requisitions **124**

Patient Preparation **124**

Preparing for the Venipuncture **127**

Performing the Venipuncture **127**

The Order of the Draw **128**

Venipuncture with the Evacuated Tube Method **128**

Venipuncture with the Syringe Method **132**

Venipuncture with the Butterfly Set (Winged Infusion Set) **133**

Performing Capillary Puncture **134**

Routine Capillary Puncture **134**

Heel Puncture in Infants **134**

Finger Punctures **136**

Postcollection Specimen Handling **137**

Routine Blood Film (Smear) **139**

Specimen Recollection **139**

Summary **139**

Critical Thinking **139**

Websites **139**

Review Questions **140**

Chapter 13 Specimen Collections and Special Procedures 141

Outline **141**

Objectives **141**

Key Terms **141**

Introduction **142**

Glucose Testing **142**

Glucose Tolerance Testing **142**

Fasting Blood Glucose Test **143**

A 2-h Postprandial Blood Glucose Level Test **144**

Hemoglobin (HbA1c) Testing **144**

Timed Specimens **144**

Fasting **145**

Platelet Function Assay **145**

Blood Donation **146**

Therapeutic Collection **147**
Chain of Custody **147**
Specimen Tampering **147**
Blood Alcohol Testing **147**
Employee Testing **147**
Athletic Testing **149**
Forensic Specimens **149**
Toxicology **149**
Therapeutic Drug Monitoring **149**
Alternative Collection Sites **150**
  Arterial Punctures **150**
  Venous Access Devices **150**
Summary **151**
Critical Thinking **151**
Websites **151**
Review Questions **151**

Chapter 14 Specialized Phlebotomy 153
Outline **153**
Objectives **153**
Key Terms **153**
Introduction **153**
Pediatric Phlebotomy **154**
Special Neonatal Blood Collection and
  Screening **154**
Blood Spot Collection **155**
Geriatric Phlebotomy **155**
  Venipuncture Procedures **155**
Blood Cultures **156**
Arterial Blood Gases **156**
Phlebotomy for Anticoagulated
  Patients **158**
Phlebotomy for Obese Patients **159**
Phlebotomy for Psychiatric
  Patients **159**
Summary **159**
Critical Thinking **159**
Websites **159**
Review Questions **159**

Chapter 15 Complications of
Phlebotomy 161
Outline **161**
Objectives **161**
Key Terms **161**
Introduction **161**
Complications of Phlebotomy **161**
  Hematoma **162**
  Hemoconcentration **162**

Nerve Damage **162**
Fainting **162**
Seizures **162**
Allergic Response **163**
Collapsed Vein **163**
Excessive Bleeding **163**
Accidental Artery Puncture **163**
Uncooperative Patients **163**
Summary **164**
Critical Thinking **164**
Websites **164**
Review Questions **164**

Chapter 16 Urinalysis and Other
Specimens 167
Outline **167**
Objectives **167**
Key Terms **167**
Introduction **168**
Anatomy of the Urinary System **168**
Urine Formation **169**
Collecting the Urine Specimen **169**
Transporting the Urine
  Specimen **171**
Urine Characteristics **171**
Pregnancy Testing **176**
Urine Toxicology **176**
Sputum Specimens **176**
Cerebrospinal Fluid Specimens **177**
Amniotic Fluid Specimens **177**
Semen Specimens **177**
Fecal Specimens **177**
Summary **177**
Critical Thinking **178**
Websites **178**
Review Questions **178**

Chapter 17 Specimen Handling and
Transport 179
Outline **179**
Objectives **179**
Key Terms **179**
Introduction **179**
Handling Specimens after
  Venipuncture **179**
Delivery Methods **181**
Clinical Laboratory Specimen
  Processing **182**

Reporting of Laboratory
    Results **182**
Summary **182**
Critical Thinking **184**
Websites **184**
Review Questions **184**

Chapter 18 Compliance 187
Outline **187**
Objectives **187**
Key Terms **187**
Introduction **187**
The Need for Compliance in
    Phlebotomy **187**
Compliance Regulations **188**
The Laboratory Compliance
    Plan **189**
Effects of Compliance **189**
Legal Actions and Phlebotomy **190**
Lawsuit Prevention **190**
Summary **190**
Critical Thinking **190**
Websites **190**
Review Questions **191**

Chapter 19 Computer Technology 193
Outline **193**
Objectives **193**
Key Terms **193**
Introduction **194**
Computers in the Clinical
    Laboratory **194**
    Computer Hardware **196**
    Computer Software **196**
    Data Storage **196**

Pneumatic Tube Systems **197**
Bar Codes **197**
Radio-Frequency Identification **197**
Computer Communications **198**
Computer Security **198**
Summary **198**
Critical Thinking **198**
Websites **198**
Review Questions **198**

Appendix A Units of Measurement and
Conversion Tables 201

Appendix B Common Laboratory
Tests 203

Appendix C NAACLS Phlebotomy
Competencies 207

Appendix D Reference Laboratory
Values 211

Appendix E ABC Laboratories Blood
Transfusion Consent
Form 213

Appendix F Military Time 215

Answer Key 217

Glossary 221

Index 233

Credits 249

Reviewers

Carol Abshire, MLT, BGS
Instructor
Lamar State College–Orange

Annette E. Bednar, MSE, MT (ASCP)
Assistant Professor of Clinical Laboratory Science
College of Nursing and Health Professions
Arkansas State University–Jonesboro

Marilyn Braswell, BA, MT (ASCP), SBB
Phlebotomy Instructor
Central Piedmont Community College

Konnie King Briggs, PBT, ASCP, CPI, ACA
Allied Health Instructor
Houston Community College

Susan L. Conforti, EdD, MT (ASCP), SBB
Professor, Medical Laboratory Technology
Farmingdale State College

Sandra Cook, MS, MT (ASCP)
Assistant Professor, Clinical Laboratory Sciences
Ferris State University

Bethany J. Dowse, RN, MSN
Professor of Nursing
White Mountains Community College

Jessica Lasiter, MHIM, MLS (ASCP), CM
Assistant Professor
University of Louisiana–Monroe

James R. McGee, MA, MT (ASCP)
Instructor of Phlebotomy
Central Piedmont Community College

Sandy Perotto, BS, MT (ASCP)
Program Director Emeritus
Idaho State University

Joyce Stone, H (ASCP), SH
Assistant Program Director
Medical Laboratory Science Program
University of New Hampshire

About the Author

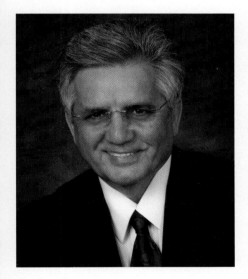

Dr. Moini was assistant professor at Tehran University School of Medicine for 9 years, where he taught medical and allied health students. He is a professor and former director (for 15 years) of allied health programs at Everest University (EU). Dr. Moini established several programs at EU's Melbourne, Florida campus.

As a physician and instructor for the past 35 years, he taught phlebotomy to medical assistants in order for them to become certified. Phlebotomists play very important roles in allied health, assisting healthcare providers in the diagnosis of various disorders and conditions.

Dr. Moini is actively involved in teaching and helping students prepare for service in various health professions. He has been an internationally published author of various allied health books since 1999.

Dedication

This book is dedicated to
my granddaughter, Laila Jade Mabry.

Acknowledgments

I acknowledge the following individuals for their time and efforts in aiding me with their contributions to this book.

Morvarid Moini, Designer
Nova Southeastern University

Greg Vadimsky, Manuscript Assistant
Melbourne, Florida

I would like to acknowledge Holmes Regional Medical Center and Melbourne Internal Medicine Associates for providing facilities, equipment, and personnel for photographs that appear in this book.

Also, I thank the entire staff of Jones & Bartlett Learning, especially David Cella, Cathy Esperti, Joseph Morita, Maro Gartside, Tracey McCrea, Grace Richards, and Sarah Cebulski.

I also thank the reviewers who gave their time and guidance in helping me to complete this book.

Preface

After 24 years of teaching allied health students and 10 years teaching phlebotomy to medical assistants, I realized that a phlebotomist has a special role as a health care provider. Phlebotomists must be skillful and knowledgeable about drawing blood from different types of patients. Communication skills are vital. Non-skilled phlebotomists may cause many complications during phlebotomy procedures, for which they may be liable.

Therefore, I have attempted to write a thorough book, *Phlebotomy: Principles and Practice*. For phlebotomists, the material must be easy to understand while simultaneously focusing on the day-to-day requirements of their jobs. This textbook contains 19 chapters, 6 appendices, an answer key, a glossary, and an index. Each chapter contains an outline, learning objectives, bolded medical terms, an introduction, many tables and full-color figures, a summary, critical thinking questions, relevant website addresses, and multiple choice review questions.

Instructors can also request access to an Instructor Manual, PowerPoints, and an extensive test bank of many review questions (including case studies and critical thinking questions). The student companion website also features activities, which include crossword puzzles, flashcards, an interactive glossary, chapter quizzes, matching exercises, and web links.

Introduction to Phlebotomy

OUTLINE

Introduction
The History of Phlebotomy
Becoming a Successful Phlebotomist
Roles and Responsibilities of Phlebotomists
Phlebotomy Education and Certification
Legal and Ethical Issues
Rules and Regulations
    Clinical and Laboratory Standards Institute
    Clinical Laboratory Improvement Act
    National Accrediting Agency for Clinical Laboratory
        Sciences
    Joint Commission
    College of American Pathologists
    State Board of Health
Classifications of Law
    Civil Law
    Criminal Law
    Preventive Law
    Ethics
Patient Self-Determination Act
Patient's Bill of Rights
Quality Assurance and Quality Control
    Quality Assurance Guidelines
    Quality Control Guidelines
Summary
Critical Thinking
Websites
Review Questions

OBJECTIVES

After reading this chapter, readers should be able to:
1. Briefly discuss the history of phlebotomy as a profession.
2. Explain why continuing education is so important to the phlebotomist.
3. Describe how a phlebotomist becomes successful.
4. Discuss the Joint Commission and the National Accrediting Agency of Clinical Laboratory Sciences.
5. Distinguish which type of civil law deals with medical professional liability.
6. Explain the two basic categories of criminal law.
7. Differentiate among malfeasance, misfeasance, and nonfeasance.
8. Describe the value of listening.
9. Describe the Patient's Bill of Rights.
10. Explain the Patient Self-Determination Act.

KEY TERMS

Bioethics: The study of ethical and moral implications of new discoveries and advances in medicine.
Bloodletting: The removal of blood as a therapeutic measure.
Chain of custody: A "paper trail"; a chronological documentation of activities.
Civil law: The type of law that deals with the rights of private citizens.
Criminal law: The type of law that deals with crimes against society.
Defense mechanisms: Unconscious psychological strategies used to cope with stressors.
Ethics: Moral principles, qualities, or practices.
Hemolysis: The destruction or dissolution of red blood cells.
Laws: Rules of conduct established by custom, agreement, or authority.
Malpractice: A type of negligence wherein a professional fails to follow acceptable standards, resulting in injury to a person or group of persons.
Phlebotomy: Opening of a blood vessel by incision or puncture in order to obtain blood.
Quality assurance: A formal monitoring program that assesses the level of health care being provided by healthcare professionals or institutions.
Quality control: A process that assesses all factors involved in the healthcare process.
Stressors: Events that provoke stress.

Introduction

Trained phlebotomists practice in a very adaptable, rewarding career focused on helping other people. Phlebotomy skills are highly valuable, and employment is readily available nearly anywhere in the world. Advances in medicine and therefore phlebotomy have increased dramatically in the past few decades. Laboratory testing to analyze blood specimens is a vital tool in assisting physicians in the diagnosis of disease. Phlebotomists play a special role in this process.

The History of Phlebotomy

The history of **phlebotomy** can be traced back to documentation of **bloodletting**. This practice has been traced back to the ancient Mayan culture, and a representation of the procedure exists in an Egyptian tomb (circa 1400 B.C.). Often, leeches were used to consume some of a patient's blood in the belief that the practice would cause the body to produce new, healthy blood. Veins were often punctured with sharpened stones and sticks in order to start blood flow. Bloodletting was intended as a therapy, but was also related to religious beliefs. In medieval times, it was believed that bloodletting allowed "evil spirits" to be bled out of the patient's body. Many people thought that the presence of evil spirits caused illnesses (see **Figure 1–1**). Others believed that bloodletting actually could remove "bad" blood and therefore remove disease.

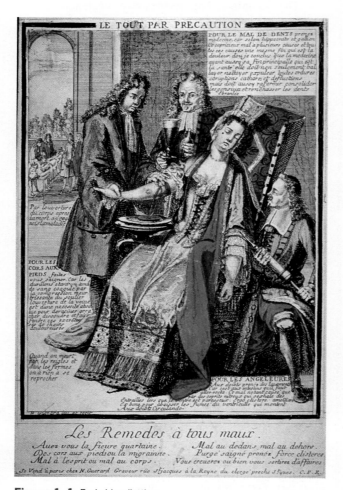

Figure 1–1 Early bloodletting.

Hippocrates (460–377 B.C.) documented the benefits of phlebotomy (then known as *venesection*). Another practice of the time was *scarification*—the removal of large amounts of blood, which was done very quickly to produce fainting. This dangerous practice often caused the death of the patient when the amount of blood removed was too great. A student of Hippocrates, Galen, recorded that specific amounts of blood should be extracted to treat certain conditions. In general, this meant between 6 oz and 1½ lb of blood, but usually 16 to 30 oz was drained. Once the patient fainted, the blood withdrawal was supposed to be stopped.

In the 12th century, barbers practiced bloodletting. The origination of the barber's red and white pole came from this practice, with the red signifying blood and the white signifying bandages. Another practice, known as *cupping*, utilized a heated glass placed on the patient's back. As it cooled, suction was created to pull capillary blood upward. Next, a spring-loaded box with multiple blades was used to cut the area to produce massive bleeding. Both venesection and cupping scarred patients very badly.

As late as the 18th century, bloodletting was considered as a major therapeutic treatment. It was widely believed that because blood was a carrier of impurities, bleeding the patient would cause new, healthy blood to replace what was lost. In the United States, former president George Washington died (in 1799) from complications related to repeated bloodlettings. He was being treated for a throat infection, and approximately 9 pt of blood was drained over a 24-h period. Instruments used at this time for bloodletting included lancets (or knives), cups, and leeches. In the 19th century, phlebotomy became a diagnostic tool, and its use as therapeutic medicine became increasingly referred to as *quackery*.

Phlebotomy has evolved with modern laboratory testing via the obtaining of blood in specific tubes containing certain ingredients. The process of bloodletting has not stopped entirely, however. After certain surgeries, leeches may still be used to reduce swelling and promote healing. Examples of procedures in which leeches are still used include the restoration of circulation to grafted tissue and reattached digits. Today, therapeutic phlebotomy is also used to treat *polycythemia* (overproduction of red blood cells) and *hemochromatosis* (excessive absorption and accumulation of iron). The term *therapeutic phlebotomy* has essentially replaced the term *bloodletting*.

Becoming a Successful Phlebotomist

Phlebotomists draw blood to be submitted for various tests. They need to know which tubes are needed for each specific type of blood draw. These tubes are prepared and color-coded differently from one another. Phlebotomists work in a variety of medical settings, including physicians' offices, hospitals, reference laboratories, and blood/plasma donor centers. Rates of pay for phlebotomists differ depending on the work location and the state in which work is performed.

To have the desired effect upon patients, a phlebotomist should be well groomed, clothed in appropriate attire, and in good health. Trained phlebotomists must have certain knowledge and skills. Education continues after formal training has been completed. Every year, large amounts of new information must be absorbed and retained. Constant changes in the practice of phlebotomy must be kept up with. Continuing education enhances the effectiveness of the professional phlebotomist.

Phlebotomists must develop good communication skills in order to interact with others, put them at ease, and develop trust and increased comfort levels. Good listening skills are essential, which involve receiving both verbal and nonverbal signals.

Stress has many effects on the human body, and some people handle **stressors** better than others. Individuals may use **defense mechanisms** as protective measures.

Roles and Responsibilities of Phlebotomists

The phlebotomist's primary responsibility is to collect blood samples via venipuncture or dermal puncture. Other duties include transporting specimens to the laboratory. Good phlebotomy practice requires efficient, accurate, and patient-friendly technique. Phlebotomists help to control both quality and costs. Specialized training and continuing education help them to remain up to date and fully competent in their duties.

Phlebotomists are increasingly involved in patient care. They must also be skilled in testing in point-of-care scenarios, performing procedures such as cardiopulmonary resuscitation (CPR) and automated external defibrillation (AED). They should be trained in medical record documentation and in the use of computer software employed in the laboratory. Sometimes a phlebotomist may be needed to assist with the taking of vital signs and in the procedure known as an *electrocardiogram* (EKG). However, most phlebotomists are not trained in performing EKGs.

Clinical skills are enhanced by the ability to perform well under pressure while maintaining professionalism, compassion, and empathy. Additional roles and responsibilities of phlebotomists include appropriate interaction with patients and clients, the use of medical terminology, an awareness of legal aspects of phlebotomy, compliance with safety standards and standard precautions, knowledge of frequently ordered lab tests, the ability to prioritize tasks and schedules, clerical skills, and (less frequently today) the preparation of blood film slides.

Phlebotomy Education and Certification

Those who work in phlebotomy must be formally trained in order to gain employment. Most employers require phlebotomy certification, as well as licensure in many cases. It is important to understand that licensure varies from state to state. Some nonlicensure states do not require that a phlebotomist become certified prior to employment, using on-the-job training instead. Other healthcare workers may perform phlebotomy, but only if they are also certified as phlebotomists. To gain certification, you must demonstrate a specific level of skill and competence by successfully completing a phlebotomy certification exam. There are a variety of phlebotomy and related certifications, including the following:

- Certified Phlebotomy Technician (CPT) via the National Phlebotomy Association (NPA), the American Society of Phlebotomy Technicians (ASPT), the National Healthcareer Association (NHA), the American Association of Allied Health Professionals (AAAHP), or the American Certification Agency (ACA)
- Registered Phlebotomy Technician (RPT) via American Medical Technologists (AMT)
- Phlebotomy Technician (PBT) via the American Society for Clinical Pathology (ASCP)
- Medical Laboratory Scientist (MLS), a new designation, via the merger of the ASCP with the American Society for Clinical Laboratory Science (ASCLS); the ASCLS along with the Association of Genetic Technologists (AGT) has ratified the uniting of the ASCP with the National Credentialing Agency for Laboratory Personnel (NCA); a medical laboratory scientist must obtain a bachelor of science in clinical laboratory science (which was formerly called medical technology)
- Nationally Certified Phlebotomy Technician (NCPT) via the National Center for Competency Testing (NCCT)

Certification exams are usually given on a national level. Most certifying agencies require continuing education to maintain certification. This keeps phlebotomists up to date with the latest medical advances and technology. Continuing education units (CEUs) may be obtained via workshops, seminars, in-service training, and even online sources.

Many hospitals, independent organizations, colleges, and universities offer phlebotomy technician training, education, and certification. Accreditation of these various outlets ensures that they meet minimum education levels and program standards. Accreditation is maintained through the National Accrediting Agency for Clinical Laboratory Sciences (NAACLS). Standards in phlebotomy are also influenced by the College of American Pathologists (CAP), which functions as a laboratory review committee. For CAP certification, laboratories undergo routine inspections, which conform to guidelines of the Joint Commission.

Legal and Ethical Issues

Laws are regulations or rules that should be observed for the protection of the safety and welfare of society. They resolve conflicts in a nonviolent, orderly manner and are continually evolving. **Ethics** are moral standards of behavior or conduct governing the actions of individuals. Good ethical standards in health care provide safety and fairness to all patients. Questions that may be asked to ensure ethical practices include the following:

- Is the practice correct?
- Is the practice legal and in compliance with the institutional policy?
- Does the practice create a "win-win" situation for the patient, supervisor, and other individuals?
- Does the practice allow you to take pride in carrying it out?

The term **bioethics** refers to moral problems and issues that may result from medical procedures, research, or technology. Bioethics often concerns issues of life and death as well as the donation of organs.

Rules and Regulations

A variety of organizations and acts regulate the practice of phlebotomy, as well as other disciplines in medicine. When rules and regulations are followed, it helps to qualify people and groups of people for the ability to continue practice, insurance reimbursement, and participation in programs such as Medicare and Medicaid.

Clinical and Laboratory Standards Institute

The Clinical and Laboratory Standards Institute (CLSI) is a nonprofit educational organization that helps laboratories to maintain high levels of performance so that they can pass regular inspections. It replaced the National Committee for Clinical Laboratory Standards (NCCLS). CLSI releases various publications concerned with guidelines for laboratory procedures, evaluation protocols, and bench and reference. The organization continually upgrades and improves its information so that it becomes and remains standardized within the medical field. Its publications are a constant, reliable source of reference for laboratory practice.

Clinical Laboratory Improvement Act

Enacted by Congress, the Clinical Laboratory Improvement Act of 1988 (CLIA, '88) mandated regulation of laboratories involved in interstate commerce. CLIA applies to all laboratories that test human patients, and it came about as a result of complaints of inaccurate testing and illegal payment practices in the reference laboratory system. CLIA, along with the Joint Commission and the College of American Pathologists, established regulated methods for inspections. Further amendments to CLIA both increased quality assurance requirements over other types of laboratories and added physician office laboratories to those regulated by the act. Clinical laboratories must now perform quality testing that can be statistically verified, always with patient protection a first priority. Through CLIA, laboratories are monitored by the Centers for Medicare and Medicaid Services (CMS), formerly the Health Care Financing Administration (HCFA), part of the U.S. Department of Health and Human Services (HHS).

The four testing categories designated by the CMS are as follows:

- Waived tests, requiring a minimum of judgment and interpretation and including test kits that are approved for home use
- Physician-performed microscopy tests, in which the physician actually uses the microscope to make judgments and interpretations
- Moderate-complexity tests, requiring more complex methods and education
- High-complexity tests, requiring additional levels of education and skill

National Accrediting Agency for Clinical Laboratory Sciences

The National Accrediting Agency for Clinical Laboratory Sciences (NAACLS) accredits and approves educational programs for clinical laboratories and other medical professions. The NAACLS conducts inspections of school facilities to ascertain that specific standards are being met. Each educational program must meet certain competencies of performance for each course of study.

Joint Commission

Hospitals may be accredited by the Joint Commission or the American Osteopathic Association (AOA), substituting for meeting most Medicare requirements. Most hospitals, however, prefer the Joint Commission, which sends a team of inspectors to each hospital. Hospitals are accredited for a 3-year period, with follow-up inspections occurring for reaccreditation. Any deficiencies must be corrected, and reinspection should occur once they are complete.

College of American Pathologists

Hospital laboratories may request voluntary inspections, which are conducted by the College of American Pathologists (CAP). CAP will explain how each laboratory compares and ranks with similar facilities throughout the United States. An approved proficiency-testing program run by CAP sends unknown samples to subscribing laboratories for testing. The obtained results are sent back to CAP, where they are evaluated and graded against peer groups. Also, the Joint Commission will frequently accept CAP approval and not conduct inspections itself. Successful participation in a CLIA-approved proficiency-testing program is an essential part of the certification or accreditation process for laboratories.

State Board of Health

Each state's individual board of health also monitors the activities of hospitals and laboratories. Inspections conducted by a state board of health may range from walk-throughs to very detailed inspections. Usually, the state board of health will accept Joint Commission or CAP approval for part of an inspection process and then will look into additional areas of practice itself.

Classifications of Law

There are two broad divisions of law that affect healthcare providers, including phlebotomists. These are civil law and criminal law.

Civil Law

Civil law is based on *tort law*, which is based on acts committed without just cause. Most healthcare cases involve civil law, which is defined as the law of private rights between persons or parties. There are three basic types of torts: intentional torts, negligence torts, and strict liability torts.

Intentional torts relate to intentional acts or willful breaches of duty. These include abandonment, assault, battery, duty of care, false imprisonment, fraud, intentional infliction of emotional distress, invasion of privacy, libel, and slander. *Duty of care* is defined as the responsibility not to infringe on another person's rights by causing intentional or careless harm.

Negligence torts result when a duty of care is unintentionally breached, causing patient harm. For negligence to occur, there must be a breach of duty, harm done as a direct result of the action, and a legal obligation owed by one person to another. Healthcare providers must take precautions that are prudent to prevent foreseeable harm to another person. If a provider fails to take such precautions and a patient is harmed, negligence can be charged. Negligence is often unintentional. Another form of negligence occurs when a healthcare provider is not fully trained in a certain procedure, but performs the procedure nevertheless, resulting in patient harm.

When negligence occurs, the responsible healthcare provider is charged, and often so is the facility he or she works for. The Latin term *respondeat superior*, meaning "let the master answer," means that the employer is ultimately responsible for the actions of all employees. However, if the employee acts outside the scope of training or duties, he or she may be held solely responsible.

Improper treatment or negligence may result in a **malpractice** claim in a civil lawsuit. Most medical malpractice lawsuits are brought against hospitals or physicians, but phlebotomists are also sometimes named. A person or group of people bringing charges in a lawsuit is called the *plaintiff*. Employers usually obtain malpractice (liability) insurance to cover all employees, but phlebotomists may purchase their own malpractice insurance as well.

Medical professional liability (commonly called *medical malpractice*) is governed by the law of torts. The term *medical professional liability* includes all possible civil liability that may be incurred during the delivery of medical care. Medical professional liability is more easily prevented than defended. Professional negligence in medicine falls into these three general classifications:

- *Malfeasance*, which is the performance of an act that is wholly wrongful and unlawful
- *Misfeasance*, which is the improper performance of a lawful act
- *Nonfeasance*, which is the failure to perform an act that should have been performed

The final type of torts, *strict liability torts*, usually concerns product liability. This relatively uncommon type of tort involves a healthcare provider being found guilty even though he or she did not actually commit a tort, but utilized products such as medical equipment that were faulty and caused patient harm. Since phlebotomy involves the use of many types of equipment and other supplies, the potential for manufacturing defects in these supplies is real and may result in patient harm even though the phlebotomist follows procedures exactly. The Safe Medical Devices Act of 1990 was designed to protect healthcare workers and patients from injuries caused by healthcare devices.

Criminal Law

Criminal law is concerned with the violation of laws that protect the general public. These violations are called *crimes*. Although many torts are considered crimes, torts are actually wrongs against individuals whereas crimes are wrongs against society. Criminal laws are divided into *felonies* (punishable by fines and more than 1 year in prison) and *misdemeanors* (punishable by fines and/or up to 1 year in jail). Examples of felonies include murder, rape, and burglary, and examples of misdemeanors include disorderly conduct, simple assault, and reckless endangerment.

Preventive Law

Preventive law is the avoidance of legal conflicts through education and planning. Lawsuits that relate to preventive law may be prevented through accurate documentation of all procedures, acquisition of informed consent prior to procedures, continuing education participation, maintenance of accepted standards of care, use of proper safety measures, and adherence to all policies and procedures.

Proving malpractice or negligence places the *burden of proof* upon the plaintiff (the party bringing the lawsuit). In phlebotomy, most cases involve malpractice or negligence. Common negligent actions include improper patient identification, mislabeling, lack of sterile techniques, reusing needles, improperly performed testing, injury to veins and other body structures, breach of confidentiality, and failure in controlling the **chain of custody**. The *chain of custody* is defined as the procedure that ensures that materials obtained from diagnosis have been taken from the correct patient, have proper labeling, and have not been tampered with while being taken to the laboratory.

Negligence can only be proved under these four conditions:

- A standard of care exists.
- The standard of care is breached.
- An injury is sustained.
- The injury can be proved to have been caused by acts that resulted from the breach of the standard of care.

Ethics

The term *ethics* comes from the Greek word *ethos*, meaning custom or practice. Ethics focus on values, actions, and choices used to determine right and wrong. The medical profession's rules of right and wrong are referred to as the *medical code of ethics*. These commonly include the following:

- Delivering quality laboratory services in a cost-effective manner
- Continuing to study, apply, and advance medical laboratory knowledge and skills while sharing them with others
- Performing all duties with accuracy, preciseness, timeliness, and responsibility
- Using laboratory resources prudently
- Keeping patient information confidential within the limits of the law
- Treating patients and colleagues with care, respect, and thoughtfulness
- Working within the boundaries of laws and regulations
- Disclosing improper or illegal behavior to appropriate authorities

Patient Self-Determination Act

The Patient Self-Determination Act requires healthcare facilities to develop and maintain written procedures that ensure all adult patients will receive information about durable powers of attorney for health care, *advance directives*, and living wills. Advance directives allow patients to make choices about their end-of-life care ahead of time. This puts the decision-making power of each patient's health care directly into his or her hands, or into the hands of the family. It provides written notification of the right to consent to or refuse medical treatment. Consent is unnecessary in emergency situations.

Patient's Bill of Rights

The Patient's Bill of Rights is officially known as the *Consumer Bill of Rights and Responsibilities*. Today, it may also be referred to as the *Patient Care Partnership*. It has three specific goals:

- To strengthen consumer confidence by ensuring a fair healthcare system that is responsive to consumer needs, providing credible and effective mechanisms to address concerns, and encouraging consumers to take an active role in improving and ensuring their health
- To reaffirm the importance of strong relationships between patients and healthcare professionals
- To reaffirm the critical role consumers play in safeguarding health by establishing the rights and responsibilities of all participants to improve their own health

This bill contains eight sections, and most healthcare facilities have adopted their own smaller versions of it. Patients are usually given this information upon admittance to facilities. Patients who do not speak English should be carefully dealt with in order to help them understand their rights fully. The use of interpreters may be required so that these patients understand their rights.

Quality Assurance and Quality Control

Phlebotomists, like other healthcare professionals, must work to achieve the highest possible degree of excellence regarding the care of every patient. Quality assurance and quality control guidelines are the most important elements in achieving this goal. **Quality assurance** is the attempt to achieve the utmost excellence in health care. It includes **quality control**, laboratory documentation, personnel orientation, proficiency-testing programs, and adequate laboratory instrumentation. Quality assurance uses many operating procedures that produce reliable laboratory results.

Quality Assurance Guidelines

Activities and programs designed to give optimal patient care are called *quality assurance* (QA). It is achieved by evaluating the adequacy, suitability, and timeliness of patient care. Problems are identified and corrected by continual evaluations. The Public Health Act offers funding to hospitals and laboratories when they have appropriate QA programs in place. The Joint Commission requires all hospitals to have QA programs in place, which are a subset of larger Total Quality Management (TQM) programs. TQM utilizes all employees' efforts to continually improve client care and services and is directed at customer satisfaction.

There are three phases of the QA testing process:

- *Preanalytical*, which identifies the right patient by age, gender, address, etc., and double-checks the physician's order to see if there are special procedures required, such as fasting. This is the phase that includes the collection of blood (phlebotomy).

- *Analytical*, which involves the analysis of collected samples, which must be accurate and error free. Examples of analytical procedures include correct tube selection, spinning of tubes for serological tests, etc.
- *Postanalytical*, which concerns the outcome of the analysis of collected samples. This also includes observing patients for signs of fainting or bleeding after blood collection, instructing patients to alert the healthcare provider if they experience any complications such as hematomas, etc.

Quality assurance program goals seek to minimize errors in all three areas of the testing process. All processes for testing and reporting must be listed in the laboratory's policies and procedures manual.

Quality assurance includes quality control, personnel orientation, laboratory documentation, knowledge of laboratory instrumentation, and enrollment in a proficiency-testing program. As a phlebotomist, you must work effectively along with the guidelines of your facility's QA program to provide accurate and reliable test results and quality specimens. You should always consider possible sources of errors and how your work can be continually improved regarding accuracy. A component of QA, quality control (QC) uses ordered steps to obtain proper test results. Other quality assurance procedures are used to maintain base levels of testing accuracy, including documentation, error checking, and preventive maintenance.

Quality Control Guidelines

Quality control is used in the laboratory setting to ensure test result accuracy and precision, while detecting and eliminating error. *Accuracy* is defined by how close the obtained value is to the real, true value. *Precision* refers to the reproducibility of a testing procedure. Quality control monitors every aspect of laboratory activity. These include specimen collection, processing, testing, and reporting. Actual test performance, supplies, reagents, machinery, and personnel are all checked for quality. QC is important because undetected laboratory errors may result in patient harm.

Special QC samples (controls) are tested daily along with patient samples. With the control samples, results must be within a preestablished range. Control samples are usually prepackaged in kits, and they should be analyzed at specified intervals. For example, controls used in the laboratory may be part of pregnancy test kits, urinalysis, and automated chemistry analyses. Consistent results of controls ensure that the testing sequence has constant, reliable conditions.

Laboratory instruments must be standardized. This involves testing samples with specific, known values as well as adjusting instrumentation until it displays that value. These samples are called *standards*. Calibrations of laboratory equipment must be made and verified at least every 6 months. Calibration ensures that the equipment is operating correctly. Each calibration must be recorded in a quality control log (see **Figure 1–2**).

Daily cleaning of equipment as well as adjustment and replacement of parts helps to prolong the life of equipment and reduce breakdowns. Logs or worksheets for each piece

QUALITY CONTROL RECORD

	PRACTICE NAME
	Precision Health Care Inc.

DEPARTMENT	Glucose Monitor-Institution #55			NAME/LEVEL
CONTROL LOT #	H542A	EXPIRATION DATE	01/29/XX	
DIRECTOR SIGNATURE DATE:				

TEST										UNITS
LOWER LIMIT				MEAN			UPPER LIMIT			
DATE	No.	VALUE	TECH	COMMENT	DATE	No.	VALUE	TECH	COMMENT	
12/8/XX	1	99	KBH			17				
12/9/XX	2	103	KBH	prev. maintenance		18				
12/10/XX	3	100	KBH			19				
12/11/XX	4	100	KBH			20				
12/14/XX	5	105	KBH			21				
12/15/XX	6	97	KBH			22				
12/16/XX	7	95	KBH			23				
12/17/XX	8	96	KBH	new battery		24				
12/18/XX	9	103	KBH			25				
12/19/XX	10	100	KBH			26				
12/20/XX	11	103	KBH			27				
12/21/XX	12	97	KBH			28				
	13					29				
	14					30				
	15					31				
	16									

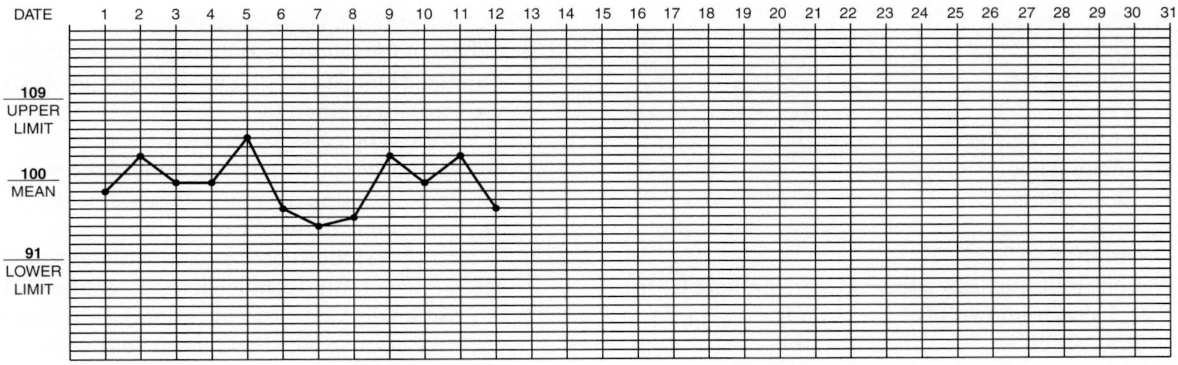

Figure 1–2 Quality control log.

of equipment should record all changes as well as daily maintenance.

Accurate record keeping is important for quality control, and today it is usually computerized. If hard copies are still used, they will usually be kept in a master logbook in the laboratory. It is important to remember that every day that the patient tests are performed, QC tests must also be performed. Results of standardization tests, dates when new control vials are begun, and expiration dates of the controls must all be entered. These records should be kept for several years, as determined by state law and CLIA mandates.

Summary

Phlebotomy evolved over thousands of years from the ancient procedure known as bloodletting. It is now an extremely useful diagnostic tool. Phlebotomists and phlebotomy technicians are very important in modern health care, and they must follow strict guidelines for practice. Phlebotomy practice requires formal education and certification. Continuing education in phlebotomy is usually required across the United States in order to continue to practice. Standards of professional phlebotomy practice are set by the Joint Commission, the Occupational Safety and Health Administration (OSHA), CLIA, and CAP. Quality assurance is the attempt to achieve the utmost excellence in health care. It includes quality control, laboratory documentation, personnel orientation, proficiency-testing programs, and adequate laboratory instrumentation. Quality assurance uses many operating procedures that produce reliable laboratory results.

CRITICAL THINKING

Anthony went to a 79-year-old male patient's room to collect blood specimens, as ordered by the patient's physician. He explained to the patient that his physician ordered several blood tests. The patient, however, refused to allow him to collect the blood. Anthony insisted that the tests were needed and that blood had to be drawn immediately. The patient continued to deny Anthony.

1. In this case, what is the first thing that Anthony should do?
2. If Anthony were to attempt to take the blood by force, which law would he be ignoring, and what could he potentially be charged with?

WEBSITES

http://phlebotomists.com/html/article_1.html

http://phlebotomycert.com/

http://www.apa2.com/exam.html

http://www.bd.com/vacutainer/labnotes/pdf/
  Volume8Number2.pdf

http://www.museumofquackery.com/devices/phlebo.htm

http://www.nationalphlebotomy.org/

http://www.phlebotomy.org/how_to_be_a_phlebotomist
  .htm

http://www.phlebotomypages.com/index.htm

REVIEW QUESTIONS

Multiple Choice

1. Who said that specific amounts of blood should be extracted to treat certain conditions?
   A. Hippocrates
   B. Galen
   C. Mithridates
   D. Proctor

2. Professional negligence is also called
   A. malpractice
   B. malfunction
   C. malice
   D. arbitration

3. A crime punishable by a fine or imprisonment for less than 1 year is known as a
   A. mitigation
   B. felony
   C. mutual assent
   D. misdemeanor

4. All of the following are parts of the Patient's Bill of Rights, EXCEPT
   A. privacy
   B. confidentiality
   C. refusing discharge from the hospital
   D. refusing treatment

5. Intentional torts
   A. include assault, defamation, and invasion of privacy
   B. are always forms of negligence
   C. are always considered misdemeanors
   D. are forms of abandonment

6. Performing venipuncture of a patient without the patient's consent would be considered
   A. rape
   B. assault
   C. abuse
   D. battery

7. A license to practice medicine is
   A. required by local law
   B. required by the local medical society
   C. required by law in each state
   D. required by federal law

8. A person or group bringing charges in a lawsuit is called a(n)
   A. defendant
   B. plaintiff
   C. arbitrator
   D. lawyer

9. The failure to perform an act that should have been performed is called
   A. malfeasance
   B. misfeasance
   C. nonfeasance
   D. feasance

10. *Respondeat superior* is a Latin term meaning
    A. "Let the master answer"
    B. "Respond as soon as possible"
    C. "Buyer, beware"
    D. "The thing speaks for itself"

11. Which of the following statements is true about computerized blood testing? It has brought phlebotomy to the fore as a method of
    A. decreasing costs for patients
    B. diagnosing many different conditions
    C. demonstrating the phlebotomist's skills
    D. doing none of the above

12. Which of the following organizations offers the Registered Phlebotomy Technician (RPT) credential?
    A. Nationally Certified Phlebotomy Technicians
    B. American Society for Clinical Pathology
    C. National Phlebotomy Association
    D. American Medical Technologists

13. Most certifying agencies require that phlebotomists complete which of the following?
    A. Drawing blood more than 150 times during externship
    B. Continuing education to maintain certification
    C. Demonstrating skills and ethics
    D. Applying for promotions

14. Improper treatment or negligence may result in
    A. fraud
    B. slander
    C. malpractice
    D. libel

15. Which of the following laws offers quality assurance to hospitals and laboratories?
    A. Public Health Act
    B. Occupational Safety and Health Act
    C. Health Insurance Portability and Accountability Act
    D. Poison Prevention Packaging Act

CHAPTER 2

Fundamentals of the Medical Laboratory

OUTLINE

Introduction
The Medical Laboratory
    Laboratory Divisions
    Laboratory Staff
    Laboratory Hazards
Professionalism
Record Keeping
Summary
Critical Thinking
Websites
Review Questions

OBJECTIVES

After reading this chapter, readers should be able to:
1. List the divisions of the medical laboratory.
2. Describe lipid profiles and sensitivity testing.
3. Define serology.
4. Describe clinical pathology and the society that regulates clinical phlebotomy training.
5. Discuss chemical hazards in the laboratory.
6. Define professionalism and how it affects phlebotomists.
7. Describe various tests that can be done in the chemistry department.
8. Compare a pathologist with a certified medical laboratory scientist.
9. Define the terms *hematology* and *immunology*.
10. Describe the importance of record keeping in the medical laboratory.

KEY TERMS

Caustic: Irreversibly damaging to body tissues or corroding anything else with which it comes in contact.
Certified medical laboratory scientists: Degreed individuals who have been accredited as proficient in the performance of complex chemical, biological, hematological, immunologic, microscopic, and bacteriological analyses.
Hematology: The study of the blood and tissues that form blood.
Immunology: The study of the immune system and immune disorders.
In vitro: Literally means "in glass"; this term is used for processes, tests, or procedures that take place outside the body.
Pathologists: Doctors who study the cause and development of disease.
Sensitivity testing: Procedures that determine how sensitive specific microorganisms are to various substances, such as antibiotics.

Introduction

The laboratory testing of patient specimens is an integral component of health care. Phlebotomists have many opportunities to work in small medical laboratories or in larger ones, such as in hospital settings. Hospital laboratories consist of several departments, each with its own specific tasks. Phlebotomists must be familiar with each of these departments and their roles. They will interact with a variety of staff members in the laboratory, each with her or his own roles and specialties.

The Medical Laboratory

The medical laboratory is where collected specimens are analyzed. Tests may be performed manually or via the use of automation. *Clinical pathology* involves applying clinical laboratory science and technology to patient care. Medical laboratories may be located in many places, including hospitals, physicians' offices, clinics, public health facilities, health maintenance organizations, and private facilities. *Anatomical pathology* is focused on the diagnosis of disease based on the gross, microscopic, chemical, immunologic, and molecular examination of organs, tissues, and whole bodies (via autopsy).

Laboratory Divisions

The divisions of the medical laboratory include chemistry, hematology, serology, blood bank, microbiology, and toxicology. In a physician's office, a medical laboratory usually performs hematology, urinalysis, and chemistry. Smaller laboratory settings usually have all of the various activities occurring in one area, while larger laboratories are divided into separate departments. Phlebotomists working in smaller laboratories usually send specimens to larger, specialized laboratories for analysis. The primary divisions of the medical laboratory are explained as follows.

Hematology

Hematology is the scientific study of blood and blood-forming tissues. Manual or automated counts may be performed of red blood cells (RBCs), white blood cells (WBCs), or platelets. Qualitative tests determine cell characteristics such as maturity, shape, and size. The hematology department also tests blood to determine how its components are able to coagulate. Common tests conducted in the hematology lab include the following:

- *Complete blood count* (CBC), also called a *full blood count*, a test a doctor or other medical professional requests that gives information about the cells in a patient's blood.
- *Blood differential*, which measures the percentage of each type of WBC in the blood and reveals any abnormal or immature cells.
- *Hematocrit*, also called the *packed cell volume* (PCV), which is the fraction of whole blood volume that consists of red blood cells.
- *Hemoglobin*, which is the oxygen-carrying compound of red blood cells.
- *Coagulation studies:*
  - *Prothrombin time* (PT), which evaluates the blood's ability to clot. Often it is done before surgery or to determine a patient's likelihood of having a bleeding or clotting problem.
  - *Partial thromboplastin time* (PTT), which is done to determine if heparin therapy is effective or to detect a clotting disorder. It is not affected by low-molecular-weight heparins.
- *International normalization ratio* (INR), which is a measure of the extrinsic pathway of coagulation. This test is used in the measure of warfarin dosage, liver damage, and vitamin K status.

Serology

Serology is the branch of laboratory medicine that studies blood serum for evidence of infection. It evaluates the antigen-antibody reaction **in vitro**. Serology is also called **immunology**. A medical laboratory scientist who prepares or supervises the preparation and testing of serum is called a *serologist*. A primary role of the serological lab is to diagnose infectious diseases by observing the presence of an immune antibody in a patient resulting from infection or entry of a pathogen into the body.

The most common serological and immunological tests include the following:

- Bacterial studies
  - Antistreptolysin O (ASO) titer—*Streptococcus* bacteria infections
  - Cold agglutinins—atypical pneumonia
  - Febrile agglutinins—antibodies to specific organisms that indicate certain diseases (such as tularemia)
  - Fluorescent treponemal antibody absorption test—syphilis
  - Rapid plasma reagin (RPR)—syphilis
- Viral studies
  - Anti-HIV—screening for human immunodeficiency virus
  - Cytomegalovirus antibody (CMV)—confirmation test
  - Epstein-Barr virus (EBV)—infectious mononucleosis
  - Hepatitis B surface antigen (HbsAg)—presence of hepatitis antigen on the surface of red blood cells
- General studies
  - Antinuclear antibody (ANA)—autoimmune disorders such as systemic lupus erythematosus
  - C-reactive protein (CRP)—increased levels in inflammatory conditions
  - Human chorionic gonadotropin (HCG)—present in pregnancy (urine and serum)
  - Rheumatoid factor (RF)—rheumatoid arthritis

Blood Bank

A blood bank is an organizational unit responsible for the collection, processing, and storing of blood for transfusion and other purposes. It is usually a subdivision of a hospital laboratory. The blood bank also commonly is responsible for serologic testing.

The most common blood bank tests include the following:

- *Blood typing*—tests for classifications of blood based on the presence or absence of inherited antigenic substances on the surface of red blood cells
- *Blood cross-matching*—prior to a blood transfusion, tests that either determine if the donor's blood is compatible with the recipient's blood or identify matches for organ transplants
- *Fetal blood screening*—test used to screen for hemolytic disease of the newborn (HDN)
- *Anti-A or anti-B titers*—tests that measure the presence and amount of these antibodies in the blood
- *Platelet antibodies*—for autoimmune conditions
- *Human leukocyte antigens* (HLA)—tests to look for specific proteins found on the surfaces of white blood cells
- *Direct antiglobin test*—formerly known as Coomb's test, in which an antiglobulin reaction is used both to detect the presence of immunoglobulin or complement on the red cell membrane and to determine the specific class of immunoglobulin or complement present

Chemistry

The chemistry department of a medical laboratory analyzes blood, cerebrospinal fluid, synovial (joint) fluid, and urine. Single tests are conducted, as are *profiles* (tests for many related substances, or *analytes*). For example, total cholesterol, triglycerides, and both high-density lipoprotein (HDL) and low-density lipoprotein (LDL) are tested in a *lipid profile*.

Urinalysis involves the examination of the chemical, physical, and microscopic properties of urine. Urinalysis tests examine levels of glucose, protein, blood, ketones, bilirubin, urobilinogen, nitrites, and pH. Under the microscope, the urine may be examined for the presence of blood cells, epithelial cells, casts, mucus, crystals, yeasts, and bacteria.

Blood chemistry tests are often ordered before surgeries or other procedures to examine a patient's overall state of health. The "Chem 8" test looks at eight specific blood substances and is often performed following surgery. The eight components are blood urea nitrogen (BUN), calcium, carbon dioxide (CO_2), creatinine, glucose, serum chloride (Cl), serum potassium (K), and serum sodium (Na). The Chem 8 test is also known as a *basic metabolic panel* (BMP).

Iron studies are also conducted in the chemistry laboratory, to measure the amount of iron in the blood; total iron binding capacity, which indirectly measures the transferrin level in the bloodstream (transferrin is a protein that carries iron); and ferritin, which measures the amount of ferritin in the blood (this is a better estimate of total body iron than the serum iron test). Other common chemistry tests include those for bicarbonate.

Microbiology

Although microorganisms are only rarely seen in a physician's office laboratory, microbiology studies bacteria, fungi, viruses, spirochetes, and rickettsiae. Microorganisms may be cultured (grown) from many different body fluids. Proper antibiotic therapies are determined by performing **sensitivity testing** upon microorganisms. Microbiological specimens require aseptic collection in containers that are sterile.

Common microbiological tests include the following:
- *Gram stain*—test that identifies specific types of pathogenic microorganisms, permitting antimicrobial therapy to begin before culture results are known
- *Culture and sensitivity* (C&S)—test that indicates infection (culture) and in vitro inhibition by an antibiotic (sensitivity), helping to select a correct treatment
- *Blood culture*—for bacteremia or septicemia
- *CLO test*—for *Helicobacter pylori*; CLO is the acronym for *Campylobacter-like organism*
- *Occult blood*—test that indicates blood in the stool, associated with gastrointestinal bleeding from carcinoma
- *Acid-fast bacilli* (AFB)—for tuberculosis (TB)
- *Fungus culture and identification*—test for presence and type of fungi
- *Ova and parasites* (O&P)—test that identifies many "etiology unknown" intestinal disorders

Note: Testing for TB, fungi, and O&P is often performed in specialty areas of the laboratory. These tests are not typically included in routine microbiology testing. For example, TB requires strict respiratory precautions, and all work is performed under a laminar airflow hood.

Toxicology

Toxicology is the study of toxins (poisons). Clinical toxicology focuses on detecting toxins and treating the effects they cause. Forensic toxicology focuses on the legal outcomes of exposure to toxins, whether accidental or intentional. Toxicology tests examine blood, hair, urine, and other body substances for toxins, which may be present in only tiny amounts. In the hospital laboratory, toxicology plays a very small role. Testing usually measures only alcohol intoxication, drug overdose, and the presence of illegal drugs. Advanced toxicology testing is not done in the hospital, but is handled by poison control centers.

Laboratory Staff

Medical laboratories may employ the following personnel:
- **Pathologists**—doctors who study the cause and development of disease. Many choose a specialty such as genetic or forensic pathology.
- Clinical laboratory scientists—also known as medical or laboratory technologists. They are responsible for verifying and performing a variety of diagnostic tests and reporting the results to doctors who use the information to treat diseases; this title requires a 4-year bachelor of science degree.
- **Certified medical laboratory scientists**—certified healthcare professionals who perform chemical, hematological, immunologic, microscopic, and bacteriological diagnostic analyses on body fluids and other specimens. This title also requires a 4-year bachelor of science degree.
- Certified medical laboratory technicians—lab technicians who perform less complex tests and laboratory procedures than medical technologists, and still may prepare specimens, operate automated analyzers, and perform supervised manual tests. Clinical laboratory scientists or laboratory managers supervise these technicians.
- Medical laboratory assistants—lab assistants who prepare (and sometimes process) samples within a pathology laboratory. They also utilize preanalytical systems needed for work by biomedical scientists or medical laboratory scientists. The term *medical laboratory scientist* is now also used interchangeably with *medical technologist*.
- Certified medical assistants—certified healthcare providers who perform administrative and clinical tasks that support the work of medical doctors and other healthcare professionals. Most facilities do not have separate job descriptions or categories for certified and noncertified medical assistants.
- Laboratory-trained phlebotomists—those responsible for drawing, transporting, and studying the anatomy and physiology of blood in the laboratory.

Many laboratory employees are required to complete 1 to 4 years of specialized training and must pass a registry examination. Medical laboratory scientists require 4-year degrees, while technicians only need 2-year degrees.

In the laboratory, phlebotomists provide specimens for accurate and reliable test results. Today, speed and accuracy are essential. This requires phlebotomists to have specialized classroom and clinical training, which the American Society of Clinical Pathologists may regulate. Many hospitals and clinics offer their own additional training to help phlebotomists enhance their working knowledge.

Laboratory Hazards

Laboratory hazards may be classified as electrical, fire, or mechanical. Many chemical hazards may be present in the laboratory. Often, these may be **caustic**, flammable, carcinogenic, poisonous, or teratogenic. Workers may be exposed to chemicals via direct absorption through the skin or mucous membranes, inhalation, ingestion, or entry into the body through an open wound. Chemical exposure is regulated by the Occupational Safety and Health Administration (OSHA).

Professionalism

Professionalism in the clinical laboratory includes proper attitude and behavior as well as grooming. Appearance should be kept within the standards of the laboratory, as defined in its policies and procedures manual. Clothing should be professional and clean, with casual attire or blue jeans being unacceptable. Hair and fingernails should be neat and trimmed, and items such as body piercing should be avoided, except for simple earrings. Tattoos should not be visible.

Record Keeping

Accurate record keeping is essential for the medical laboratory. Besides recording information about equipment maintenance, it is important to record test results in patient records. This way, it is possible to keep track of every specimen that passes through your hands. Today, this commonly involves the use of computerization. Each procedure performed is logged with dates and times included. Results are entered in great detail. Records are maintained for a minimum of several years, as determined by state law and the mandates of CLIA.

Summary

Manual or automated tests are performed upon specimens in the medical laboratory. Divisions of the medical laboratory include chemistry, hematology, serology, blood bank, microbiology, and toxicology. Medical laboratories employ pathologists, clinical laboratory scientists, certified medical laboratory scientists, certified medical laboratory technicians, medical laboratory assistants, certified medical assistants, and laboratory-trained phlebotomists. OSHA regulates laboratory hazards such as chemical exposures. Accurate record keeping is essential for the medical laboratory.

CRITICAL THINKING

The blood serum of a 26-year-old female was sent to the clinical laboratory to be tested to diagnose her symptoms of fatigue, lack of appetite, and vomiting. The test came back as positive for pregnancy. The physician knew this could not be the case because of her history.

1. What could have caused a false-positive test result for pregnancy?
2. What should the laboratory technicians do to verify the accuracy of the test?

WEBSITES

http://www.ascp.org/mainmenu/laboratoryprofessionals/careercenter.aspx

http://www.bls.gov/oco/ocos096.htm

http://www.cdc.gov/labstandards/

http://www.cdc.gov/ncidod/dhqp/worker.html

http://www.ehow.com/list_6293458_requirements-certified-laboratory-phlebotomist.html

http://www.hematology.org/

http://www.ilpi.com/msds/ref/engineeringcontrols.html

http://www.lbl.gov/ehs/chsp/html/work_practices.shtml

http://www.osha.gov/SLTC/bloodbornepathogens/index.html

http://www.osha.gov/SLTC/personalprotectiveequipment/

REVIEW QUESTIONS

Multiple Choice

1. Which of the following divisions of the medical laboratory involves the study of fungi and viruses?
   A. chemistry
   B. histology
   C. microbiology
   D. cytology
2. A blood culture and sensitivity test is most likely performed in which division of the clinical laboratory?
   A. urinalysis
   B. chemistry
   C. serology
   D. microbiology
3. The percentage of each type of leukocyte is called which of the following?
   A. complete blood count
   B. blood differentiation
   C. hematocrit
   D. coagulation study
4. The study of platelets is done in which division of the medical laboratory?
   A. serology
   B. hematology
   C. microbiology
   D. cytology
5. Urinalysis may determine the presence of
   A. mucus
   B. yeasts
   C. ketones
   D. all of the above
6. A pathologist is a
   A. certified medical laboratory technician
   B. clinical laboratory scientist

C. medical laboratory scientist

D. specialist physician

7. The organization that regulates clinical training and specialized classrooms for phlebotomists is the
   A. American Medical Association
   B. American Society of Clinical Pathologists
   C. American Association of Medical Assistants
   D. American Medical Technologists

8. Chemical hazards and exposure are regulated by
   A. OSHA
   B. AAMA
   C. FDA
   D. AMT

9. Which of the following evaluates the blood's ability to clot?
   A. prothrombin time
   B. direct antiglobin test
   C. antinuclear antibody
   D. cold agglutinins

10. Which of the following laws mandates that records be maintained for a minimum of several years?
    A. CLIA
    B. OSHA
    C. FDA
    D. MSDS

11. Which of the following blood tests may confirm infectious mononucleosis?
    A. cytomegalovirus antibody
    B. C-reactive protein

C. human chorionic gonadotropin

D. Epstein-Barre virus

12. All of the following are among the most common blood bank tests, EXCEPT
    A. platelet antibodies
    B. human leukocyte antigens
    C. acid-fast bacilli
    D. anti-A or anti-B titers

13. CLO test is used for which of the following conditions?
    A. tuberculosis
    B. bacteremia
    C. *Helicobacter pylori*
    D. ova and parasites

14. Which of the following terms is used for packed cell volume?
    A. hematocrit
    B. hemoglobin
    C. complete blood count
    D. iron studies

15. The antinuclear antibody test is used for which of the following diseases?
    A. atypical pneumonia
    B. tularemia
    C. syphilis
    D. systemic lupus erythematosus

Communication Skills for Phlebotomists

OUTLINE

Introduction
The Communication Cycle
Types of Communication
    Verbal Communication
    Nonverbal Communication
    Written Communication
    Telephone and Computer Communication
Improving Your Communication Skills
Interactions with Other Individuals
Barriers to Communication
Defense Mechanisms
Summary
Critical Thinking
Websites
Review Questions

OBJECTIVES

After studying this chapter, readers should be able to:
1. Describe the elements of the transactional communication process.
2. Discuss the value of eye contact in the communication process.
3. Differentiate between verbal and nonverbal communication.
4. Explain why first impressions are critically important.
5. Explain comfort zones in nonverbal communication.
6. Describe cultural diversity.
7. Explain some of the barriers to effective communication.
8. Discuss defense mechanisms and recognize commonly used defense mechanisms.
9. Describe the value of listening.
10. Explain how to improve communication skills.

KEY TERMS

Active listening: A form of listening wherein the receiver pays complete attention to the speaker's verbal and nonverbal communication and then provides feedback about what was received.
Confidentiality: Keeping information private and away from individuals who are not authorized to receive it.
Defense mechanisms: Reactions often seen when people feel attacked or pressured that help them to deal with difficult events.
Feedback: A response from the receiver back to the sender that signifies the message has been received and understood.
Pitch: The frequency of sound emitted by the voice; it is used in verbal communication to indicate various types of information such as questions, statements, and continuation of ideas.
Stereotype: To establish a preconceived image or opinion about someone.

Introduction

Communication skills for phlebotomists are vital. A first impression involves much more than your clothing or physical appearance. The most important factors that help you make a good first impression include attitude, compassion, and smile. Professional phlebotomists must primarily strive to care for patients and offer them the best customer service possible. Patients must be warmly welcomed and called by name, which will give them confidence that staff members care about them.

The Communication Cycle

For effective interpersonal interactions, a transactional communication cycle must exist (see **Figure 3–1**). This cycle involves the following components:
- The sender (or *source*) sends the message using his or her voice, facial expression, tone, and other factors.

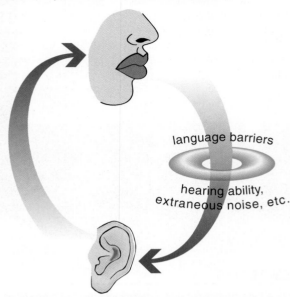

The sender (or source) sends the message using his or her voice, facial expression, tone, and other factors

language barriers

hearing ability, extraneous noise, etc.

The receiver decodes the message and provides feedback to the sender signifying that it has been received and understood.

Figure 3–1 The communication cycle.

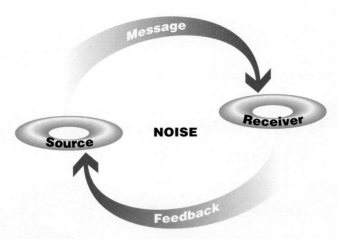

Figure 3–2 Levels of effectiveness of different types of communication.

- The message is filtered through extraneous noise, hearing ability, language barriers, etc.
- The receiver decodes the message and provides **feedback** to the sender signifying that it has been received and understood.

Feedback is essential for completing the communication loop so that both parties know whether the message was successfully communicated.

Face-to-face communication is the most effective form of communication, and it is the method that phlebotomists should strive to practice every day. **Figure 3–2** depicts the various levels of effectiveness of different types of communication.

Types of Communication

Communication can be verbal, nonverbal, or written. It can also be positive or negative.

Verbal Communication

Messages are conveyed through language, which may be written, spoken, or communicated in other ways. Verbal communication requires words and sounds. The **pitch** of the voice is a part of verbal communication, such as when the voice lifts at the end of a question or drops at the end of a statement. Usually, when a speaker intends to continue a statement, the voice will remain at the same pitch. At the same time, the speaker's head will usually remain straight, and the eyes and hands will remain in one position. This signifies to

the listener that the message is continuing and should not be interrupted. If it is interrupted, the speaker's train of thought may be incomplete. Tone of voice and the actual words used also affect messages.

Verbal communication may be compromised by a variety of different factors, including age, different cultures, and gender. This includes communications with patients, their families, coworkers, and other individuals. The desired goal is clear, cooperative, and harmonious communication. Patients should be treated with as much compassion and empathy as possible. Respect for patient privacy, the patient's health condition, and the needs of patients themselves (as well as family members) must be demonstrated. Building trust and establishing a rapport between patients and their supporters create a climate of openness. To listen actively, healthcare workers should always face the patient, maintain an open and relaxed posture, lean toward the patient, maintain eye contact, and listen intently. The providing of positive feedback encourages patients to communicate honestly.

Languages

When healthcare workers are dealing with people whose first language is not English, with children, with the elderly, and with anyone who may have difficulty interpreting instructions and information, it is vital to communicate in a simple, straightforward fashion. Complex medical terms should be avoided because many people are not literate when it comes to medical terminology. Various words may mean different things to people from different generations and backgrounds. To facilitate understanding, each patient's language abilities should be understood.

Healthcare workers who speak other languages may be needed to help with patient education about medications, treatments, procedures, and other information. It is important to ask the patients and their families whether they understand the information provided. A good way to do this is to have them confirm the information in their own words. All patients, regardless of their language abilities, should be treated with fairness, compassion, and dignity.

Hearing-Impaired Patients

It is important to treat hearing-impaired patients carefully to ensure their understanding of information. They should be asked whether they would like anything repeated rather than being asked if they "understand." Always speak slowly and clearly with the hearing impaired. You may also provide written instructions or use sign language, if you are knowledgeable about that form of communication. If a patient still appears to not fully understand the information being provided, a coworker who has the ability to use sign language should be asked to help. It is important to ask the patient to respond in her or his own words (either verbal or written) as to the information the patient is required to understand.

Visually Impaired Patients

Visual ability often decreases with age. Patients with decreased visual ability may be referred to (based on the amount of their vision loss) as visually impaired, low vision, or *blind*. Sightless or visually impaired individuals may be knowledgeable about using the *Braille* system, which utilizes patterns of raised dots that can be read by touch alone. When healthcare workers are dealing with visually impaired patients, it is important to do the following:

- Speak directly to the patient and not to anyone assisting the patient unless the visually impaired patient has designated this other person to communicate directly with you.
- It is important to introduce yourself in a clear, positive voice because the patient cannot see your face or your smile.
- If the patient uses a cane or guide dog, advise the patient of any impediments in the office as he or she moves through—you can offer the patient your arm for assistance, but you should not grab the patient's arm without warning.
- Make sure that no supplies are in any area that the patient may come into contact with due to lack of visual ability.
- Introduce anyone else in the room to the patient before any procedure begins.
- Assist the patient with sitting, standing, lying down, etc.
- Do not dwell on the patient's lack of visual ability—handle her or his medical situation as you would that of any other patient.
- Always communicate who you are and what procedures you will be doing.

Young Patients

Children are more receptive to phlebotomists' requests and suggestions once they realize that their feelings are being taken seriously. You should always explain any procedure in very simple terms, regardless of how basic it is. Always be truthful with young patients, and use praise for their good behavior.

Speaking Clearly

Speaking clearly and articulating carefully are called *enunciation*. Clear speech involves a variety of different components.

These include *pace* (the speed and urgency of the information spoken), *tone* (the lowering or raising of the voice pitch), and *volume* (the loudness of the voice). Pace, tone, and volume can influence the positive and negative understanding (or misunderstanding) of communication. Healthcare workers should attempt to continually speak calmly, smoothly, and confidently, avoiding any abrupt changes in pace, tone, or volume. Smiling while speaking helps the patient feel welcomed and valued. Saying *please* and *thank you* demonstrates respect and concern for the patient's well-being.

Nonverbal Communication

Both verbal and nonverbal communication are important for the exchange of thoughts and information. Nonverbal communication consists of messages that are conveyed without the use of words. They are transmitted by body language, gestures, and mannerisms that may or may not "agree" with the words being spoken. Body language consists of instincts, thoughts, and initiative. It involves eye contact, facial expressions, hand gestures, clothing, grooming, space, tone of voice, posture, and touch.

Nonverbal communication can be positive or negative, greatly influencing the outcome of the communication between individuals. Face-to-face positioning and relaxed body posture aid in communication and help to make interactions more pleasant. A poor posture, rolling of the eyes, staring, squirming, sighing, yawning, and other movements may cause discomfort and uneasiness.

Your expression tells patients a lot about your attitude toward them. Smiling is always important as it opens up communication and makes patients feel important. The most expressive parts of the face are the eyes, and eye contact is important for effective communication and promoting trust and honesty between individuals. Eye level is also important because most people are comfortable when communicating at the same eye level as another. When healthcare workers communicate with a bed ridden patient, it is important to sit beside the patient, more on the patient's eye level, rather than stand above the patient.

Another consideration arises when healthcare workers deal with patients from different cultures. Certain people from Asian, Native American, and Muslim cultures may feel that too much direct eye contact is rude, invasive, or immodest. You should take cues from the patient—obvious signs of discomfort may result from eye contact, body posture, proximity to the patient, and other factors.

Comfort Zones

A *comfort zone* is the area of space around a patient that he or she considers "private territory." If you "invade" that space, the patient may feel uncomfortable. In the United States, there are generally four zones of interpersonal space:

- *Intimate space* (up to 18 in away)—close relationships and for healthcare procedures that require touching of the patient
- *Personal space* (18 in to 4 ft)—between friends and for certain patient encounters
- *Social space* (4 to 12 ft)—for most everyday interactions

- *Public space* (12 ft and above)—for speeches, lectures, etc.

A proximity that is too close may cause a patient to feel nervous or anxious, and healthcare workers should never move toward a patient in a quick or threatening manner. This is especially true for pediatric patients who may be fearful of unknown adults. Your manner should always appear calm, professional, and confident. Always talk to the patient in a friendly manner if you sense any discomfort—this will help to convince the patient that your actions are focused on his or her comfort and well-being.

Cultural Diversity

Systems of realistic beliefs, practices, and values all combine to form a person's *culture*. Phlebotomists must learn about the various cultures of patients whom they may be treating. It is best to follow the patient's "lead," observing how he or she interacts, so that your actions do not seem abrupt or offensive to the patient. By observing the patient's gestures, mannerisms, and facial expressions, it will be relatively simple for you to determine how the patient interacts comfortably and to mimic his or her actions. Always respect the patient's needs and dignity.

Negative Communication

The following body language examples may result in negative communication and distractions:

- Breathing patterns—sighing (may convey boredom), moaning (may convey fear, anxiety, or a feeling of inadequacy)
- Nervous behaviors—squirming or tapping (may show or actually increase anxiety and nervousness)
- Eye movements—rolling the eyes (may convey boredom, unwillingness to comply, or inattentiveness), gazing or staring (may convey an uncaring attitude)
- Other behaviors—crossed arms, looking at your watch, wrinkling the forehead, yawning, stretching, gum chewing, and other behaviors (may indicate negativity or defensive attitudes)

Positive Communication

Positive communication promotes patients' comfort and well-being and is essential in medical facilities. Examples of positive communication include the following:

- Smiling naturally
- Remaining friendly, warm, and attentive
- Verbalizing your concern for patients
- Encouraging patients to ask questions
- Looking directly at patients when speaking to them
- Speaking slowly and clearly
- Listening carefully
- Asking patients to repeat instructions to make sure that they understand them
- Remaining calm with an angry patient
- Remaining calm if mentally disabled patients become confused
- Addressing elderly patients as "Mr." or "Mrs." unless they tell you otherwise

Active listening ensures that the receiver understands the sender's message. Listening skills can easily be improved by practicing them. Carefully listening improves the interpretation of patients' needs and other information. It is important to ask patients if they have followed instructions and if they have had any problems or difficulties with what they were required to do. *Active listening* is defined as complete attention to a speaker's verbal message, body language, and the provision of feedback about these forms of communication. It differs from passive listening, which involves no replies and is employed when attending a lecture.

Steps for active listening include the following:

- Getting ready to listen by clearing your mind of distracting thoughts
- Facing the speaker
- Using the speaker's pauses to summarize the information
- Verifying that you are listening by short "return" comments to the speaker
- Avoiding judging the speaker until the communication is finished
- Verifying the conversation with feedback
- Paying attention to body language and asking for clarification
- Maintaining eye contact, showing interest and concern
- Using encouragement to expand the speaker's thoughts
- Practicing active listening at work and at home

Written Communication

Written communication may involve a variety of different types of paperwork. Always use clear, correct wording and grammar and proofread all documents. Make sure handwriting is legible and, if possible, write in permanent ink.

Telephone and Computer Communication

Similar to other forms of communication, use of the telephone or computer still involves a sender and a receiver. The telephone utilizes exclusively verbal communication via the voices of the participants. Enunciation, pitch, and quality of the voice become more important than in face-to-face encounters. On the phone, speakers should use a conversational, confident, and warm tone. Proper phone etiquette must always be practiced to ensure continually strong patient relationships. The phone should be answered within a maximum of three rings. You should smile as you answer the phone as this will actually influence the positive tone of your voice. Speak expressively, not in a flat monotone. The conversation should be upbeat and professional, and you should never interrupt the patient.

It is good business practice to greet callers with the time of day ("good morning" or "good afternoon"), identify the place of employment, and then identify yourself. Ask the caller, "How may I help you?" Make sure you write down the caller's name and use it throughout the conversation. If you are unable to help the caller, redirect the call to someone who may be able to do so.

In the case of multiple phone lines, answer calls as they come in and put callers on hold in order to answer additional lines. Do not finish one call before attempting to answer another, or the other callers may hang up before you can get to them. When it seems that a call will be lengthy, return to the other callers and ask for their information so that you can call them back shortly. Always attempt to let callers know how long it may be before they receive a return phone call. When you are attempting to put a caller on hold, ask the caller's permission to do so, wait for his or her response, explain why you need to put the caller on hold, and thank the caller for holding when you return to the call.

When you are taking a message, make sure to accurately record the following information:

- The caller's name, correctly spelled
- The company name, if applicable
- Telephone number with area code
- Time of call
- Exact message, as close to the caller's words as possible

Make sure to repeat all information back to the caller before you hang up. Next to the phone, you should always keep pens, pencils, and a telephone message pad (see **Figure 3–3** for an example of this type of pad).

Make sure to end calls positively, repeating any actions that were agreed upon during the call. Ask the caller if you can do anything else to help, and thank the caller for contacting you. Let the caller hang up before you do so that you do not cut him or her off. Make sure that all information is recorded correctly immediately after the call ends.

Remember that it is not appropriate to give patient information over the phone to anyone except the patient. Test results are usually not given out over the phone. Phlebotomists are never allowed to give detailed explanations about test results and are not allowed to diagnose conditions—these are solely the roles of the healthcare provider.

Most medical facilities today use computers as communication tools. They quickly and easily facilitate communication among laboratories and various types of medical facilities, and among departments inside a specific facility. The same rules of etiquette and professionalism used over the telephone apply to computer communication.

Improving Your Communication Skills

To improve your communication skills, you should follow the listening patterns that are commonly used in medical facilities. There are three basic types of listening patterns: active (described in detail previously), passive, and evaluative listening. Unlike active listening, which requires two-way communication, passive listening involves both listening without answering and offering feedback. Evaluative listening provides immediate responses and opinions, and it requires the listener to pay attention to everything the speaker says.

Improving your communication skills also involves utilizing interpersonal skills such as empathy, genuineness, consideration, sensitivity, openness, and respect. The unique needs of every patient should be addressed, and you should always attempt to make each patient feel at ease so that effective communication can occur. You should learn when to use silence (which reduces pressure on the patient), restate what the patient has said, reflect patients' questions so that they can answer their own questions and concerns, use open-ended questions that require the patient to elaborate, keep the patient focused on particular topics, and develop positive rapport with patients.

Ineffective methods of communication include the following, which should be avoided or minimized:

- Agreeing and disagreeing—try to remain as neutral as possible
- Advising the patient, which places you outside your scope of practice
- Approval of a patient's behavior, which makes the patient seek praise
- Disapproval of a patient's behavior, which decreases communication
- Defending criticisms about yourself or the workplace
- Minimizing a patient's feelings, discomfort, or concerns
- Probing a topic that the patient does not want to discuss
- Reassuring patients, which devalues their feelings and gives false hope
- Requesting explanations—asking "why" questions may intimidate the patient
- Stereotyping by using clichés instead of reasonable, thoughtful explanations

Interactions with Other Individuals

Family members and friends may be in attendance when a patient visits the healthcare facility. When they are there for support and display proper behavior, they may actually make the encounter more effective. However, when they are distracting or negative, it is your responsibility to handle the situation to the best of your ability. During certain procedures,

PHONE MESSAGE

To: _____

From: _____

Company: _____

Tel: _____

Date: _____ Time: _____

Message: _____

_____

_____

_____

Figure 3–3 A telephone message pad.

especially those requiring privacy or that may cause embarrassment, these individuals may be asked to leave the procedure room until it is completed. Children should always be accompanied by their parent or guardian. If required, the healthcare worker should allow privacy between a patient and his or her physicians and religious figures. When a procedure is stat, it is advisable to apologize for any interruptions that may be required to complete it on a timely basis. Family members and friends should not be provided with private patient information unless this has been arranged for previously through patient permission. **Confidentiality** of patient records must always be considered to ensure patient privacy and safety.

Barriers to Communication

Barriers to communication include physical impairment, language (discussed previously), prejudice, stereotyping, and perception. Physical impairments include hearing, vision, speech, and mobility problems. Although many elderly people do have health problems that impair communication, many others do not. Each patient's ability to communicate should be assessed and reacted to correctly. The patient's chart should be noted in an easily noticed area when a patient has a specific barrier to communication.

Personal or social bias (prejudice) causes discrimination, which results in unfair treatment of a person because of gender, race, religion, handicaps, or other reasons. Discrimination and prejudice are unethical and both morally and socially wrong. While creating a communication barrier, these practices may also be illegal. More *subtle* forms of discrimination may occur because of a person's appearance, lifestyle, values, weight, personal relationship status, sexual orientation, need for government financial assistance, or whether she or he has a sexually transmitted disease. Medical professionals cannot allow personal prejudice to affect how they care for their patients.

It is also unfair to **stereotype** anyone based on preconceived (and often incorrect) assumptions. Patients should not be judged before they can be understood as individuals. Stereotypic categories should not be considered when caring for patients. The perception of what a patient is saying can be distorted based on an experience with another individual from the same ethnic group. It is unfair to do this, and each patient must be communicated with as an individual, not as part of a group.

Stress is one of the greatest barriers to communication. Phlebotomists may experience high levels of stress in their daily work environment. Stress can result from feelings of being under pressure, or it may be a reaction to anger, frustration, or a change in routine. Stress can be minimized by keeping a balance among work, family, and leisure activities as well as exercising and eating a healthy diet. Stress management is important in order to prevent *burnout*, which is an energy-depleting condition that will affect your health and your career.

Defense Mechanisms

Defense mechanisms are often used when people feel attacked or pressured. They are often subconscious reactions that help individuals to deal with difficult events. Often, a person may be unaware of using defense mechanisms and may even aggressively deny that she or he is doing so. Professional phlebotomists should be familiar with defense mechanisms so that they can better communicate with patients and other people they come into contact with in the course of their daily activities. Common defense mechanisms include the following:

- Apathy—lack of emotion, feeling, concern, or interest
- Compensation—making up for one behavior by stressing another
- Denial—avoiding confrontation with a problem or reality by denying its existence
- Displacement—the redirection of an emotion or impulse from its original object to another object
- Physical avoidance—completely staying away from a person, place, object, or anything else that reminds a person of negative feelings or happenings
- Projection—attributing a person's feelings, attitudes, or ideas to others
- Rationalization—attributing actions to rational, credible motives without analyzing underlying methods
- Regression—reversion to an earlier mental or behavioral level
- Repression—blocking a problem or unwanted desire (or impulse) from conscious thought
- Sarcasm—hostile or cruel intention in verbal expression intending to cause pain or anger in another individual
- Verbal aggression—a verbal attack on another without addressing the original complaint or problem

Summary

Effective communication skills require a communication cycle, including a sender, message, and receiver. Communication can be verbal, nonverbal, written, positive, or negative. Language barriers, hearing impairments, visual impairments, young patients, and poor enunciation all combine to block verbal communication. Nonverbal communication includes body language, comfort zones, cultural diversity, and both negative and positive communication. Written communication should always be clear, with correct wording and grammar that has been proofread for errors. Telephone and computer communication requires positive, professional communication skills so that messages are not misinterpreted. Proper phone etiquette makes callers feel appreciated and important. Improving communication skills requires utilization of active, passive, and evaluative listening. Aside from language, barriers to communication include physical impairment, prejudice, stereotyping, and perception. People may use defense mechanisms when they feel attacked or pressured. These include denial, projection, rationalization, and many others.

CRITICAL THINKING

Ashley is a phlebotomist who was attempting to draw blood from an elderly person. She called the patient by his first name. While drawing blood from this patient, Ashley was completely silent and did not explain the procedure as it occurred. When she finished the procedure, Ashley misspelled the patient's last name in the computer and did not correct it. The patient was not happy with his interactions with Ashley.

1. Why are communication skills essential for phlebotomists?
2. Give some suggestions about dealing with different age groups of patients.
3. Why is computer communication important for phlebotomists?

WEBSITES

http://www.aafp.org/afp/2008/0515/p1431.html

http://www.blatner.com/adam/level2/nverb1.htm

http://www.effective-communicating.com/written-communication.html

http://www.hodu.com/barriers.shtml

http://www.media-visions.com/communication.html

http://www.nursinglaw.com/deafpatient.pdf

http://www.phlebotomypages.com/job_description.htm

http://www-usr.rider.edu/~suler/defenses.html

REVIEW QUESTIONS

Multiple Choice

1. Nonverbal communication is also known as
   A. true feelings
   B. touching
   C. body language
   D. nodding
2. The three types of listening are evaluative, active, and
   A. responsive
   B. selective
   C. two-way
   D. passive
3. Which of the following is NOT part of the communication cycle?
   A. message
   B. witness
   C. sender
   D. feedback
4. Which of the following is the definition of the term *prejudice*?
   A. holding a negative opinion about an individual because of his or her beliefs
   B. respecting an individual as a human being
   C. refusing to acknowledge something
   D. recognizing that the patient is nervous
5. When dealing with a seriously ill patient, you should
   A. judge the patient's statements
   B. avoid empty promises
   C. abandon the patient
   D. isolate the patient
6. One of the greatest barriers to communication is
   A. poor communication skills
   B. complaining
   C. assertiveness
   D. stress
7. When communicating with very young patients, you should
   A. treat them the same as adults
   B. explain any procedure in very simple terms
   C. show them videotapes of procedures
   D. mimic their behaviors
8. Which of the following defense mechanisms is defined as putting unpleasant events, feelings, or thoughts out of one's mind?
   A. repression
   B. displacement
   C. dissociation
   D. compensation
9. Which of the following types of materials should you use when dealing with visually impaired patients?
   A. large print
   B. nonverbal
   C. infrared
   D. Braille
10. Positive communication includes
    A. discussing payment history
    B. smiling at all times
    C. encouraging patients to ask questions
    D. listening to patients and other staff simultaneously
11. Which of the following is NOT an example of negative communication?
    A. speaking sharply
    B. showing boredom
    C. rushing through
    D. looking directly at patients when you speak to them
12. Speaking clearly and articulating carefully are known as
    A. pronunciation
    B. enunciation
    C. intonation
    D. salutation
13. The redirection of an emotion or impulse from its original object to another object is referred to as
    A. displacement
    B. compensation
    C. regression
    D. repression
14. An example of negative communication is
    A. speaking slowly
    B. verbalizing
    C. mumbling
    D. smiling naturally
15. Good communication techniques include
    A. not looking directly at the patient
    B. having only the doctor talk to the patient
    C. watching only your own body language
    D. demonstrating respect

Terminology and Abbreviations

OUTLINE

Introduction
The Language of Medicine
    Word Roots
    Prefixes
    Suffixes
    Combining Forms
Common Medical Terminology Related to the
Cardiovascular System
    Common Terms Related to the Cardiovascular System
    Common Terms Related to Anatomy and Physiology
    Cardiovascular System—Abbreviations
    Laboratory and Phlebotomy—Abbreviations
Summary
Critical Thinking
Websites
Review Questions

OBJECTIVES

After reading this chapter, readers should be able to:

1. List the three basic component parts of a word.
2. Define the terms *prefix* and *suffix*.
3. Define the terms *word root* and *combining form*.
4. Correctly identify at least 15 combining forms related to the cardiovascular system.
5. Identify at least 10 prefixes related to phlebotomy.
6. Identify at least 10 suffixes related to laboratory procedures.
7. List 10 common terms related to cardiovascular diseases.
8. Define the terms *antigen, hemostasis, homeostasis, metabolism,* and *phagocytosis.*
9. Identify at least 10 common laboratory abbreviations.
10. Define the terms *coarctation of the aorta, bradycardia, dysrhythmia,* and *pericarditis.*

Introduction

Medicine has its own language, which can be learned by memorizing word parts and learning how they fit together to create medical terms. Learning medical terminology allows health professionals to understand the language of medicine and communicate with one another. Therefore, phlebotomists and laboratory technicians must learn word parts in order to understand complex medical terminology.

The Language of Medicine

All medical fields utilize the language of medicine, which is primarily based on Greek and Latin terms. Medical terminology is broken down into word roots, prefixes, suffixes, and combining forms. It is relatively easy to learn medical terminology as long as you understand the basics of how medical terms are constructed.

Word Roots

All medical terms are derived from *word roots*, which establish the meaning of each term. In general, word roots are used to signify body systems, organs, tissues, and even colors. When word roots are used with prefixes, suffixes, and combining forms, new words can be created.

Prefixes

Prefixes are placed in front of word roots to create a new term. Prefixes usually indicate amounts, locations, times, sizes, or other descriptive information. **Table 4–1** shows commonly used prefixes.

Suffixes

Suffixes are added after word roots or combining forms. Like prefixes, suffixes also change the meaning of the new term, but they often indicate conditions, diseases, disorders, or procedures. Note that there are several suffixes that mean "pertaining to" or "relating to" (see **Table 4–2**).

■ Table 4–1 Commonly Used Prefixes

Prefix	Meaning	Prefix	Meaning
A-, ab-, an-	Away from	Mal-	Bad, evil, poor
Ac-, ad-, af-, as-, at-	To, toward	Med-, mes-	Middle
Al-	Like, similar	Mega-	Great, large
Ante-	Before, forward	Meta-	After, behind, change, hindmost, next, subsequent to, transformation
Anti-	Against, counter		
Bi-	Double, twice, two	Multi-	Many, much
Brachy-	Short	Neo-	New, strange
Brady-	Slow	Nitro-	Nitrogen
Cent-	Hundred	Non-	No
Circum-	About, around	Nuli-	None
Co-, com-, con-	Together, with	Ortho-	Correct, normal, straight
Contra-	Against, counter, opposite	Os-	Bone, mouth
Cort-	Covering	Pan-	All, entire, every
Cyst-	Bag, bladder	Para-	Abnormal, apart from, beside, near
De-	Down, from, lack of, not	Per-	Excessive, through
di-	Double, twice, twofold	Peri-	Around, surrounding
Dia-	Apart, between, complete, through	Poly-	Many
Dis-	Absence, apart, negative	Post-	After, behind
Dys-	Bad, difficult, painful	Pre-	Before, in front of
Ecto-	Out, outside	Re-	Again, back
En-, endo-	In, into, within	Retro-	Back of, backward, behind
Epi-	Above, on, upon, upper	Semi-	Half
Eu-	Easy, good, well	Sub-	Below, less, under
Ex-, exo-	Away from, out of, outside	Super-	Above, excessive, higher than
Extra-	Beyond, on the outside, outside	Sym-	Together, with
Fore-	Before, in front of	Syn-	Association, union
Hem-	Relating to the blood	Tachy-	Fast, rapid
Hemi-	Half	Tetra-	Four
Hydra-	Relating to water	Trans-	Across, through
Hyper-	Above, excessive, increased, over	Tri-	Three
Hypo-	Below, decreased, deficient, under	Ultra-	Beyond, excess
In-	In, into, not, without	Un-	Not
Infra-	Below, beneath, inferior to	Uni-	One
Inter-	Among, between	Venter-	Abdomen
Intra-, intro-	Inside, into, within		

■ Table 4–2 Commonly Used Suffixes

Suffix	Meaning	Suffix	Meaning
-able	Able to, capable of	-agra	Attack of severe pain, excessive pain, seizure
-ac, -al, -ar, -ary, -eal, -iac, -ic, -ous, -tic	Pertaining to		
		-aise	Comfort, ease
-ago	Attack	-algesic	Painful

Table 4–2 Commonly Used Suffixes *(Continued)*

Suffix	Meaning	Suffix	Meaning
-arche	Beginning	-oid	Like, resembling
-ase	Enzyme	-ologist	Specialist
-blast	Embryonic, immature stage	-ology	Science or study of
-cele	Cyst, hernia, tumor	-oma	Neoplasm, tumor
-centesis	Surgical puncture to remove fluid	-osis	Abnormal condition, disease
-cidal	Pertaining to death	-ostomy	Surgically creating a mouth or opening
-cide	Causing death	-otomy	Cutting, surgical incision
-clasis, -clast	Break	-paresis	Partial or incomplete paralysis
-clysis	Irrigation, washing	-penia	Deficiency, lack, abnormal reduction
-crasia	A blending or mixture	-pexy	Surgical fixation, to put in place
-crit	Separate	-phage	A cell that destroys, one that eats
-cytic	Pertaining to a cell	-phagia	Eating, swallowing
-cytosis	Abnormal condition of cells	-phasia	Speak or speech
-dema	Swelling with fluid	-pheresis	Removal
-desis	Bind, surgical fixation, tie together	-phoresis	Carrying, transmission
-duct	Opening	-phoria	Carry, feeling, mental state, to bear
-dynia	Pain	-phylactic	Preventive, protective
-ectasia, -ectasis	Dilation, enlargement, stretching	-phylaxis	Protection
-ectomy	Cutting out, excision, surgical removal	-physis	To grow
-emesis	Vomiting	-plasia	Formation, growth, development
-emia	Blood, blood condition	-plasm	Formative material of cells
-esis	Abnormal condition or state	-plasty	Surgical repair
-esthesia	Feeling, sensation	-plegia	Palsy, paralysis, stroke
-exia, -exis	Condition	-plegic	One affected with paralysis, paralysis
-ferent	Carrying	-pnea	Breathing
-form	Figure, form, shape	-poiesis	Formation
-fuge	To drive away	-porosis	Passage, porous condition
-gene	Formation, origin, production	-praxia	Action, condition concerning performance of movements
-genesis, -genic	Forming, producing		
-globin	Protein	-ptosis	Drooping, dropping down, prolapse, sagging
-grade	Degree, rank, step		
-gram	Picture, record, tracing	-ptysis	Spitting
-graph	Instrument for recording, picture	-rrhaphy	Stitching, suturing
-graphy	Process of recording	-rrhea	Discharge, flow
-ia	Condition, state	-rrhexis	Rupture
-iasis	Abnormal condition, pathologic state, condition	-sarcoma	Cancer, tumor
		-scope	Instrument for visual examination
-ile	Able to, capable of being, pertaining to	-scopic	Pertaining to visual examination
-ism	Condition, state of	-scopy	See, visual examination
-itis	Inflammation	-stasis	Controlling, stopping
-kinesis	Motion	-stenosis	Narrowing, stricture, tightening of a duct or canal
-lith	Calculus, stone		
-lithiasis	Presence of stones	-stomy	Furnish with a mouth, new opening, or outlet
-lysis	Break down, destruction, separation, setting free		
		-tomy	Cutting, incision
-lytic	Destroy, reduce	-tripsy	Crushing stone
-mania	Obsessive, preoccupation	-tropic	Having an affinity for, turning toward
-megaly	Enlargement, extreme, great, large	-uresis	Urination
-meter	Measure	-uria	Urination, urine
-necrosis	Tissue death	-version	To turn

Combining Forms

Combining forms utilize the combining vowels *o* or *i*. These vowels may be added as extensions of word roots to modify spellings. If a suffix begins with a vowel, a combining vowel is not added between the word root and the suffix. They are used when a suffix begins with a consonant. The word root *cardi* means "heart." The combining form *cardi/o* may be combined with a suffix such as *-pathy* to form the new term *cardiopathy*, which means "heart disease." In this case, the combining vowel is included in the final term because the suffix begins with a consonant. In the term *carditis*, which utilizes the suffix *-itis*, the suffix begins with a vowel.

Therefore, the *o* in the combining form *cardi/o* is dropped when the word root and suffix are combined. See **Table 4–3** for commonly used combining forms related to the cardiovascular system.

Common Medical Terminology Related to the Cardiovascular System

Table 4–4 lists common medical terms that are related to the cardiovascular system.

Common Terms Related to the Cardiovascular System

Table 4–5 lists common terms related to cardiovascular system.

Table 4–3 Commonly Used Combining Forms Related to the Cardiovascular System

Combining Form	Meaning
Agglutin/o	Clumping, sticking together
Aneurysm/o	Aneurysm
Aort/o	Aorta
Arteri/o	Artery
Ather/o	Fatty substance, plaque
Brachi/o	Arm
Cardi/o	Heart
Cholesterol/o	Cholesterol
Coagulat/o	Congeal, curdle, fix together
Corpuscul/o	Little body
Cyan/o	Blue
Dilat/o	Expand, spread out
Ecchym/o	Pouring out of fluid
Eosin/o	Dawn-colored, red, rosy
Erythem/o	Flushed, redness
Erythr/o	Red
Fibrin/o	Fibers, fibrin, threads of a clot
Hem/o	Relating to the blood
Hemangi/o	Blood vessel
Hemat/o	Relating to the blood
Hepat/o	Liver
Jugul/o	Throat
Lip/o	Fat, lipid
Myocardi/o	Heart muscle, myocardium
Occlud/o	To shut or close
Occult/o	Concealed, hidden
Phleb/o	Vein
Plasm/o	Formed or molded
Pulm/o	Lung
Syring/o	Tube
Thromb/o	Clot
Varic/o	Dilated or swollen vein
Vascul/o	Little vessel
Ven/o	Vein
Ventricul/o	Ventricle of heart or brain
Venul/o	Venule, small vein

Table 4–4 Common Medical Terms Related to the Cardiovascular System

Term	Meaning
Apnea	Temporary cessation of breathing
Arrhythmia	Irregularity or loss of heart rhythm
Assay	The analysis of a substance or mixture to determine the components and relative proportion of each
Auscultate	To examine by listening for sounds within the body
Brachial	Pertaining to the arm
Bradycardia	A slow heartbeat characterized by a pulse rate below 60 beats per minute throughout one 10-min period
Bradypnea	Abnormally slow breathing
Carotid	Pertaining to the right and left common carotid arteries, which comprise the principal blood supply to the head and neck
Diastole	The normal "rest period" in the heart cycle during which the muscle fibers lengthen, the heart dilates, and the cavities fill with blood
Febrile	Feverish; abnormal elevation of temperature
Hypertension	A condition of higher than normal blood pressure (usually, in adults, this is greater than 140/90)
Hypotension	A condition of lower than normal blood pressure (usually, in adults, this is less than 90/60)
Hypothermia	The state in which an individual's body temperature is reduced below the normal range; less than 96 degrees Fahrenheit (96°F)
Palpate	To examine by touch; to feel
Preexisting condition	Any illness that began before an insurance policy was written
Pulse	Rate, rhythm, and condition of arterial walls
Radial pulse	Pulse palpated over the radial artery of the arm
Respiration	The act of inhaling and exhaling (breathing)
Systole	Contractions of the chambers of the heart, in which blood is pumped from the chambers
Tachycardia	An abnormally rapid heartbeat, usually defined as 100 or more beats per minute (in adults)
Tachypnea	Abnormal rapidity of respiration
Vital signs	Heartbeat, body temperature, respiration, blood pressure, and other traditional signs of life

Table 4–5 Common Terms Related to the Cardiovascular System

Term	Meaning
Aneurysm	Ballooning of an artery wall due to weakness in the wall
Angina pectoris	Chest pain, usually due to lowered oxygen or blood supply to the heart
Aortic regurgitation	Backward flow or leakage of blood through a faulty aortic valve
Aortic stenosis	Narrowing of the aorta
Arrhythmia	Irregularity of the heartbeat rhythm
Arteriosclerosis	Hardening of the arteries, causing thickening of the walls and loss of elasticity
Arteritis	Inflammation of an artery or arteries
Asystole	Cardiac arrest
Atheroma	A fatty deposit (plaque) in the wall of an artery
Atherosclerosis	Hardening of the arteries caused by deposits of fatlike material in the lining of the arteries
Atrial fibrillation	Irregular, usually rapid heartbeat caused by overstimulation of the atrioventricular node
Atrioventricular block	Heart block; partial or complete blockage of electrical impulses from the atrioventricular node to the ventricles
Benign	Noncancerous
Bradycardia	Heart rate of fewer than 60 beats per minute
Bruit	Sound or murmur, especially an abnormal heart sound heard on auscultation of (commonly) the carotid artery
Cardiac arrest	Sudden stopping of the heart; also called asystole
Cardiac tamponade	Compression of the heart due to fluid accumulation in the pericardial sac
Cardiomyopathy	Disease of the heart muscle
Claudication	Limping caused by inadequate blood supply during activity; usually subsides during rest
Coarctation of the aorta	Abnormal narrowing of the arch of the aorta
Congenital heart disease	Heart disease that exists at birth, usually due to a malformation
Congestive heart failure	Inability of the heart to pump enough blood out during the cardiac cycle, resulting in a collection of fluid in the lungs
Constriction	Compression or narrowing caused by contraction, as of a vessel
Coronary artery disease	A condition that reduces the flow of blood and nutrients through the arteries of the heart
Cyanosis	Bluish or purplish coloration (often, of the skin) as a result of inadequate oxygenation of the blood
Deep vein thrombosis	Formation of a thrombus (clot) in a deep vein, such as a femoral vein
Degeneration	Change of tissue to a less functionally active form
Dysrhythmia	Abnormal heart rhythm
Embolus	A mass of lipid plaques attached to the inside of blood vessels or as part of a thrombus (blood clot) blocking a vessel
Endocarditis	Inflammation of the endocardium, especially due to a bacterial or fungal agent
Essential hypertension	High blood pressure without any known cause
Etiology	Cause of a disease
Fibrillation	Random irregular heart rhythm
Flutter	Regular but very rapid heartbeat
Hemorrhoids	Varicose condition of veins in the anal region
Hypertension	A chronic condition with blood pressure greater than 140/90
Hypertensive heart disease	Heart disease caused or worsened by high blood pressure
Hypotension	A chronic condition with blood pressure below normal
Infarct	Area of necrosis caused by a sudden drop in the supply of arterial or venous blood
Infarction	Sudden drop in the supply of arterial or venous blood, often due to an embolus or thrombus
Infection	The presence and growth of a microorganism that produces tissue damage
Intermittent claudication	Attacks of limping, particularly in the legs, due to ischemia of the muscles
Ischemia	A temporary reduction of blood supply to an organ or tissue due to obstruction of a blood vessel

(Continues)

Table 4–5 Common Terms Related to the Cardiovascular System *(Continued)*

Term	Meaning
Malaise	Not feeling well; the first indication of illness
Malignant	Cancerous
Microorganism	A microscopic living organism
Mitral insufficiency or reflux	Backward flow of blood due to a damaged mitral valve
Mitral stenosis	Abnormal narrowing at the opening of the mitral valve
Mitral valve prolapse	Backward flow of blood into the left atrium due to protrusion of one or both mitral cusps into the left atrium during contractions
Murmur	A consistent, repeating, abnormal heart sound usually heard only with the aid of a stethoscope
Myocardial infarction	Sudden drop in the supply of blood to an area of the heart muscle, usually due to a blockage in a coronary artery
Myocarditis	Inflammation of the myocardium
Necrosis	Death of tissue or an organ or part due to irreversible damage, usually due to oxygen deprivation
Nosocomial	An infection acquired in a hospital or other institution
Occlusion	Closing of a blood vessel
Palpitations	Uncomfortable pulsations of the heart felt as a thumping in the chest
Patent ductus arteriosus	A condition at birth in which the ductus arteriosus between the aorta and pulmonary artery remains abnormally open
Pathogen	An organism capable of causing a disease, condition, or infection
Pathogenic	Capable of causing disease
Pericarditis	Inflammation of the pericardium
Peripheral vascular disease	Vascular disease in the lower extremities, usually due to blockages in the arteries of the groin or legs
Petechiae	Minute hemorrhages in the skin
Phlebitis	Inflammation of a vein
Plaque	Buildup of solid material, such as a fatty deposit, on the lining of an artery
Prognosis	Prediction about the outcome of a disease
Prophylaxis	Protection against disease
Pulmonary artery stenosis	Narrowing of the pulmonary artery, preventing the lungs from receiving enough blood from the heart to oxygenate
Pulmonary edema	Abnormal accumulation of fluid in the lungs
Raynaud's phenomenon	Spasm in the arteries of the fingers causing numbness or pain
Remission	Cessation of signs and symptoms
Rheumatic heart disease	Heart valve and/or muscle damage caused by an untreated streptococcal infection
Risk factor	Anything considered to increase the probability that a disease will occur
Septal defect	Congenital abnormality consisting of an opening in the septum between the atria or ventricles
Stenosis	Narrowing of blood vessels, cardiac valves, or other structures
Tachycardia	Heart rate over 100 beats per minute
Tetralogy of Fallot	A set of four congenital heart abnormalities that cause deoxygenated blood to enter the systemic circulation: ventricular septal defect, pulmonary stenosis, incorrect position of the aorta, and right ventricular hypertrophy
Thrombophlebitis	Inflammation of a vein with a thrombus
Thrombosis	Presence of a thrombus in a blood vessel
Thrombotic occlusion	Narrowing caused by a thrombus
Thrombus	A blood clot that forms in the cardiovascular system. Thrombi may form in a blood vessel inside one of the heart's chambers.
Tricuspid stenosis	Abnormal narrowing of the opening of the tricuspid valve
Varicose vein	Dilated, enlarged, or twisted vein, usually on the leg

Common Terms Related to Anatomy and Physiology

Table 4–6 lists common terms related to anatomy and physiology as used in phlebotomy.

Cardiovascular System—Abbreviations

Abbreviations are commonly used to simplify medical terms, but they should always be used with caution. Many abbreviations have multiple meanings—and these may cause confusion

▪ Table 4–6 Common Terms Related to Anatomy and Physiology

Term	Meaning
Agranulocyte	A nongranular white blood cell
Anatomy	The study of the structure of an organism
Antecubital fossa	The triangular area lying anterior to and below the elbow; location of the major veins for venipuncture
Anterior	Before or in front of; the ventral or abdominal side of the body
Antigen	A protein that identifies a cell as "self" or "nonself"
Arteriole	A small branch of an artery
Basophils	White blood cells that are essential to nonspecific immune response to inflammation
Cerebrospinal fluid	CSF; a water cushion that protects the brain and spinal cord from physical impact
Deoxygenated	The state of having oxygen removed from a compound (such as blood) or tissue
Dermis	The true skin, lying immediately beneath the epidermis
Distal	The farthest from point of origin of a structure; opposite of proximal
Elasticity	The quality of returning to original size and shape after compression or stretching
Eosinophils	White blood cells that increase in an allergic response
Epidermis	The outermost layer of skin
Erythrocyte	A mature red blood cell (RBC)
Granulocyte	A white blood cell having granules in its cytoplasm
Hematuria	Blood in the urine
Hemoglobin	The oxygen-carrying pigment of the blood
Hemolysis	The bursting of red blood cells
Hemopoiesis (hematopoiesis)	Production and development of blood cells, normally in the bone marrow
Hemostasis	A stoppage of bleeding or of circulation
Homeostasis	The state of dynamic equilibrium of the internal body environment
Inferior	Beneath; lower; referring to the underside of an organ or indicating a structure below another
Interstitial fluid	Fluid between the tissues that surrounds cells
Lateral	Toward the side of the body
Leukocyte	A white blood cell or corpuscle (WBC)
Lymph	Watery fluid in the lymphatic vessels
Lymphocytes	White blood cells that either directly attack infected cells (T cells) or produce antibodies (B cells)
Medial	Toward the midline of the body
Mediastinum	Part of the thoracic cavity containing the heart and blood vessels and lying between the sternum and vertebral column as well as between the lungs
Meninges	Membranes that cover the spinal cord and brain (dura mater, arachnoid, and pia mater)
Metabolism	Sum of the processes of digestion, absorption, and the resulting release of energy
Monocytes	Large mononuclear leukocytes that ingest pathogens which become macrophages when they leave the bloodstream
Neutrophil	A white blood cell with a many-lobed nucleus that phagocytizes bacteria; sometimes called *polys* or *segs*
Phagocytosis	The ingestion of foreign substances or other particles, such as worn-out cells, by certain white blood cells
Physiology	The study of the functions of a living organism and its components
Posterior	Behind or at the back; opposite of anterior
Prone	The position of lying on the stomach with the face downward

(Continues)

■ **Table 4–6 Common Terms Related to Anatomy and Physiology** *(Continued)*

Term	Meaning
Proximal	Nearest the point of attachment, center of the body, or point of reference
Subcutaneous	Beneath the skin
Superficial	Pertaining to or situated near the surface
Superior	Higher; denoting upper of two parts
Supine	The position of lying on the back with the face upward
Thrombocyte	Platelet
Tunica adventitia	The outermost fibroelastic layer of a blood vessel
Tunica intima	The lining of a blood vessel, composed of an epithelial layer and the basement membrane, a connective tissue layer; usually an internal elastic lamina
Tunica media	The middle layer in the wall of a blood vessel, composed of circular or spiraling smooth muscle and some elastic fibers
Universal donor	An individual with type O blood, which can be donated to all blood types because it lacks A and B antigens
Universal recipient	An individual belonging to the AB blood group who can accept blood from all blood types
Uremia	The presence of urea and excess waste products in the blood
Vasoconstriction	A decrease in the caliber of blood vessels

or medical errors. It is wise to remember this warning: *When in doubt, spell it out.* Any time that you feel a term may be mistaken for another, spell out the term in its entirety. **Table 4–7** lists common cardiovascular system abbreviations.

Laboratory and Phlebotomy—Abbreviations

Table 4–8 lists common abbreviations that relate to the laboratory and phlebotomy.

■ **Table 4–7 Common Cardiovascular System Abbreviations**

Abbreviation	Meaning	Abbreviation	Meaning
ACE	Angiotensin-converting enzyme	CAD	Coronary artery disease
ACEI	Angiotensin-converting enzyme inhibitor	CCR	Comprehensive cardiac rehabilitation
ACLS	Advanced cardiac life support	CFR	Coronary flow reserve
ADH	Antidiuretic hormone	CHD	Coronary heart disease
AED	Automated external defibrillator	CHF	Chronic heart failure or congestive heart failure
AF	Atrial fibrillation	CKD	Chronic kidney disease
AMI	Acute myocardial infarction	CO	Cardiac output
Ao	Aorta	COX	Cyclo-oxygenase
ARB	Angiotensin receptor blocker	CPR	Cardiopulmonary resuscitation
AS	Aortic stenosis	CR	Cardiac rehabilitation
ASA	Acetylsalicylic acid	CV	Cardiovascular
ASD	Atrial septal defect	CVA	Cerebrovascular accident; cardiovascular accident
ATP	Adenosine triphosphate	CVD	Cardiovascular disease
AV	Atrioventricular	DCM	Dilated cardiomyopathy
AVN	Atrioventricular node	DVT	Deep vein thrombosis
AVSD	Atrioventricular septal defect	ECG, EKG	Electrocardiogram
BAV	Bicuspid aortic valve	ECHO	Echocardiography
BB	Bundle branches	Hb	Hemoglobin
BP	Blood pressure	HCTZ	Hydrochlorothiazide
bpm	Beats per minute	HDL	High-density lipoprotein
BSA	Body surface area	HTN	Hypertension
CABG	Coronary artery bypass graft	ICA	Internal carotid artery

Table 4–7 Common Cardiovascular System Abbreviations *(Continued)*

Abbreviation	Meaning	Abbreviation	Meaning
ICD	Implantable cardioverter defibrillator	PE	Pulmonary embolism
IHD	Ischemic heart disease	PET	Positron emission tomography
IV	Intravenous	PH	Pulmonary hypertension
LA	Left atrium/atrial	PV	Pressure–volume
LCA	Left coronary artery	PVC	Premature ventricular contraction
LDL	Low-density lipoprotein	PVD	Peripheral vascular disease
LMWH	Low-molecular-weight heparin	RA	Right atrium
LV	Left ventricle/ventricular	RV	Right ventricle
MI	Myocardial infarction	SBP	Systolic blood pressure
MR	Magnetic resonance	SCD	Sudden cardiac death
MV	Mitral valve	SV	Stroke volume
MVP	Mitral valve prolapse	SVT	Supraventricular tachycardia
OH	Orthostatic hypotension	TIA	Transient ischemic attack
PA	Pulmonary artery	VF	Ventricular fibrillation
PAC	Premature atrial contraction	VLDL	Very low-density lipoprotein
PAD	Peripheral arterial disease	VSD	Ventricular septal defect
PAH	Pulmonary arterial hypertension	VT	Ventricular tachycardia
PAI	Plasminogen activator inhibitor		

Table 4–8 Common Laboratory and Phlebotomy Abbreviations

Abbreviation	Meaning	Abbreviation	Meaning
ABG	Arterial blood gas	CO_2	Carbon dioxide
ABN	Abnormal	C&S	Culture and sensitivity
ACT	Activated coagulation time	CSF	Cerebrospinal fluid
Alb	Albumin	CT, C-T	Computerized tomography
Alk	Alkaline	diag	Diagnosis
AMS	Amylase	DIC	Diffuse intravascular coagulation
Amt	Amount	diff	Differential
ant	Anterior	DNA	Deoxyribonucleic acid
A&P	Anterior and posterior	Dx	Diagnosis
aPTT	Activated partial thromboplastin time	EDTA	Ethylenediaminetetraacetic acid
aq	Aqueous	EIA	Enzyme immunoassay
bil	Bilateral	eos, eosins	Eosinophils
Bld	Blood	ESR	Erythrocyte sedimentation rate
BOLD	Blood oxygen level dependent	FBS	Fasting blood sugar
BT	Bleeding time	FOB	Fetal occult blood
BUN	Blood urea nitrogen	g, gm	Gram
bx	Biopsy	gr	Grain
CA	Cancer	GTT	Glucose tolerance test
cath	Catheter; catheterize	gtt	Drop or drops
CBC	Complete blood count	H&H	Hemoglobin and hematocrit
cc	Cubic centimeter	Hbf	Fetal hemoglobin
Ch, chol	Cholesterol	hct	Hematocrit
cm	Centimeter	H&P	History and physical

(Continues)

■ **Table 4–8 Common Laboratory and Phlebotomy Abbreviations** *(Continued)*

Abbreviation	Meaning	Abbreviation	Meaning
Hx	History	PCV	Packed cell volume
Ig	Immunoglobulin	pH	Acidity; hydrogen ion concentration
kg	Kilogram	PI	Present illness
KVO	Keep vein open	PKU	Phenylketonuria
L	Liter	PLTS	Platelets
lab	Laboratory	pos	Positive
lat	Lateral	prep	Prepare
lb	Pound	pt	Patient
lymphs	Lymphocytes	PT	Prothrombin time
lytes	Electrolytes	PTT	Partial thromboplastin time
m	Minim	qt	Quart or quiet
mcg	Microgram	RBC	Red blood cell; red blood count
MCHC	Mean corpuscular hemoglobin concentration	RBCV	Red blood cell volume
MCV	Mean corpuscular volume	Rh neg, Rh–	Rhesus factor negative
mEq	Milliequivalent	Rh pos, Rh+	Rhesus factor positive
mg	Milligram	RIA	Radioimmunoassay
mL	Milliliter	RNA	Ribonucleic acid
mm	Millimeter	RPR	Rapid plasma regain
mono	Monocytes	SCA	Sickle cell anemia
MRI	Magnetic resonance imaging	sp gr	Specific gravity
NEG, neg	Negative	SR	Sedimentation rate
NKA	No known allergies	stat	Immediately
NKDA	No known drug allergies	TIBC	Total iron binding capacity
No., #	Number	Trig	Triglycerides
O_2	Oxygen	U	Units
oz	Ounce	VP	Venipuncture; venous pressure
P	Pulse	VS	Vital signs
Path	Pathology	W	Water
PC	After meals	WBC	White blood cell; white blood count
PCO_2	Pressure of carbon dioxide in the blood	WNL	Within normal limits

Summary

Medical terminology is primarily based on Greek and Latin terms. All medical terms are derived from word roots. Prefixes are placed in front of word roots to change their meaning. Suffixes are added after word roots or combining forms, which utilize the combining vowels *o* or *i*. Abbreviations are commonly used to simplify medical terms, but they should always be used with caution to avoid confusion or medical errors.

CRITICAL THINKING

Roxanne tried to memorize medical terms in order to take her final exam. Her score was unsatisfactory, and she did not pass the exam.

1. What is the best method to learn medical terminology?

2. Why are medical terms essential for all health professionals?

WEBSITES

http://anatomyphysiology.suite101.com/article.cfm
/anatomy_and_physiology_vocabulary

http://library.med.utah.edu/WebPath/TUTORIAL/PHLEB
/PHLEB.html

http://www.labtestsonline.us/understanding/analytes/wbc
/test.html

http://www.medicinenet.com/complete_blood_count
/article.htm

http://www.medilexicon.com/medicalabbreviations.php

http://www.medterms.com/script/main/hp.asp

REVIEW QUESTIONS

Multiple Choice

1. Which of the following suffixes means "inflammation"?
   A. -iasis
   B. -osis
   C. -itis
   D. -trophy

2. The abbreviation for the word *diagnosis* is
   A. DG
   B. Dx
   C. Diag
   D. DIC

3. The prefix *ab-* means
   A. toward
   B. away from
   C. without
   D. against

4. The underlined portion of the word *hypolipemia* represents which of the following word parts?
   A. prefix
   B. root
   C. suffix
   D. combining form

5. Which of the following prefixes means "bad, difficult, painful"?
   A. ex-
   B. dis-
   C. dys-
   D. meta-

6. The prefix *milli-* means
   A. one-thousandth
   B. one-hundredth
   C. one-tenth
   D. many

7. The abbreviation *stat* means
   A. do not change
   B. immediately
   C. daily
   D. statistics

8. Which of the following contains the central meaning of a word?
   A. prefix
   B. suffix
   C. root
   D. both B and C

9. The combining form *brachi/o* refers to the
   A. face
   B. arm
   C. wrist
   D. leg

10. Hardening of the arteries, causing thickening of the walls and loss of elasticity, is called
    A. varicosis
    B. arteriosclerosis
    C. atherosclerosis
    D. achondroplasia

11. The prefix *intra-* means
    A. between
    B. above
    C. beside
    D. within

12. The suffix *-pathy* means
    A. disease
    B. excision
    C. tumor
    D. spasm

13. A prefix is
    A. the first part of a word
    B. the last part of a word that gives the word its root meaning
    C. a word structure at the beginning of a term that modifies the root
    D. a word structure at the end of a term that modifies the root

14. Which of the following prefixes is matched correctly with the meaning?
    A. hypo / above
    B. peri / around
    C. antero / back
    D. endo / over

15. When the combining form *cyan/o* is used, it means that
    A. the skin is involved
    B. the object is oily
    C. the object is blue
    D. something is poisonous

Anatomy and Physiology of the Cardiovascular System

OUTLINE

Introduction
The Heart
    Structures of the Heart
    Conduction System
    Functions of the Heart
The Blood Vessels and Circulation
    Blood Vessels
    Blood Pressure
    Blood Circulation
Summary
Critical Thinking
Websites
Review Questions

OBJECTIVES

After reading this chapter, readers should be able to:

1. Describe the organization of the cardiovascular system and the heart.
2. Identify the layers of the heart wall.
3. Describe the general features of the heart.
4. Answer the question of why the left ventricle is more muscular than the right ventricle.
5. Describe the components and functions of the conducting system of the heart.
6. Explain the events of the cardiac cycle.
7. Define cardiac output and stroke volume.
8. Distinguish among the types of blood vessels, their structures, and their functions.
9. Identify the major arteries and veins of the pulmonary circuit as well as the areas they serve.
10. Describe the hepatic portal system.

KEY TERMS

Aorta: The largest artery in the body, the aorta originates from the left ventricle of the heart and extends down to the abdomen, where it branches off.

Aortic arch: The second section of the aorta; it branches into the brachiocephalic trunk, left common carotid artery, and left subclavian artery.

Aortic valve: Located at the base of the aorta, the aortic valve has three cusps and opens to allow blood to leave the left ventricle during contraction.

Arteries: Elastic vessels able to carry blood away from the heart under high pressure.

Arterioles: Subdivisions of arteries; they are thinner and have muscles that are innervated by the sympathetic nervous system.

Atria: The upper chambers of the heart; they receive blood returning to the heart.

Atrioventricular node (AV node): A mass of specialized tissue located in the inferior interatrial septum beneath the endocardium; it provides the only normal conduction pathway between the atrial and ventricular syncytia.

AV bundle: The bundle of His; a large structure that receives the cardiac impulse from the distal AV node. It enters the upper part of the interventricular septum.

Blood volume: The sum of formed elements and plasma volumes in the vascular system; most adults have about 5 L of blood.

Capillaries: The smallest-diameter blood vessels, which connect the smallest arterioles to the smallest venules.

Cardiac conduction system: The initiation and distribution of impulses through the myocardium that coordinates the cardiac cycle.

Cardiac cycle: A heartbeat; it consists of a complete series of systolic and diastolic events.

Cardiac output: The volume discharged from the ventricle per minute, calculated by multiplying stroke volume by heart rate, in beats per minute.

Cardiac veins: Those veins that branch out and drain blood from the myocardial capillaries to join the coronary sinus.

Carotid sinuses: Enlargements near the base of the carotid arteries that contain baroreceptors and help to control blood pressure.

KEY TERMS CONTINUED

Cerebral arterial circle: The circle of Willis; it connects the vertebral artery and internal carotid artery systems.

Chordae tendineae: Strong fibers originating from the papillary muscles that attach to the cusps of the tricuspid valve.

Coronary arteries: The first two aortic branches, which supply blood to the heart tissues.

Coronary sinus: An enlarged vein joining the cardiac veins; it empties into the right atrium.

Diastole: The relaxation of a heart structure.

Diastolic pressure: The lowest pressure that remains in the arteries before the next ventricular contraction.

Electrocardiogram (EKG): The recording of electrical changes in the myocardium during the cardiac cycle. The EKG machine works by placing nodes on the skin that connect via wires and respond to weak electrical changes of the heart. The abbreviation EKG is more commonly used than ECG.

Endocardium: The inner layer of the heart wall.

Epicardium: The outer layer of the heart wall.

Functional syncytium: A mass of merging cells that functions as a unit.

Hepatic portal system: The veins that drain the abdominal viscera, originating in the stomach, intestines, pancreas, and spleen, to carry blood through a hepatic portal vein to the liver.

Inferior vena cava: Along with the superior vena cava, one of the two largest veins in the body; it is formed by the joining of the common iliac veins.

Mitral valve: The bicuspid valve; it lies between the left atrium and left ventricle, preventing blood from flowing back into the left atrium from the ventricle.

Myocardium: The thick middle layer of the heart wall that is mostly made of cardiac tissue.

Pacemaker: The term used to refer to the sinoatrial node (SA node).

Papillary muscles: Those muscles that contract as the heart's ventricles contract, pulling on the chordae tendineae to prevent the cusps from swinging back into the atrium.

Pericardium: A membranous structure that encloses the heart and proximal ends of the large blood vessels and that consists of double layers.

Peripheral resistance: A force produced by friction between blood and blood vessel walls.

Pulmonary circuit: The venules and veins, which send deoxygenated blood to the lungs to receive oxygen and unload carbon dioxide.

Pulmonary valve: Lying at the base of the pulmonary trunk, this valve has three cusps and allows blood to leave the right ventricle while preventing backflow into the ventricular chamber.

Purkinje fibers: Consisting of branches of the AV bundle that spread and enlarge, these fibers are located near the papillary muscles; they continue to the heart's apex and cause the ventricular walls to contract in a twisting motion.

Septum: A solid, wall-like structure that separates the left atria and ventricle from the right atria and ventricle.

Sinoatrial node (SA node): A small mass of specialized tissue just beneath the epicardium in the right atrium that initiates impulses through the myocardium to stimulate contraction of cardiac muscle fibers.

Stroke volume: The volume of blood discharged from the ventricle with each contraction; it is usually about 70 mL.

Superior vena cava: Along with the inferior vena cava, one of the two largest veins in the body; the superior vena cava is formed by the joining of the brachiocephalic veins.

Systemic circuit: The arteries and arterioles, which send oxygenated blood and nutrients to the body cells while removing wastes.

Systole: The contraction of a heart structure.

Systolic pressure: The maximum pressuring during ventricular contraction.

Thyrocervical arteries: Those that branch off to the thyroid and parathyroid glands, larynx, trachea, esophagus, pharynx, and muscles of the neck, shoulder, and back.

Tricuspid valve: Lying between the right atrium and ventricle, this valve allows blood to move from the right atrium into the right ventricle while preventing backflow.

Vasoconstriction: The contraction of blood vessels, which reduces their diameter.

Vasodilation: The relaxation of blood vessels, which increases their diameter.

Veins: Blood vessels that carry blood back to the atria; they are less elastic than arteries.

Ventricles: The lower chambers of the heart; they receive blood from the atria, which they pump out into the arteries.

Venules: Microscopic vessels that link capillaries to veins.

Vertebral arteries: One of the main divisions of the subclavian and common carotid arteries; the vertebral arteries run upward through the cervical vertebrae into the skull and supply blood to the vertebrae, their ligaments, and their muscles.

Viscosity: Thickness or stickiness; the resistance of fluid to flow. In a biologic fluid, viscosity is caused by the attraction of cells to one another.

Introduction

The human heart pumps blood through the arteries, which connect to smaller arterioles and then even smaller capillaries. It is here that nutrients, electrolytes, dissolved gases, and waste products are exchanged between the blood and surrounding tissues. The capillaries are thin-walled vessels interconnected with the smallest arteries and smallest veins.

Approximately 7,000 L of blood is pumped by the heart every day. In an average person's life, the heart will contract about 2.5 billion times.

Blood flow throughout the body begins its return to the heart when the capillaries return blood to the venules and then to the larger veins. The cardiovascular system, therefore, consists of a closed circuit: the heart, arteries, arterioles, capillaries, venules, and veins (see **Figure 5–1**). The venules

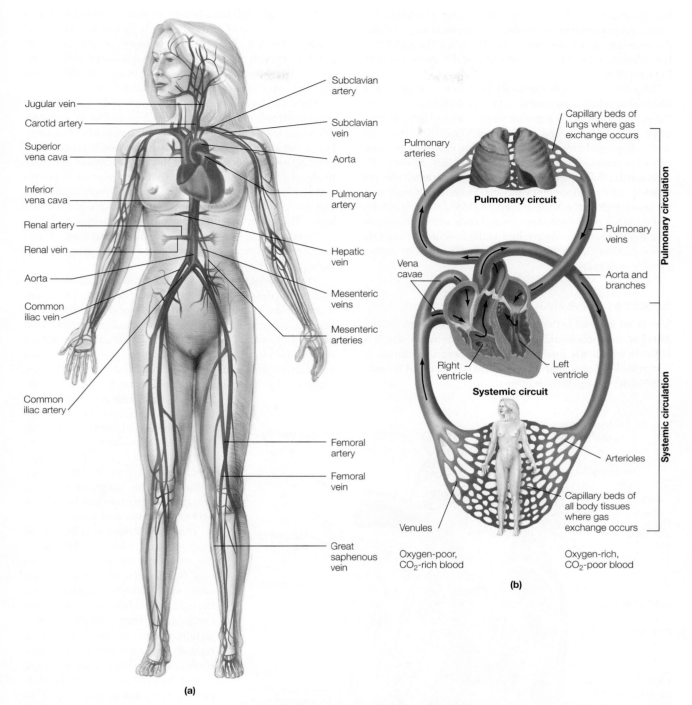

Figure 5–1 The circulatory system. (a) The circulatory system consists of a series of vessels that transport blood to and from the heart, the pump. (b) The circulatory system has two major circuits: the pulmonary circuit, which transports blood to and from the lungs, and the systemic circuit, which transports blood to and from the body (excluding the lungs).

and veins are part of the **pulmonary circuit** because they send deoxygenated blood to the lungs to receive oxygen and unload carbon dioxide. The arteries and arterioles are part of the **systemic circuit** because they send oxygenated blood and nutrients to the body cells while removing wastes. All body tissues require circulation to survive.

The Heart

The human *heart* is a muscular organ containing four chambers that is situated just to the left of the midline of the thoracic cavity. It is approximately the size of a man's closed fist. The upper two chambers (**atria**) are divided by a wall-like structure called the *interatrial septum*. The lower two chambers (**ventricles**) are divided by a similar structure called the *interventricular septum*. Between each atrium and ventricle, valves allow blood to flow in one direction, preventing backflow.

Blood flow through the heart is shown in **Figure 5–2**. Blood that is low in oxygen flows into the right atrium from the veins known as the **superior vena cava** and **inferior vena cava**. The superior vena cava carries blood from the head, neck, chest, and arms. The inferior vena cava carries blood from the remainder of the trunk and the legs. Blood in the right atrium then flows through the **right atrioventricular (tricuspid)** *valve* into the right ventricle. From here it begins the **pulmonary circuit**, with deoxygenated blood flowing into the right and left pulmonary arteries and their smaller branches. The blood becomes oxygenated while moving through the lungs' capillary beds. Also in this part of the system, carbon dioxide is released.

Structures of the Heart

The heart lies inside the thoracic cavity, resting on the diaphragm. It is hollow and cone-shaped, varying in size. The heart is within the mediastinum in between the lungs. Its posterior border is near the vertebral column, and its anterior border is near the sternum.

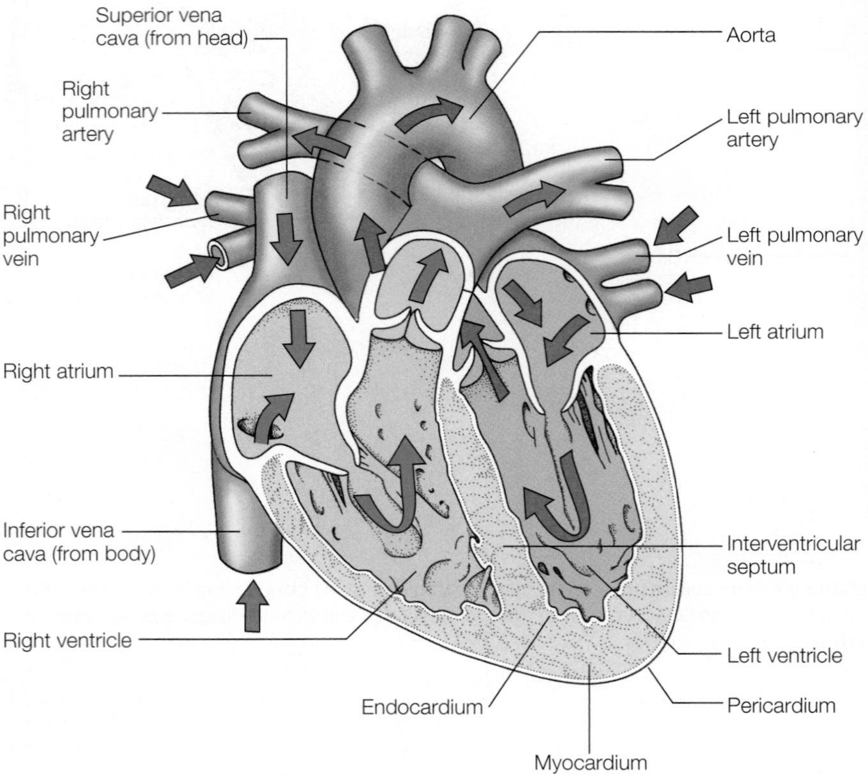

An average adult has a heart that is about 14 cm long by 9 cm wide. The *base* of the heart is actually the upper portion, where it is attached to several large blood vessels. This portion lies beneath the second rib. The distal end of the heart extends downward, to the left, ending in a blunt point called the *apex*, which is even with the fifth intercostal space.

The three layers comprising the wall of the heart are the outer **pericardium**, middle **myocardium**, and inner **endocardium** (see Figure 5–2). The pericardium consists of connective tissue and some deep adipose tissue, and it protects the heart by reducing friction. The thick **myocardium** is mostly made of cardiac muscle tissue that is organized in planes and richly supplied by blood capillaries, lymph capillaries, and nerve fibers. It pumps blood out of the chambers of the heart. The **endocardium** is made up of epithelium and connective tissue with many elastic and collagenous fibers. It also contains blood vessels and specialized cardiac muscle fibers known as **Purkinje fibers**.

The inside of the heart is divided into four hollow chambers, with two on the left and two on the right. The upper chambers are called **atria** and receive blood returning to the heart. They have *auricles*, which are small projections that extend anteriorly. The lower chambers are called **ventricles** and receive blood from the atria, which they pump out into the arteries (see Figure 5–2). The left atria and ventricle are separated from the right atria and ventricle by a solid wall-like structure (**septum**). This keeps blood from one side of the heart from mixing with blood from the other side (except in a developing fetus). The atrioventricular valve (AV valve), which consists of the **mitral valve** on the left and the **tricuspid valve** on the right, ensures one-way blood flow between the atria and ventricles.

The right atrium receives blood from two large veins called the superior vena cava and the inferior vena cava as well as a smaller vein (the **coronary sinus**), which drains blood into the right atrium from the heart's myocardium. The tricuspid valve has projections (*cusps*) and lies between the right atrium and ventricle. This valve allows blood to move from the right atrium into the right ventricle while preventing backflow. The cusps of the tricuspid valve are attached to strong fibers called **chordae tendineae**, which originate from small **papillary muscles** that project inward from the ventricle walls. These muscles contract as the ventricle contracts. When the tricuspid valve closes, they pull on the chordae tendineae to prevent the cusps from swinging back into the atrium.

The right ventricle's muscular wall is thinner than that of the left ventricle, as it only pumps blood to the

Figure 5–2 Blood flow through the heart. Deoxygenated (carbon-dioxide-enriched) blood (blue arrows) flows into the right atrium from the systemic circulation and is pumped into the right ventricle. The blood is then pumped from the right ventricle into the pulmonary artery, which delivers it to the lungs. In the lungs, the blood releases its carbon dioxide and absorbs oxygen. Reoxygenated blood (red arrows) is returned to the left atrium, then flows into the left ventricle, which pumps it to the rest of the body through the systemic circuit.

Labels: Superior vena cava (from head); Right pulmonary artery; Right pulmonary vein; Right atrium; Inferior vena cava (from body); Right ventricle; Endocardium; Myocardium; Aorta; Left pulmonary artery; Left pulmonary vein; Left atrium; Interventricular septum; Left ventricle; Pericardium

lungs with a low resistance to blood flow. The left ventricle is thicker because it must force blood to all body parts, with a much higher resistance to blood flow. As the right ventricle contracts, its blood increases in pressure to passively close the tricuspid valve. Therefore, this blood can only exit through the *pulmonary trunk*, which divides into the left and right *pulmonary arteries* that supply the lungs. At the trunk's base, there is a **pulmonary valve** with three cusps that allow blood to leave the right ventricle while preventing backflow into the ventricular chamber (see **Figure 5–3**).

Four *pulmonary veins* (two from each of the lungs) supply the left atrium with blood. Blood passes from the left atrium into the left ventricle through the mitral valve (bicuspid valve), preventing blood from flowing back into the left atrium from the ventricle. Like the tricuspid valve, the papillary muscles and chordae tendineae prevent the mitral valve's cusps from swinging back into the left atrium when the ventricle contracts. The mitral valve closes passively, directing blood through the large artery known as the **aorta**.

At the base of the aorta is the **aortic valve**, with three cusps. This valve opens to allow blood to leave the left ventricle during contraction. When the ventricle relaxes, the valve closes to prevent blood from backing up into the ventricle. The mitral and tricuspid valves are known as atrioventricular valves because they lie between the atria and ventricles. The pulmonary and aortic valves have "half-moon" shapes and are therefore referred to as *semilunar valves*. **Table 5–1** summarizes the various heart valves.

The right atrium receives low-oxygen blood through the vena cava and coronary sinus. As the right atrium contracts, the blood passes through the tricuspid valve into the right ventricle (see Figure 5–3). As the right ventricle contracts, the tricuspid valve closes. Blood moves through the pulmonary valve into the pulmonary trunk and pulmonary arteries. It then enters the capillaries of the alveoli of the lungs, where gas exchanges occur. This freshly oxygenated blood then returns to the heart through the pulmonary veins, into the left atrium.

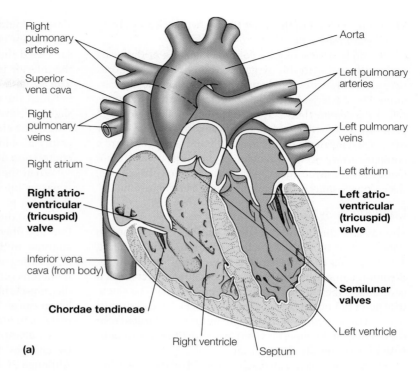

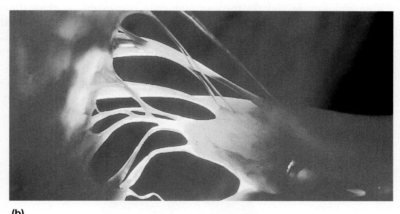

(b)

Figure 5–3 Heart valves. (a) A cross-section of the heart showing the four chambers and the location of the major vessels and valves. (b) Photograph of chordae tendineae.

The left atrium contracts, moving blood through the mitral valve into the left ventricle. When the left ventricle contracts, the mitral valve closes. Blood moves through the aortic valve into the aorta and its branches. The first two aortic branches are called the right and left **coronary arteries**.

Table 5–1 The Heart Valves

Heart Valve	Location	Action
Tricuspid valve	Between right atrium and right ventricle	During ventricular contraction, it prevents blood from moving from right ventricle into right atrium.
Pulmonary valve	At entrance to pulmonary trunk	During ventricular relaxation, it prevents blood from moving from pulmonary trunk into right ventricle.
Mitral (bicuspid) valve	Between left atrium and left ventricle	During ventricular contraction, it prevents blood from moving from left ventricle into left atrium.
Aortic valve	At entrance to aorta	During ventricular relaxation, it prevents blood from moving from aorta into left ventricle.

They supply blood to the heart tissues, with openings lying just beyond the aortic valve.

The body tissues require continual beating of the heart because they need freshly oxygenated blood to survive. Coronary artery branches supply many capillaries in the myocardium. These arteries have smaller branches with connections called *anastomoses* between vessels providing alternate blood pathways (*collateral circulation*). These pathways may supply oxygen and nutrients to the myocardium when blockage of a coronary artery occurs. Branches of the **cardiac veins** drain blood from the myocardial capillaries, joining an enlarged vein, the coronary sinus, which empties into the right atrium.

Conduction System

Strands and clumps of specialized cardiac muscle contain only a few myofibrils and are located throughout the heart. These areas initiate and distribute impulses through the myocardium, comprising the **cardiac conduction system** that coordinates the **cardiac cycle** (see **Figure 5–4**). The **sinoatrial node (SA node)** is a small mass of specialized tissue just beneath the **epicardium**, in the right atrium. It is located near the opening of the superior vena cava, with fibers continuous with those of the atrial syncytium.

The SA node's cells can reach threshold on their own, initiating impulses through the myocardium, stimulating contraction of cardiac muscle fibers. Its rhythmic activity occurs 70 to 80 times per minute in a normal adult. Since it generates the heart's rhythmic contractions, it is often referred to as the **pacemaker**.

The path of a cardiac impulse travels from the SA node into the atrial syncytium, and the atria begin to contract almost simultaneously. The impulse passes along junctional fibers of the conduction system to a mass of specialized tissue called the atrioventricular node (AV node), located in the inferior interatrial septum, beneath the endocardium. The AV node provides the only normal conduction pathway between the atrial and ventricular syncytia. Impulses are slightly delayed due to the small diameter of the junctional fibers. The atria, therefore, have more time to contract and empty all of their blood into the ventricles before ventricular contraction occurs.

When the cardiac impulse reaches the distal AV node, it passes into a large **AV bundle** (*bundle of His*), entering the upper part of the interventricular septum. Nearly half-way down the septum, these branches spread into enlarged Purkinje fibers, extending into the papillary muscles. They continue to the heart's apex, curving around the ventricles and passing over their lateral walls. The Purkinje fibers have numerous small branches that become continuous with cardiac muscle fibers and irregular *whorls*. Purkinje fiber stimulation causes the ventricular walls to contract in a twisting motion, to force blood into the aorta and pulmonary trunk.

An **electrocardiogram (EKG)** is used to record electrical changes in the myocardium during the cardiac cycle. Although ECG is the correct abbreviation for *electrocardiogram*, the abbreviation EKG is more commonly used. Because phlebotomists do not generally perform this procedure, it is not discussed in depth in this chapter. The most important ions that influence heart action are potassium and calcium. Excess extracellular potassium ions (*hyperkalemia*) decrease contraction rates and forces, while deficient extracellular potassium ions (*hypokalemia*) may cause a potentially life-

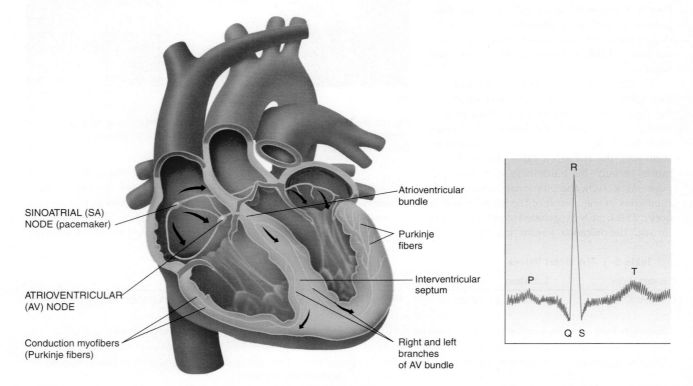

SINOATRIAL (SA) NODE (pacemaker)

ATRIOVENTRICULAR (AV) NODE

Conduction myofibers (Purkinje fibers)

Atrioventricular bundle

Purkinje fibers

Interventricular septum

Right and left branches of AV bundle

P   R   Q   S   T

Figure 5–4 The cardiac conduction system. Also shown is a tracing of an EKG. The P wave corresponds to atrial depolarization, the QRS coplex to ventricular depolarization, and the T wave to ventricular repolarization.

threatening abnormal heart rhythm (arrhythmia). Excess extracellular calcium ions (*hypercalcemia*) can cause the heart to contract for an abnormally long time, while low extracellular calcium ions (*hypocalcemia*) depress heart action.

Functions of the Heart

The heart chambers are coordinated so that their actions are effective. The atria contract (atrial **systole**) as the ventricles relax (ventricular **diastole**). Likewise, ventricles contract (ventricular systole) as atria relax (atrial diastole). Then a brief period of relaxation of both atria and ventricles occurs. This complete series of events makes up a heartbeat, also called a cardiac cycle.

One cardiac cycle causes pressure in the heart chambers to rise and fall and valves to open and close. Early during diastole, pressure in the ventricles is low, causing the AV valves to open and the ventricles to fill with blood. Nearly 70% of returning blood enters the ventricles before contraction. As the atria contract, the remaining 30% is pushed into the ventricles. As the ventricles contract, ventricular pressure rises. When ventricular pressure exceeds atrial pressure, the AV valves close and papillary muscles contract, preventing the cusps of the AV valves from bulging into the atria excessively. During ventricular contraction, the AV valves are closed, and atrial pressure is low. Blood flows into the atria while the ventricles are contracting, so that the atria are prepared for the next cardiac cycle.

As ventricular pressure exceeds pulmonary trunk and aorta pressure, the pulmonary and aortic valves open. Blood is ejected from the ventricles into these arteries, and ventricular pressure drops. When ventricular pressure is lower than in the aorta and pulmonary trunk, the semilunar valves close. When ventricular pressure is lower than atrial pressure, the AV valves open, and the ventricles begin to refill.

A heartbeat makes a characteristic double thumping sound when heard through a stethoscope. This is due to the vibrations of the heart tissues related to the valves closing. The first thumping sound occurs during ventricular contraction when the AV valves close. The second sound occurs during ventricular relaxation when the pulmonary and aortic valves close.

Cardiac muscle fibers are similar in function to skeletal muscle fibers, but are connected in branched networks. If any part of the network is stimulated, impulses are sent throughout the heart, and it contracts as a single unit. A **functional syncytium** is a mass of merging cells that functions as a unit. There are two of these structures in the heart: one in the atrial walls and another in the ventricular walls. A small area of the right atrial floor is the only part of the heart's muscle fibers that is not separated by the heart's fibrous skeleton. Here, cardiac conduction system fibers connect the atrial syncytium and the ventricular syncytium.

Newly oxygenated blood flows into the left and right pulmonary veins, returning to the left atrium (see Figure 5–3). Blood then flows through the *left atrioventricular (bicuspid* or *mitral) valve* into the left ventricle, passing through the *aortic semilunar valve* into the systemic circuit (via the *ascending aorta*). The systemic circuit moves blood to the body tissues, supplying their required oxygen. Should blood

flow backward at this point due to a valve malfunction, a *heart murmur* will result. To summarize, the right side of the heart pumps oxygen-poor blood to the lungs, and the left side pumps oxygen-rich blood toward the body tissues.

The contraction of the heart is called *systole*, and its relaxation is called *diastole*. The **systolic** blood pressure is the first number in a blood pressure reading, measuring the strength of contraction. The **diastolic** blood pressure is the second number in a blood pressure reading, measuring the strength of relaxation. The right ventricle does not need to pump blood with as much force as the left ventricle. This is so because the right ventricle supplies blood to the nearby lungs and the pulmonary vessels are wide and relatively short. This means that the walls of the right ventricle are thinner and less muscular than those of the left ventricle, which must pump blood to the entire body.

The Blood Vessels and Circulation

The blood vessels of the human body carry blood to every type of tissue and organ. Vessels decrease in size as they move away from the heart (arteries and arterioles), ending in the capillaries, and then increase in size as they move toward the heart (venules and veins). The largest artery in the body is the aorta, with the largest veins being the venae cavae, each being approximately 1 in wide.

Blood Vessels

There are five general classes of blood vessels in the cardiovascular system: arteries, arterioles, capillaries, venules, and veins (see **Figure 5–5**). **Arteries** are elastic vessels that are very strong, able to carry blood away from the heart under high pressure. They subdivide into thinner tubes that give rise to branched, finer **arterioles**. An artery's wall consists of three distinct layers, as shown in **Figure 5–6**. The innermost *tunica interna* is made up of a layer of simple squamous epithelium known as *endothelium*. It rests on a connective tissue membrane with many elastic, collagenous fibers. The endothelium helps prevent blood clotting and may also help in regulating blood flow. It releases nitric oxide to relax the smooth muscle of the vessel. Vein walls are similar but not identical to artery walls.

The middle *tunica media* makes up most of an arterial wall, including smooth muscle fibers and a thick elastic connective tissue layer. The outer *tunica externa (tunica adventitia)* is thinner, mostly made up of connective tissue with irregular fibers—it is attached to the surrounding tissues. Smooth artery and arteriole muscles are innervated by the sympathetic nervous system. *Vasomotor fibers* receive impulses to contract and reduce blood vessel diameter (**vasoconstriction**). When inhibited, the muscle fibers relax and the vessel's diameter increases (**vasodilation**). Changes in artery and arteriole diameters greatly affect blood flow and pressure.

Larger arterioles also have three layers in their walls, which get thinner as arterioles lead to capillaries. Very small arteriole walls only have an endothelial lining and some smooth muscle fibers, with a small amount of surrounding connective tissue.

The smallest-diameter blood vessels are **capillaries**, which connect the smallest arterioles to the smallest venules. The

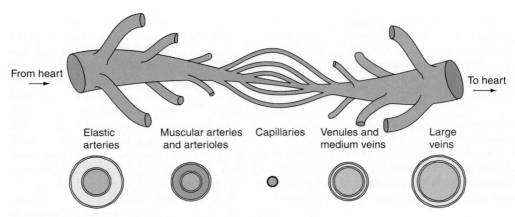

Figure 5–5 The structure and diameter of blood vessel walls.

walls of capillaries are also composed of endothelium and form the semipermeable layer through which substances in blood are exchanged with substances in tissue fluids surrounding cells of the body.

Capillary walls have thin slits where endothelial cells overlap. These slits have various sizes, affecting permeability. Capillaries of muscles have smaller openings than those of the glands, kidneys, and small intestine. Tissues with higher metabolic rates (such as muscles) have many more capillaries than those with slower metabolic rates (such as cartilage).

Some capillaries pass directly from arterioles to venules while others have highly branched networks (see **Figure 5–7**). *Precapillary sphincters* control blood distribution through capillaries. Based on the demands of cells, these sphincters constrict or relax so that blood can follow specific pathways to meet tissue cellular requirements.

Gases, metabolic by-products, and nutrients are exchanged between capillaries and the tissue fluid surrounding body cells. Capillary walls allow the diffusion of blood with high levels of oxygen and nutrients. They also allow high levels of carbon dioxide and other wastes to move from the tissues into the capillaries. Plasma proteins usually cannot move through the capillary walls due to their large size, so they remain in the blood. Blood pressure generated when capillary walls contract provides force for filtration via hydrostatic pressure.

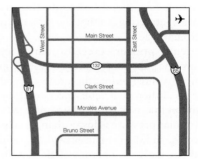

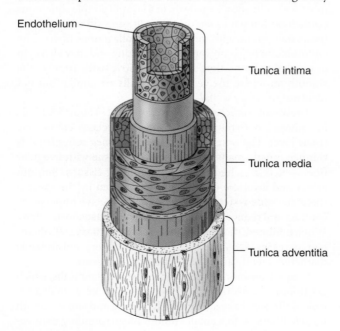

Figure 5–6 General structure of the blood vessel. The artery shown here consists of three major layers, the tunica intima, tunica media, and tunica adventitia.

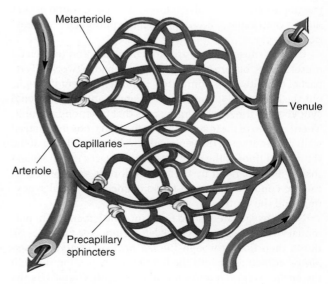

Figure 5–7 Similar to the way roadways are designed, larger arterioles and venules are interconnected with smaller capillaries.

Blood pressure is strongest when blood leaves the heart and weaker as the distance from the heart increases because of friction (peripheral resistance) between the blood and the vessel walls. Therefore, blood pressure is highest in the arteries, less so in the arterioles, and lowest in the capillaries. Filtration occurs mostly at the arteriolar ends of capillaries because the pressure is higher than at the venular ends. Plasma proteins trapped in capillaries create an osmotic pressure that pulls water into the capillaries (*colloid osmotic pressure*).

Capillary blood pressure favors filtration while plasma colloid osmotic pressure favors reabsorption. At the venular ends of capillaries, blood pressure has decreased due to resistance so that reabsorption can occur.

More fluid usually leaves capillaries than returns to them. Lymphatic capillaries have closed ends and collect excess fluid to return it via lymphatic vessels to the venous circulation. Unusual events may cause excess fluid to enter spaces between tissue cells, often in response to chemicals such as histamine. If enough fluid leaks out, lymphatic vessels can be overwhelmed, and affected tissues swell and become painful.

Venules are microscopic vessels that link capillaries to **veins**, which carry blood back to the atria. Vein walls are similar to arteries but have poorly developed middle layers. Because they have thinner walls that are less elastic than arteries, their lumens have a greater diameter.

Many veins have flaplike *valves* projecting inward from their linings. These valves often have two structures that close if blood begins to back up in the vein. They aid in returning blood to the heart, opening if blood flow is toward the heart, but closing if it reverses. Unlike the arteries, veins do not have sufficient pressure from the contractions of the heart to keep blood moving through them. To keep blood flowing, the veins rely on the movement of nearby skeletal muscles, as well as the opening and closing of the valves within them. Therefore, a major structural difference between veins and arteries is that arteries do not have valves.

Veins also act as reservoirs for blood in certain conditions, such as during arterial hemorrhage. Resulting venous constrictions help to maintain blood pressure by returning more blood to the heart, ensuring an almost normal blood flow even when up to one-quarter of the blood volume is lost. See **Table 5–2** for a summary of blood vessel characteristics.

Blood Pressure

Blood pressure is defined as the force that blood exerts against the inner walls of blood vessels. It most commonly refers to pressure in arteries supplied by the aortic branches, even though it actually occurs throughout the vascular system. Arterial blood pressure rises and falls according to cardiac cycle phases. The maximum pressure during ventricular contraction is called the **systolic pressure**.

The lowest pressure that remains in the arteries before the next ventricular contraction is called the **diastolic pressure**. Arterial blood pressure is measured with a device called a *sphygmomanometer* (blood pressure cuff). Its results are reported as a fraction of the systolic pressure over the diastolic pressure, such as 120/80. The upper (first) number indicates the arterial systolic pressure in millimeters of mercury (mm Hg), and the lower (second) number indicates the arterial diastolic pressure, also in millimeters of mercury. A millimeter of mercury is a unit of pressure that is equal to 0.001316 of normal atmospheric pressure. This means that a blood pressure of 120/80 displaces 120 mm Hg on a sphygmomanometer, showing the systolic pressure, and also displaces 80 mm Hg on the same device, showing diastolic pressure. **Figure 5–8** shows changes in blood pressure as the distance from the left ventricle increases.

The artery walls are distended as blood surges into them from the ventricles, but they recoil almost immediately. This expansion and recoiling can be felt as a *pulse* in an artery near the surface of the skin. Most commonly, the radial artery is used to take a person's pulse, although the carotid, brachial, and femoral arteries are also checked. Arterial blood pressure depends on heart rate, stroke volume, blood volume, peripheral resistance, and blood viscosity.

Heart action determines the amount of blood entering the arterial system with each ventricular contraction. **Stroke volume** is defined as the volume of blood discharged from the ventricle with each contraction. An average adult male's stroke volume is about 70 mL. The **cardiac output** is defined as the volume discharged from the ventricle per minute. It is calculated by multiplying the stroke volume by the heart rate, in beats per minute. So if the stroke volume is 70 mL and the heart rate is 75 beats per minute (bpm), the cardiac output is 5,250 mL/min. Blood pressure varies with cardiac output

Table 5–2 Characteristics of Blood Vessels

Type of Vessel	Vessel Wall	Actions
Artery	Three-layer thick wall (endothelial lining, middle smooth muscle and elastic connective tissue layer, and outer connective tissue layer)	Carries relatively high-pressure blood from the heart to the arterioles
Arteriole	Three-layer thinner wall (smaller arterioles have an endothelial lining, some smooth muscle tissue, and a small amount of connective tissue)	Helps control blood flow from arteries to capillaries by vasoconstriction or vasodilation
Capillary	One layer of squamous epithelium	Has a membrane allowing nutrients, gases, and wastes to be exchanged between blood and tissue fluid
Venule	Thinner wall than arterioles, with less smooth muscle and elastic connective tissue	Connects capillaries to veins
Vein	Thinner wall than arteries but similar layers; poorly developed middle layer; some have flaplike valves	Carries relatively low-pressure blood from venules to the heart; valves prevent blood backflow; veins serve as blood reservoirs

and increases or decreases based upon similar changes in stroke volume or heart rate.

Blood volume is defined as the sum of formed elements and plasma volumes in the vascular system. Blood volume varies with age, body size, and gender. Most adults have approximately 5 L of blood, which makes up 8% of the body weight in kilograms. Blood pressure and volume are usually directly proportional. Any changes in volume can initially alter pressure. When measures are taken to restore normal blood volume, normal blood pressure can be reestablished. Fluid balance fluctuations may also affect blood volume.

The resistance of arteries to blood flow is defined as **peripheral resistance**. The degree of peripheral resistance is determined by the blood vessel diameter and the force of contraction exerted by vascular smooth muscle. Therefore, peripheral resistance is a factor that accounts for blood pressure.

Viscosity is defined as the resistance of a fluid to flow. In a biologic fluid, viscosity is caused by the attraction of molecules or cells to one another. The higher the viscosity, the greater the resistance to flowing. Blood viscosity is increased by blood cells and plasma proteins. The greater the resistance, the greater the force needed to move the blood. Blood pressure rises as blood viscosity increases, and vice versa.

Blood pressure (BP) is calculated by multiplying cardiac output (CO) by peripheral resistance (PR). Normal arterial pressure is maintained by regulating these two factors. Ideally, the volume of blood discharged from the heart should be equal to the volume entering the atria and ventricles. Fiber length and force of contraction are interrelated because of the stretching of the cardiac muscle cell just before contraction. This is known as the *Frank-Starling law of the heart*, and it is important during exercise when greater amounts of blood return to the heart from the veins.

Peripheral resistance also controls blood pressure. Changes in the diameters of arterioles regulate peripheral resistance. The *vasomotor center* of the medulla oblongata controls peripheral resistance. When arterial blood pressure increases suddenly, baroreceptors in the aorta and carotid arteries alert the vasomotor center, which vasodilates the vessels to decrease peripheral resistance. Carbon dioxide, oxygen, and hydrogen ions also influence peripheral resistance by affecting precapillary sphincters and smooth arteriole wall muscles.

Blood flow through the venous system depends only slightly on heart action, but more so on skeletal muscle contraction, movements of breathing, and the vasoconstriction of veins (*venoconstriction*). As skeletal muscles press on veins with valves, some blood moves from one valve section to another, helping to push blood forward through the venous system to the heart. During inspiration, thoracic cavity pressure is reduced while abdominal cavity pressure is increased. Blood is then squeezed out of abdominal veins and forced into thoracic veins. When venous pressure is low, the walls of the veins contract to help force blood out toward the heart.

Blood Circulation

Blood enters the *pulmonary circuit* from the right ventricle through the pulmonary trunk, which extends upward posteriorly from the heart. It divides into right and left pulmonary

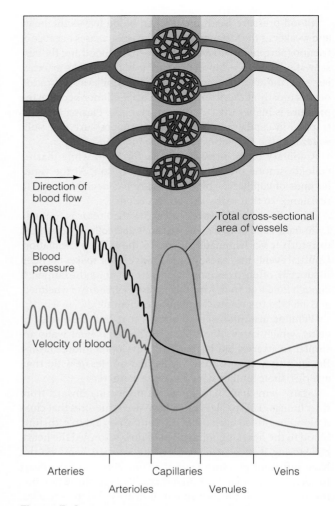

Figure 5–8 Blood pressure in the circulatory system. Blood pressure declines in the circulatory system as the vessels branch. Arterial pressure pulses because of the heartbeat, but pulsation is lost by the time the blood reaches the capillary networks, creating an even flow through body tissues. Blood pressure continues to decline in the venous side of the circulatory system.

arteries, which enter the right and left lungs, respectively. Repeated divisions connect to arterioles and capillary networks associated with the walls of the alveoli, where gas is exchanged between blood and air. The pulmonary capillaries lead to venules and then veins. Four pulmonary veins, two from each lung, return blood to the left atrium, completing the vascular loop of the pulmonary circuit.

The *systemic circuit* involves the movement of freshly oxygenated blood from the left atrium to left ventricle, then into the aorta and its branches, leading to all body tissues. Eventually it makes its way to the companion vein system that returns blood to the right atrium.

The Arteries

The largest-diameter artery in the body is the aorta, extending upward from the left ventricle to arch over the heart to the left, descending anterior and to the left of the vertebral column. The first portion of the aorta is called the *ascending aorta*. It begins at the aortic valve of the left ventricle. The left and right coronary arteries originate in the aortic sinus.

This origination occurs at the base of the ascending aorta, slightly superior to the aortic valve.

The **aortic arch** curves across the superior surface of the heart. It connects the ascending aorta with the *descending aorta* (see **Figure 5–9**). Three arteries originate along the aortic arch. They deliver blood to the head, neck, shoulders, and upper limbs. These arteries are as follows:

1. The brachiocephalic trunk
2. The left common carotid artery
3. The left subclavian artery

The brachiocephalic trunk ascends only for a short distance before it branches to form the right subclavian and right common carotid arteries. The descending aorta is continuous with the aortic arch. The diaphragm divides the descending aorta into a superior *thoracic aorta* and an inferior *abdominal aorta*. The branches of the thoracic aorta include the bronchial, pericardial, esophageal, mediastinal, and intercostal arteries.

The abdominal aorta, beginning immediately inferior to the diaphragm, is a continuation of the thoracic aorta (see Figure 5–9). It delivers blood to the abdominopelvic organs and structures. The abdominopelvic branches of the aorta include the following: celiac, phrenic, superior mesenteric, suprarenal, renal, gonadal, inferior mesenteric, lumbar, middle sacral, and common iliac arteries. **Table 5–3** summarizes the major branches of the aorta.

The subclavian and common carotid arteries supply blood to the neck, head, and brain. The main divisions of these arteries are the vertebral and thyrocervical arteries. The **vertebral arteries** run upward through the cervical vertebrae into the skull and supply blood to the vertebrae and to their ligaments and muscles. They unite in the cranial cavity to form the *basilar artery*, which branches to the pons, midbrain, and cerebellum. It ultimately divides into the two *posterior cerebral arteries*.

The posterior cerebral arteries help form the **cerebral arterial circle** (also known as the *circle of Willis*), connecting the vertebral artery and internal carotid artery systems (see **Figure 5–10**). These united systems provide alternate blood pathways to circumvent blockages and reach brain tissues and to equalize blood pressure in the brain's blood supply.

The **thyrocervical arteries** give off branches to the thyroid and parathyroid glands, larynx, trachea, esophagus, pharynx, and muscles of the neck, shoulder, and back. The left and right *common carotid arteries* separate into the internal and external carotid arteries. **Table 5–4** discusses these arteries. Near the base of the carotid arteries are enlargements (**carotid sinuses**) that contain baroreceptors and help to control blood pressure.

The subclavian artery, which is a branch of the brachiocephalic artery, continues into the arm, passing between the clavicle and first rib to become the *axillary artery*. It becomes the *brachial artery* and gives rise to a *deep brachial artery*. The *ulnar artery* leads down to the lower arm, on the ulnar side of the forearm to the wrist. Some of its branches supply the elbow joint, while others supply the muscles of the forearm. The *radial artery* provides blood to the wrist and hand, traveling along the radial side of the forearm to the wrist. It also supplies the lateral muscles of the forearm. Near the wrist, it approaches the surface, providing a point where the radial pulse may easily be taken.

The *internal thoracic artery* branches into two *anterior intercostal arteries* supplying the intercostal muscles and mammary glands. The *posterior intercostal arteries* supply other intercostal muscles as well as the vertebrae, spinal cord, and deeper back muscles. The *internal thoracic artery* and *external iliac artery* provide blood to the anterior abdominal wall while the *phrenic artery* and *lumbar artery* supply blood to posterior and lateral abdominal wall structures. The major vessels of the arterial system include the *common iliac*

Table 5–3 Major Branches of the Aorta

Branch	Area of Aorta	Main Regions or Organs Supplied
Right and left coronary arteries	Ascending aorta	Heart
Brachiocephalic artery Left common carotid artery Left subclavian artery	Arch of the aorta	Right upper limb and right side of head Left side of head Left upper limb
Descending aorta: Bronchial artery Pericardial artery Esophageal artery Mediastinal artery Posterior intercostal artery	Thoracic aorta	 Bronchi Pericardium Esophagus Mediastinum Thoracic wall
Descending aorta: Celiac artery Phrenic artery Superior mesenteric artery Suprarenal artery Renal artery Gonadal artery Inferior mesenteric artery Lumbar artery Middle sacral artery Common iliac artery	Abdominal aorta	 Upper digestive tract organs Diaphragm Small and large intestines Adrenal gland Kidney Ovaries or testes Lower large intestine Abdominal wall (posterior) Sacrum and coccyx Lower abdominal wall, pelvic organs, lower limbs

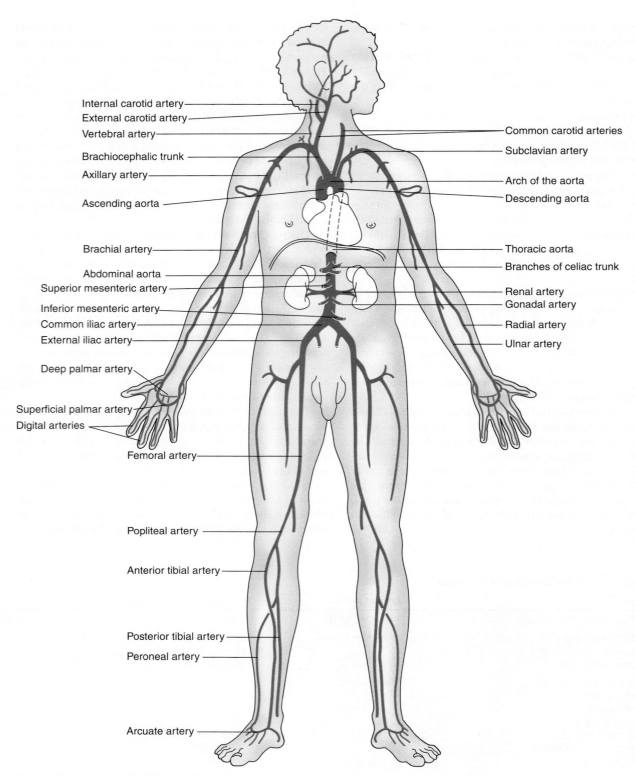

Figure 5–9 Overview of the arteries.

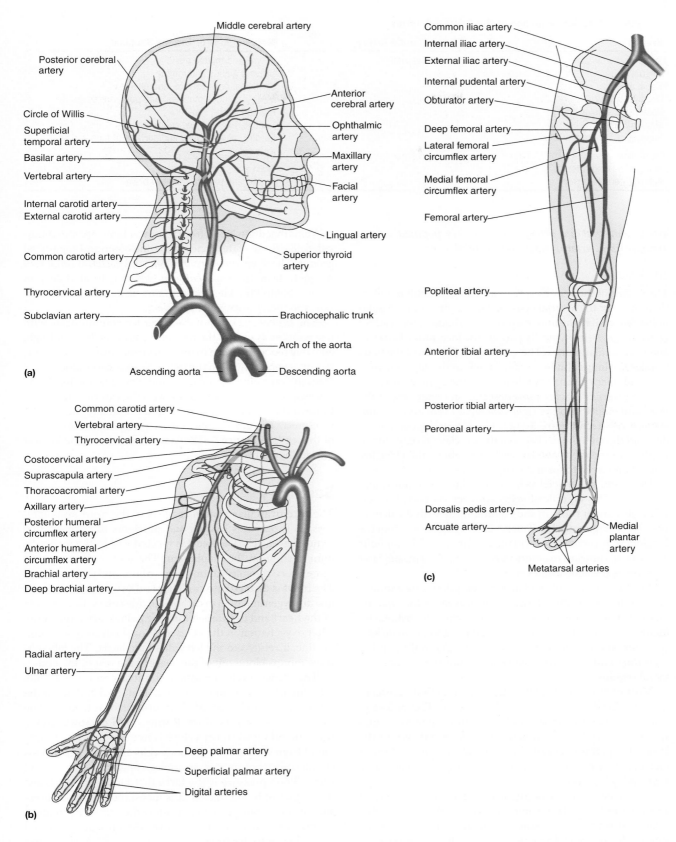

Figure 5–10 Detailed views of the arteries in the body.

■ **Table 5–4 Major Branches of the Carotid Arteries**

Branch	Carotid Artery	Main Regions or Organs Supplied
Superior thyroid artery	External	Larynx and thyroid gland
Lingual artery		Salivary glands and tongue
Facial artery		Chin, lips, nose, palate, and pharynx
Occipital artery		Meninges, neck muscles, and posterior scalp
Posterior auricular artery		Ear and lateral scalp
Maxillary artery		Cheeks, eyelids, jaw, and teeth
Superficial temporal artery		Parotid salivary gland and surface of face and scalp
Ophthalmic artery	Internal	Eyes and eye muscles
Anterior choroid artery		Brain and choroid plexus
Anterior cerebral artery		Frontal and parietal lobes of brain

arteries, internal iliac artery, femoral artery, popliteal artery, anterior tibial artery, and *posterior tibial artery*.

The Veins

The vessels of the venous system are more difficult to follow than those of the arterial system. They connect in irregular networks, with many unnamed vessels joining to form larger veins. Larger veins typically parallel the locations of arteries and have similar names. The veins from all parts of the body besides the lungs and heart converge into the superior vena cava and inferior vena cava, leading to the right atrium.

The *external jugular veins* descend on either side of the neck and empty into the *right subclavian vein* and *left subclavian vein* (see **Figure 5–11**). The *internal jugular veins* descend through the neck to join the subclavian veins, forming *brachiocephalic veins* on each side, above the clavicles. They then merge to form the superior vena cava.

Deep and superficial veins drain the upper limbs and shoulders. The superficial veins connect via complex networks just under the skin and communicate with the deeper vessels (see **Figure 5–12**). The *basilic vein* ascends to join the *brachial vein*, merging to form the *axillary vein*. The *cephalic vein* ascends upward to empty into the axillary vein, and later it becomes the subclavian vein.

The brachiocephalic and azygos veins drain the abdominal and thoracic walls. The *azygos vein* ascends through the mediastinum to join the superior vena cava. Its tributaries include the *posterior intercostal veins, superior hemiazygos veins,* and *inferior hemiazygos veins*. The right and left *ascending lumbar veins* have vessels from the lumbar and sacral regions.

Most veins carry blood directly to the heart's atria, except for veins that drain the abdominal viscera (see **Figure 5–13**). They originate in the stomach, intestines, pancreas, and spleen to carry blood through a *hepatic portal vein* to the liver. This pathway is called the **hepatic portal system**. It includes the right and left *gastric veins, superior mesenteric vein,* and *splenic vein*.

The liver helps to regulate blood concentrations of absorbed amino acids and lipids. It modifies them into usable cells, oxidizes them, or changes them into forms that can be stored. Hepatic portal venous blood usually contains bacteria from intestinal capillaries. Large *Kupffer cells* in the liver phagocytize microorganisms before they can leave the liver. This blood then travels through merged vessels into *hepatic veins*, emptying into the inferior vena cava.

Veins that drain blood from the lower limbs are also subdivided, like those of the upper limbs, into deep and superficial groups. The deep *anterior tibial vein* and *posterior tibial vein* merge to from the *popliteal vein* (which is located deep in the leg, behind the knee), continuing upward as the *femoral vein* and then the *external iliac vein*.

The *saphenous veins* of the lower leg communicate with one another as well as the deeper veins of the leg and thigh, allowing blood to return to the heart from the lower extremities by several routes. In the pelvis, vessels carry blood away from the reproductive, urinary, and digestive organs via the *internal iliac veins*. These unite with the external iliac veins to form the *common iliac veins* and eventually the inferior vena cava. The great saphenous vein runs the entire length of the leg (see **Figure 5–12c**) and is considered the longest vein in the body.

Summary

The cardiovascular system consists of the heart and blood vessels. It provides oxygen and nutrients to tissues while removing wastes. The heart is located within the mediastinum, resting on the diaphragm. The wall of the heart has three layers: the epicardium, myocardium, and endocardium. The heart is divided into two atria and two ventricles. Blood low in oxygen and high in carbon dioxide enters the right side of the heart and is pumped into the pulmonary circulation. After oxygenation in the lungs and some removal of carbon dioxide, it returns to the left side of the heart. The left ventricle pumps blood out of the heart to the rest of the body.

The cardiac cycle consists of the atria contracting while the ventricles relax, and vice versa. Electrical activity of the cardiac cycle can be recorded via an electrocardiogram. The cardiac cycle consists of the P wave, QRS complex, and T wave. Blood vessels form a closed circuit of tubes that carry blood from the heart to the body cells and back again. This circuit consists of arteries, arterioles, capillaries, venules, and veins. Blood pressure is the force that blood exerts against the insides of blood vessels. It is measured as systolic pressure over diastolic pressure, meaning the pressure produced during ventricular contraction over the pressure produced when the ventricles relax.

The pulmonary circuit consists of vessels that carry blood from the right ventricle to the lungs and back to the left atrium. The systemic circuit consists of vessels that lead from the left ventricle to the body cells and back to the heart,

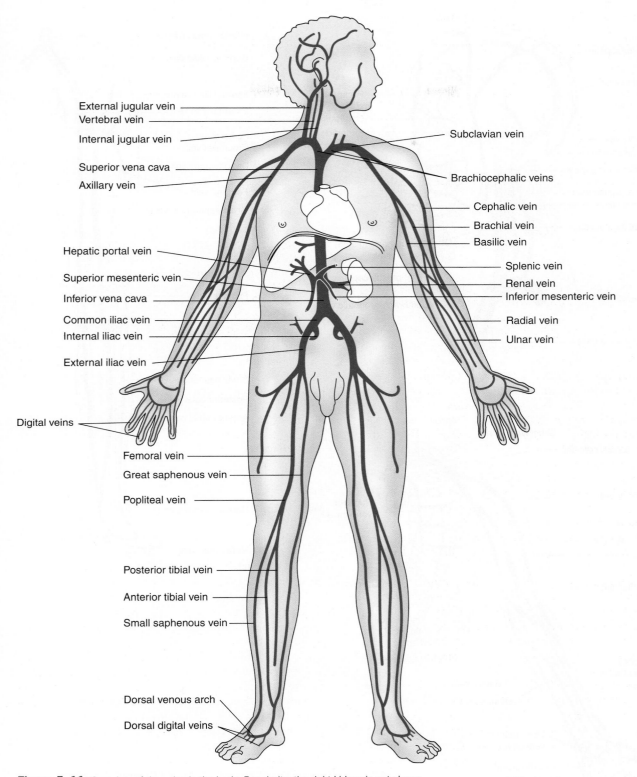

External jugular vein
Vertebral vein
Internal jugular vein
Superior vena cava
Axillary vein
Subclavian vein
Brachiocephalic veins
Cephalic vein
Brachial vein
Basilic vein
Hepatic portal vein
Superior mesenteric vein
Inferior vena cava
Common iliac vein
Internal iliac vein
External iliac vein
Splenic vein
Renal vein
Inferior mesenteric vein
Radial vein
Ulnar vein
Digital veins
Femoral vein
Great saphenous vein
Popliteal vein
Posterior tibial vein
Anterior tibial vein
Small saphenous vein
Dorsal venous arch
Dorsal digital veins

Figure 5–11 Overview of the veins in the body. For clarity, the right kidney is not shown.

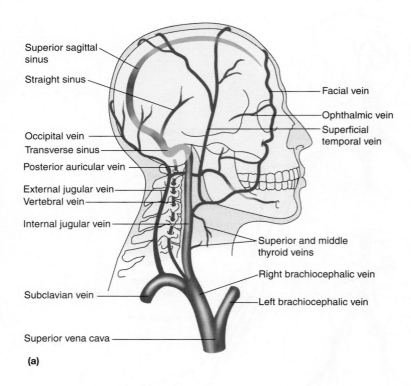

(a)

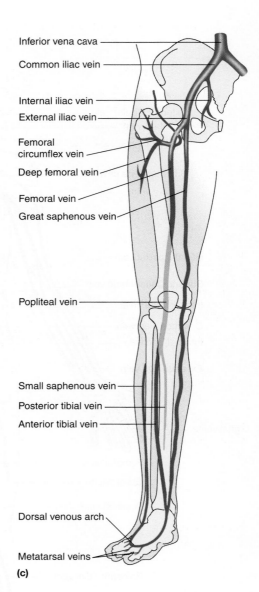

(c)

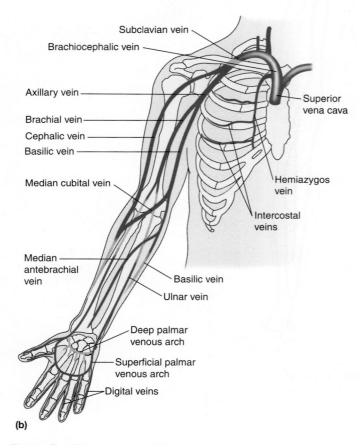

(b)

Figure 5–12 Detailed views of the arteries.

including the aorta and its branches. The aorta is the largest artery in the body, with respect to diameter.

CRITICAL THINKING

Two phlebotomists were studying together to take the National Certification Exam. One of them was questioning the other about the anatomy and physiology of the heart and circulatory system. The questions that follow were what he asked.

1. How many veins return blood to the right atrium? Name these veins.
2. Where in the heart are the Purkinje fibers located?
3. Where is the lowest blood pressure found in the blood vessels?

WEBSITES

http://lsa.colorado.edu/essence/texts/heart.html

http://www.americanheart.org/presenter.
  jhtml?identifier=4473

http://www.ivy-rose.co.uk/HumanBody/Blood/Heart
  _Structure.php

http://www.nhlbi.nih.gov/health/dci/Diseases/hhw/hhw
  _circulation.html

http://www.texasheart.org/hic/anatomy/

http://www.thic.com/conduction.htm

http://www.tpub.com/content/medical/14295/css/14295_36
  .htm

REVIEW QUESTIONS

Multiple Choice

1. Blood leaving the left ventricle enters the
   A. pulmonary trunk
   B. pulmonary artery
   C. inferior vena cava
   D. aorta
2. The right ventricle pumps blood to the
   A. systemic circuit
   B. lungs
   C. left atrium
   D. right atrium
3. The visceral pericardium is the same as the
   A. epicardium
   B. endocardium
   C. myocardium
   D. parietal pericardium
4. The mitral valve is located between the
   A. right atrium and right ventricle
   B. left atrium and left ventricle
   C. left ventricle and aorta
   D. right ventricle and pulmonary trunk
5. The heart wall is composed of how many layers?
   A. two
   B. three
   C. four
   D. five

6. The function of an atrium is to
   A. pump blood to the lungs
   B. pump blood into the systemic circuit
   C. pump blood to the heart muscle
   D. collect blood
7. The left and right pulmonary arteries carry blood to the
   A. brain
   B. liver
   C. lungs
   D. kidneys
8. The pacemaker cells of the heart are located in the
   A. SA node
   B. AV node
   C. left ventricle
   D. left atrium
9. Which of the following blood vessels returns blood to the left atrium?
   A. inferior vena cava
   B. superior vena cava
   C. pulmonary vein
   D. pulmonary trunk
10. Each of the following factors will increase cardiac output, EXCEPT
    A. increased parasympathetic stimulation
    B. increased sympathetic stimulation
    C. increased venous return
    D. increased heart rate
11. The difference between the systolic and diastolic pressures is referred to as
    A. a pulse
    B. circulatory pressure
    C. blood pressure
    D. mean arterial pressure
12. Blood from the brain returns to the heart via a vein called the
    A. external jugular
    B. internal jugular
    C. vertebral vein
    D. azygos vein
13. Branches off of the aortic arch include the
    A. brachio and right axillary arteries
    B. right and left subclavian arteries
    C. right and left common carotid arteries
    D. left subclavian and left common carotid arteries
14. Nutrients from the digestive tract enter the
    A. hepatic vein
    B. hepatic portal vein
    C. inferior vena cava
    D. azygos vein
15. The longest vein in the human body is the
    A. inferior vena cava
    B. superior vena cava
    C. saphenous vein
    D. femoral vein

Common Disorders and Conditions Related to Phlebotomy

OUTLINE

Introduction
Cardiovascular Disorders
    Coronary Artery Disease
    Angina Pectoris
    Myocardial Infarction
    Cardiac Arrhythmias
    Hypertension
    Cardiomyopathy
    Carditis
    Heart Failure
    Cardiac Arrest
    Pulmonary Edema
    Rheumatic Fever
    Valvular Heart Disease
    Mitral Valve Prolapse
    Shock
Blood Vessel Disorders
    Atherosclerosis
    Arteriosclerosis
    Emboli
    Aneurysms
    Phlebitis
    Thrombophlebitis
    Varicose Veins
Blood Disorders
    Anemias
    Polycythemia
    Hemochromatosis
    Leukemias
    Lymphatic Diseases
    Transfusion Incompatibility Reaction
    Clotting Disorders
Summary
Critical Thinking
Websites
Review Questions

OBJECTIVES

After studying this chapter, readers should be able to:

1. Describe the condition known as angina pectoris.
2. Explain major factors that cause myocardial infarction.
3. Describe primary hypertension.
4. Compare arteriosclerosis with atherosclerosis.
5. Distinguish among endocarditis, myocarditis, and pericarditis.
6. Explain the various types of anemias.
7. Compare polycythemia and leukemias.
8. Describe the various types of shock.
9. Explain the possible consequences of emboli.
10. Describe disseminated intravascular coagulation.

KEY TERMS

Abruptio placentae: A complication of pregnancy wherein the placental lining has separated from the uterus of the mother, causing late pregnancy bleeding, fetal heart rate effects, and potential fetal or maternal death.

Angina pectoris: Sharp pain usually felt in the chest or arm that occurs when the heart does not receive enough oxygen to support its workload.

Anoxia: Absence of oxygen supply to an organ or tissue.

Arrhythmia: An irregular heartbeat, which can range from mild to life-threatening; also called *dysrhythmia*.

Arthralgia: Joint pain.

Atherosclerosis: A form of arteriosclerosis characterized by deposits of cholesterol and other fats on the sides of the arteries.

Celiac disease: An autoimmune disorder of the small intestine that causes diarrhea, failure to thrive (in children), fatigue, and other effects upon multiple body systems; it is triggered by a reaction to wheat gluten.

Dysrhythmia: Also called *arrhythmia*, meaning "irregular heartbeat."

KEY TERMS CONTINUED

Eclampsia: An acute, life-threatening complication of pregnancy wherein the mother may experience tonic-clonic seizures and coma.

Gastrectomy: Partial or complete surgical removal of the stomach.

Graves' disease: An autoimmune condition caused by overactive thyroid (hyperthyroidism), causing "bulging" eyes, bone damage, and central or peripheral nervous system symptoms.

Hemarthrosis: Blood accumulation or hemorrhage in a joint.

Hematopoietic stem cells: Stem cells that develop into all the different types of blood cells.

Hemochromatosis: Iron overload caused by either repeated transfusions or a genetic disorder.

Hemoglobin S: An inherited type of abnormal adult hemoglobin, which mostly affects African Americans, causing sickle-cell anemia.

Hemophilia A: The most common form of hemophilia; it is an inherited condition primarily affecting males wherein coagulation is much more prolonged than normal.

Hypertrophied: Enlarged, due to an increase in cell size.

Hypoplasia: Lack of development of a tissue or organ.

Hypoplastic anemia: Aplastic anemia; actually a variety of related anemias that result from destruction of or injury to stem cells in the bone marrow or its matrix.

Ischemia: A temporary reduction of blood supply to an organ or tissue due to obstruction of a blood vessel.

Lymph: Part of the interstitial fluid, which is referred to as *lymph* when it enters a lymph capillary; it picks up and carries bacteria to the lymph nodes to be destroyed.

Lymphoblasts: Immature cells that form lymphocytes; in acute lymphoblastic leukemia, lymphoblasts proliferate uncontrollably and are found in large numbers in the peripheral blood.

Mastectomy: Partial or complete removal of one or both breasts.

Megaloblastic anemia: An anemia that results from inhibition of DNA synthesis in red blood cell production; it is characterized by megaloblasts in the bone marrow.

Myocardial infarction: A heart attack; sudden death of cells in the heart muscle caused by an abrupt interruption of blood flow (and lack of oxygen) to part of the heart.

Myxedema: A type of cutaneous and dermal edema secondary to hypothyroidism and Graves' disease.

NSAID: Nonsteroidal anti-inflammatory drug; common examples include aspirin and ibuprofen.

Pancytopenia: A combination of anemia, leukopenia (decreased white blood cells), and thrombocytopenia (decreased platelets).

Proliferation: Growth and reproduction of cells.

Reed-Sternberg cells: Cells usually derived from B lymphocytes that are much larger than surrounding cells and are found via light microscopy in cases of Hodgkin's disease and certain other disorders.

Respiratory acidosis: A condition in which decreased respiration increases blood carbon dioxide and decreases pH.

Sepsis: The presence of pathogenic bacteria in tissue.

Thalassemia: An inherited autosomal recessive blood disorder in which hemoglobin chains are not synthesized normally, leading to anemia.

Thrombus: A blood clot that forms in the cardiovascular system.

Ventricular asystole: The absence of contraction of the ventricles.

Ventricular fibrillation: Abnormal discharge of electrical nerve impulses that cause the heart to stop beating.

Introduction

Common disorders and conditions that are related to phlebotomy include cardiovascular disorders such as coronary artery disease, myocardial infarction, and hypertension as well as blood vessel disorders and blood disorders. Heart attack (myocardial infarction) is the leading cause of death in the United States. Hypertension is a major cause of cardiac disease, renal failure, and stroke. Atherosclerosis (hardening of the arteries) causes most myocardial and cerebral infarctions. Anemias are defined as conditions of reduced blood cells or hemoglobin as well as the reduced ability to carry oxygen to the cells. Leukemias are malignant neoplasms of the bone marrow, spleen, and lymph nodes. Diseases of the lymphatic system include lymphedema, lymphangitis, and various lymphomas.

Cardiovascular Disorders

Cardiovascular disease is described as any abnormal condition characterized by heart or blood vessel dysfunction. Cardiovascular disease is the leading cause of death in the United States.

Coronary Artery Disease

Coronary artery disease is an abnormal condition that may affect the arteries of the heart and produce varying pathologic effects, primarily reduced flow of oxygen and nutrients to the myocardium. **Atherosclerosis** is the most common type of coronary artery disease (see **Figure 6–1**). Angina pectoris is the classic symptom of coronary artery disease; it results from myocardial ischemia.

Angina Pectoris

Angina pectoris is a sudden outburst of chest pain frequently caused by myocardial **anoxia** as a result of atherosclerosis or coronary artery spasm.

Angina pectoris attacks are often related to emotional stress, eating, exertion, and exposure to intense cold. Complications of angina pectoris include arrhythmias, myocardial infarction, and ischemic cardiomyopathy.

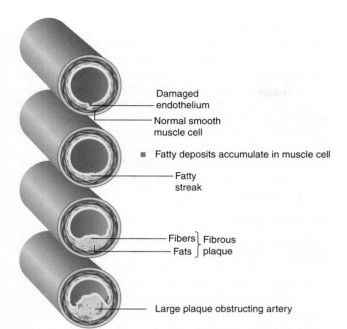

Figure 6–1 Development of a deposition of fat-containing substances that form plaque and lead to arterial occlusion.

Myocardial Infarction

When coronary blood flow is interrupted for extended periods, necrosis (tissue death) of part of the cardiac muscle occurs. Necrosis results in **myocardial infarction** (see **Figure 6–2**). When the coronary arteries are obstructed, this may result in atherosclerosis, a spasm, or a **thrombus**. Myocardial infarction (MI) is also called *heart attack*.

Heart attack is the leading cause of death in the United States. When treatment is delayed, mortality is high. Nearly one-half of sudden myocardial infarction deaths occur before the patient can be hospitalized, usually within 1 h of the onset of symptoms. Risk factors for myocardial infarction include the following:

- Family history of MI
- Aging
- Gender
- Hypertension
- Elevated total cholesterol
- Obesity
- Lifestyle
- Smoking
- Stress or *type A personality*
- Drug use (especially cocaine and amphetamines)

Cardiac Arrhythmias

A **dysrhythmia** (an **arrhythmia**) is a disturbance of heart rhythm caused by abnormal electrical conduction or automaticity. Normally, the sinoatrial (SA) node generates heart rhythms that travel through the heart's conduction system. This causes the atrial and ventricular myocardium to contract and relax at a regular rate. This rate maintains circulation during various levels of physical activity. Arrhythmias range from mild and asymptomatic such as sinus arrhythmia to catastrophic ventricular fibrillation (which requires immediate resuscitation).

Common causes of arrhythmias include the following:

- Congenital defects
- Drug toxicity
- Electrolyte imbalances
- Myocardial infarction or **ischemia**
- Organic heart disease
- Degeneration of the conductive tissue
- Connective tissue disorders
- Cellular hypoxia
- Hypertrophy of the heart muscle
- Acid–base imbalances
- Emotional stress

Hypertension

Hypertension is an elevation in either systolic or diastolic blood pressure. It occurs as either essential (primary) hypertension or secondary hypertension. Primary hypertension is the most common type and is of unknown cause. Secondary hypertension results from renal disease or other identifiable causes. Malignant hypertension is a severe form of hypertension that may be either primary or secondary. Hypertension is a major cause of cardiac disease, renal failure, and stroke.

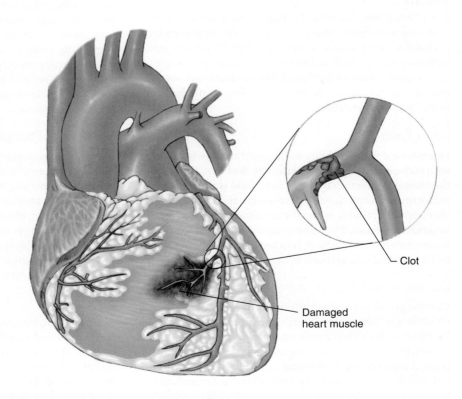

Figure 6–2 Damage caused by myocardial infarction.

Risks for hypertension increase with age. Hypertension is more prevalent in the black population than in the white population. It is also more prevalent in people with less education and lower income. During young and middle adulthood, men have a higher incidence of hypertension, but thereafter, women have a higher incidence.

Risk factors for essential hypertension include the following:

- The aging process
- Family history
- Obesity
- High intake of sodium
- High intake of saturated fat
- Sleep apnea
- Stress
- Excessive alcohol consumption
- Sedentary lifestyle
- Diabetes mellitus
- Tobacco use

Cardiomyopathy

Cardiomyopathy is a term that generally applies to a disease of the heart muscle fibers. It is the second most common direct cause of sudden death (after coronary artery disease). The most common type of cardiomyopathy is the dilated form. Men and blacks have the greatest risk for dilated cardiomyopathy. Other risk factors include coronary artery disease, hypertension, pregnancy, viral infections, and the use of alcohol or illegal drugs. Hypertrophic cardiomyopathy is different in that it is caused by a genetic abnormality.

Carditis

Carditis is defined as inflammation of the heart and its surrounding structures. The several types of carditis include pericarditis, myocarditis, and endocarditis. Common causes of the various forms of carditis include viral infections, bacterial infections, fungal infections, immune conditions, myocardial infarction, trauma, uremia, cancers, certain medications, radiation, and other causes.

Heart Failure

Heart failure is the inability of the heart muscle to contract with enough force to properly circulate the blood throughout the body. Dysfunction of the left ventricle is the most common cause of heart failure. However, the right ventricle may also be dysfunctional, especially in pulmonary disease (right ventricular failure). The most common form of heart failure is congestive heart failure. It is called this because of the collection of fluid (congestion) in the lungs and extremities.

Cardiac Arrest

Cardiac arrest is a sudden cessation of cardiac output and effective circulation. It is usually precipitated by **ventricular fibrillation** or **ventricular asystole**. When cardiac arrest occurs, the delivery of oxygen and removal of carbon dioxide cease. Tissue cell metabolism becomes anaerobic, and metabolic acidosis and **respiratory acidosis** occur. Immediate initiation of cardiopulmonary resuscitation (CPR) is required. Cardiac arrest is also called *cardiopulmonary arrest.*

Pulmonary Edema

Pulmonary edema involves fluid that shifts into the extravascular spaces of the lungs. Pulmonary circulation becomes overloaded with excessive blood volume. It causes dyspnea; coughing; orthopnea; raised cardiac and respiratory rates; and bloody, frothy sputum. Blood pressure may be reduced, and the skin feels cold and clammy. Symptoms often occur after a patient goes to bed. Pulmonary edema is caused by left-sided heart failure, mitral valve disease, pulmonary embolus, arrhythmias, renal failure, or systemic hypertension. Other causes include drug overdose, exposure to high altitudes, and head trauma.

Rheumatic Fever

Rheumatic fever affects the joints and cardiac tissue, and it is a systemic inflammatory and autoimmune disease. It follows a sore throat that is caused by group-A beta-hemolytic streptococcus. This usually occurs in children, resulting in fever and polyarthritis. The joints most affected include the knees, ankles, and fingers. Other symptoms include carditis, cardiac murmurs, cardiomegaly, and congestive heart failure. Symptoms occur within 5 weeks after the upper respiratory tract infection. Prompt assessment is required. Rheumatic fever develops as antibodies against the bacteria cross-react with normal tissues. The body attacks its own cells to initiate an inflammatory reaction, which migrates to the endocardium and heart valves.

Valvular Heart Disease

Valvular heart disease can affect all heart valves, and it may be acquired or congenital. If insufficient, the valves do not close completely, and blood is forced back into the previous chamber as the heart contracts. This increases the heart's workload. Stenosis occurs when the cusps of the valves harden, preventing complete opening. Diagnosis of valvular heart disease requires electrocardiogram, echocardiogram, cardiac catheterization, and radiographic chest studies. Treatment involves digitalis or quinidine, to treat arrhythmias, and prophylactic antibiotics.

Mitral Valve Prolapse

Mitral valve prolapse is defined as one or both cusps of the mitral valve protruding back into the left atrium when the ventricles contract. It is usually a benign condition, with patients being asymptomatic. When symptoms do exist, they include dyspnea, chest pain, fatigue, dizziness, and syncope. It affects all age groups and often results in severe anxiety. Mitral valve prolapse is usually diagnosed during a routine physical examination, although a physician should evaluate any reports of chest pain promptly.

Shock

Shock is defined as cardiovascular system collapse. It includes fluid shifts and vasodilation along with inefficient cardiac output. The organs and tissues experience inadequate perfusion, and the patient appears pale, cold, and clammy. The pulse is rapid (tachycardia), weak, and thready, and there is rapid breathing as well as an altered level of consciousness. Drops in blood pressure may cause anxiety, irritability, and restlessness. Other symptoms include dizziness, extreme thirst, profuse sweating, and then dilation of the pupils, shaking, and trembling. Shock is a true medical emergency.

Shock may be caused by anaphylaxis, hemorrhage, respiratory distress, **sepsis**, heart failure, neurologic failure, emotional catastrophe, or severe metabolic insult. The vital organs eventually do not receive enough oxygen and nutrients to sustain life. Rapid blood loss or fluid loss, with hypovolemia, precipitates shock. Another cause of shock is failure of the heart to pump adequately.

Types of shock include the following:

- *Cardiogenic*—decreased cardiac output with tissue hypoxia in the presence of adequate intravascular volume; it is caused by heart failure (usually after myocardial infarction)
- *Hypovolemic*—develops when intravascular volume has decreased by approximately 15%; it is caused by hemorrhage, burns, or loss of interstitial fluid
- *Neurogenic*—widespread vasodilation due to parasympathetic overstimulation or sympathetic understimulation; it is caused by spinal cord or medulla trauma, depressants, anesthetics, pain, or severe emotional stress
- *Anaphylactic*—results from a widespread hypersensitivity reaction (anaphylaxis); often caused by allergies and poisons—it may lead to death quickly if untreated
- *Septic*—part of the systemic inflammatory response syndrome; it begins with an infection that progresses to bacteremia and sepsis, resulting in multiple organ dysfunction syndrome

Blood Vessel Disorders

The vascular system contains the arteries, arterioles, capillaries, venules, and veins. These vessels supply the tissues with oxygen and nutrients, which are carried in the blood. This system also moves carbon dioxide and waste products to the appropriate organs for excretion. The arteries carry oxygenated blood away from the heart, and in general, the veins carry deoxygenated blood back to the heart. The capillaries are the point of exchange at the cellular level. Blood vessel disorders include atherosclerosis, arteriosclerosis, emboli, aneurysms, phlebitis, thrombophlebitis, and varicose veins.

Atherosclerosis

Atherosclerosis is defined as a form of arteriosclerosis characterized by deposits of cholesterol and other fats on the sides of blood arteries (see Figure 6–1). Atherosclerosis causes most myocardial and cerebral infarctions. Risk factors include heredity, a sedentary lifestyle, a diet high in fats and cholesterol, smoking cigarettes, hypertension, diabetes mellitus, and obesity. Infarction becomes more likely as plaque forms and thickens the arterial walls. Blood tests will indicate elevated cholesterol, triglyceride, and lipid levels, and hypertension is usually noted. Treatment consists of changes in diet and exercise as well as stopping smoking. Drug therapies are quite varied, including hyperlipidemic agents and those that inhibit cholesterol absorption in the intestine.

Arteriosclerosis

Arteriosclerosis is actually a group of diseases characterized by the hardening of the arteries. The most common form of arteriosclerosis is atherosclerosis. Some types of arteriosclerosis involve the destruction of muscle and elastic fibers as well as deposits of calcium. Arteriosclerosis occurs when the walls of the arterioles thicken, and a loss of elasticity and contractility occurs.

Emboli

Emboli are (usually) blood clots that lodge in blood vessels to inhibit blood flow. Symptoms vary, but usually include severe pain in the area of the embolus. If an embolus lodges in an extremity, paleness, numbness, or coldness may develop. If nausea, vomiting, fainting, or shock occurs, the patient is in an emergency state. Emboli may also be composed of air bubbles, clumps of bacteria, globules of fat, or pieces of tissue. Venous thrombosis in the deep veins of the legs is most common. When a portion of a thrombus breaks loose, it travels through the veins until it lodges in a narrow vessel, such as a vessel in the lungs. Thrombi can form in the heart because of cardiac arrhythmias. This can result in a myocardial infarction, or the thrombus can travel to the brain, which results in a stroke.

Aneurysms

Aneurysms are defined as abnormal dilations of blood vessels located in distinctly limited areas (see **Figure 6–3**). Symptoms vary with location, and abdominal aortic aneurysm is the most common type. Aneurysms are often caused by a buildup of atherosclerotic plaque that weakens vessel walls. If the aneurysm is abdominal, a "bruit" sound is heard on auscultation.

Phlebitis

Phlebitis is defined as inflammation of a vein. It occurs usually in the lower legs, but it can affect any veins in the body. Pain and tenderness in the affected area develop first, followed by intensifying discomfort, swelling, redness, and warmth. Phlebitis can develop into thrombophlebitis. Although the exact cause is unknown, it is possible that venous stasis, blood disorders, obesity, injury to a vein during phlebotomy, and surgery may be related.

Thrombophlebitis

Thrombophlebitis results from phlebitis, with a thrombus forming on the vessel wall. It interferes with blood flow and causes edema, pain, swelling, heaviness, warmth in the affected area, and chills and fever. It is also influenced by venous stasis, blood disorders that cause hypercoagulability, and injury to the venous wall. The tunica intima is affected, allowing the formation of clots. Often, there will be gross edema in one leg, with tenderness to the touch. Thrombophlebitis is confirmed with radiographic venography and ultrasonography. It requires immediate treatment, with immobilization of the affected part. Heparin is given to prevent enlargement of the clot, and antibiotics are used to prevent infection. Surgery may be used to ligate the affected vessel so that collateral circulation can develop. Prevention of deep vein thrombosis during immobilization or reduced physical activity is essential.

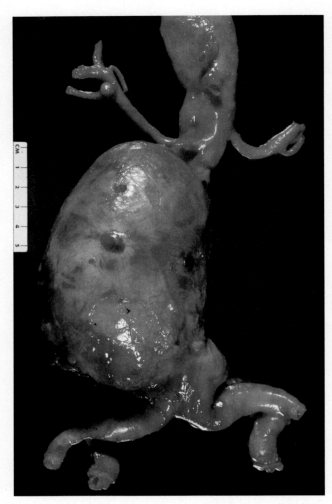

Figure 6–3 Large arteriosclerotic aneurysm extending from renal arteries (above) to iliac arteries (below).

Varicose Veins

Varicose veins usually occur in the lower legs and appear swollen, tortuous, and knotted. They usually develop gradually, causing leg fatigue and then a continuous dull ache. Eventually, the veins become harder and thicker, with pain worsening. They are easily diagnosed by their appearance. Although the cause is not clearly identified, absent or defective valves in the veins are suspected. When the patient has adequate exercise, the blood in the legs moves normally. When the patient is standing or sitting for extended periods, gravity causes the blood to be pushed downward, causing pressure on the valves. When advanced, varicosities cause skin around the affected vessels to become brownish. Treatment involves frequent rest with the legs raised, exercise, submergence in warm water, and wearing support stockings. Surgery may be indicated if these treatments are not adequate.

Blood Disorders

The common blood disorders include anemias, leukemias, lymphatic diseases, transfusion incompatibility reaction, and clotting disorders.

Anemias

Anemias are defined as conditions of reduced red blood cells or hemoglobin as well as the reduced ability to carry oxygen to the cells. Types of anemias include iron deficiency, folic acid deficiency, pernicious, aplastic, sickle cell, hemorrhagic, and hemolytic. Most anemic patients are pale and fatigued. Progressive symptoms include dyspnea, tachycardia, and the pounding of the heart, which a physician should promptly assess. Various causes include hemorrhage, heavy menstrual flow, the insufficient intake of iron, the insufficient intake of folic acid, oversized immature RBCs, autoimmune conditions, damaged stem cells, and exposure to certain cytotoxic agents. Diagnosis shows reduced numbers of RBCs, hemoglobin, and hematocrit. Treatment is based on the etiology of the anemia.

Iron Deficiency Anemia

Iron deficiency anemia is a disorder of oxygen transport. Hemoglobin synthesis is deficient in this disease, which affects between 10 and 30% of adults in the United States. It is the most common type of anemia, and IT occurs in all ages. Replacement therapy usually reverses the condition. Possible causes of iron deficiency anemia include the following:

- Inadequate dietary intake of iron
- Blood loss (due to drugs, heavy menses, hemorrhaging, peptic ulcers, etc.)
- Iron malabsorption (from chronic diarrhea, gastrectomy, **celiac disease**, etc.)
- Various types of hemoglobinuria (the presence of free hemoglobin in the urine)
- Pregnancy (wherein iron is carried from the mother to the fetus)
- Mechanical red blood cell trauma (due to prosthetic heart valves or vena cava filters)

Folic Acid Deficiency Anemia

Folic acid deficiency anemia is a slowly progressing form of **megaloblastic anemia**. It is very common, usually occurring in infants, adolescents, pregnant or lactating women, alcoholics, elderly people, and patients with malignancies or intestinal diseases. It is caused by the following:

- Alcohol abuse, which suppresses the metabolic effects of folate
- Poor diet
- Impaired absorption due to intestinal dysfunction or diseases
- Overcooking of food, destroying much of the contained folic acid
- Prolonged drug therapy (including anticonvulsants and estrogens)
- Increased need for folic acid (during pregnancy, increased periods of growth throughout life, and in patients with skin diseases or neoplastic diseases)

Pernicious Anemia

Pernicious anemia is the most common form of megaloblastic anemia. It is mainly caused by malabsorption of vitamin B_{12}. It usually affects people between the ages of 50 and 60, and incidence increases with age. It is a fatal condition if not treated. When treated properly, its signs and symptoms subside, although certain neurologic deficits may be permanent. Possible causes of pernicious anemia include the following:

- Genetic predisposition
- Thyroiditis, **myxedema**, or **Graves' disease**
- Partial **gastrectomy**
- Lack of adequate dietary consumption of vitamin B$_{12}$ (usually in the elderly)

Aplastic Anemia

Aplastic anemia is also called **hypoplastic anemia**. These terms actually describe a variety of related anemias. Aplastic anemia results from the destruction of or injury to stem cells in the bone marrow or its matrix. It causes **pancytopenia** and bone marrow **hypoplasia**. Pancytopenia actually results from the decreased functioning of hypoplastic fatty bone marrow. Aplastic anemia usually results in fatal bleeding or infection, with the death rate for severe cases being between 80 and 90% of patients. Possible causes of aplastic anemia include the following:

- Drugs (antibiotics, anticonvulsants) or toxic agents
- Radiation (nearly one-half of all cases are related to radiation exposure)
- Severe disease (especially hepatitis)
- Preleukemic and neoplastic infiltration of bone marrow
- Congenital (idiopathic) causes

Sickle-Cell Anemia

Sickle-cell anemia is a congenital condition caused by defective hemoglobin molecules. The sickle-cell trait results from mutations of the **hemoglobin S** gene. The disease is initially asymptomatic. However, about 50% of patients die by their early twenties from this condition. Very few will live to middle age. Sickle-cell anemia mainly affects people of African or Mediterranean descent. It is also commonly seen in Puerto Rico, India, the Middle East, and Turkey.

Hemorrhagic Anemia

A hemorrhage is a loss of a large amount of blood in a short period, either externally or internally. Hemorrhaging may occur in arteries, veins, or capillaries. An untreated hemorrhage may result in anemia. This is referred to as *hemorrhagic anemia*. Hemoglobin levels are lowered severely due to rapid, massive hemorrhage. Most commonly, hemorrhagic anemia is seen after car accidents, major surgery, gunshot or stab wounds, and other severe forms of tissue damage. Surgery to repair the bleeding tissues or organs is usually indicated, as are blood transfusions. If prompt treatment is not given, the patient goes into shock, which leads to coma and death.

Hemolytic Anemia

Hemolytic anemia is a disorder characterized by the chronic premature destruction of red blood cells. Anemia may be minimal or absent and may reflect the ability of bone marrow to increase red blood cell production. The process of the destruction of red blood cells is called *hemolysis*. The condition may be associated with an infectious disease, certain inherited red blood cell disorders, or neoplastic diseases. Hemolytic anemia occurs when the bone marrow cannot produce more red blood cells than are being destroyed. Hemolytic anemias are seen in disorders such as malaria and **thalassemia**. These may be due to protein abnormalities or differences.

Polycythemia

Polycythemia is an abnormal increase in the number of erythrocytes in the blood. It may be primary or secondary to pulmonary disease, heart disease, or prolonged exposure to high altitudes. It may also be idiopathic. Symptoms include headaches, dyspnea, irritability, mental sluggishness, dizziness, syncope, night sweats, and weight loss. Diagnosis is made via blood tests, spleen enlargement, and total RBC mass evaluation. Periodic phlebotomy is used to reduce blood volume, as are myelosuppressive drugs and radiation.

Hemochromatosis

Hemochromatosis is defined as an iron overload that may be caused by either repeated transfusions or a genetic condition. When related to heredity, the disorder causes the small intestine to absorb excessive iron. Symptoms include **arthralgia**, decreased libido, and fatigue, followed by cirrhosis of the liver, diabetes, excessive melanin-related skin pigmentation, and heart failure. The excess iron is stored in muscles and organs such as the liver, pancreas, and heart. Liver damage may result in liver carcinoma. Symptoms usually develop in the fifth or sixth decade of life, with clinical signs being more prevalent in males.

Leukemias

Leukemias are malignant neoplasms of the bone marrow, spleen, and lymph nodes. They produce an abnormal proliferation of certain lymphoid or myeloid cells, causing reduced production and function of normal blood cells. They are classified by the proliferating cell type and degree of differentiation of the neoplastic cells. Leukemias may be acute or chronic. Common types of leukemias include acute lymphocytic leukemia, chronic lymphocytic leukemia, acute myelogenous leukemia, and chronic myelogenous leukemia.

Acute Lymphocytic Leukemia

Acute lymphocytic leukemia causes an overproduction of immature lymphoid cells (**lymphoblasts**) in the lymph nodes and bone marrow. Common signs and symptoms include bone pain, sore throat, fatigue, night sweats, weakness, and weight loss. Prompt assessment by a physician is required. This type of leukemia usually affects children and people over age 65. It is the most common childhood leukemia.

Chronic Lymphocytic Leukemia

Chronic lymphocytic leukemia is a neoplasm that usually affects the B lymphocytes. It progresses slowly, resulting in mature-appearing but hypofunctional lymphocytes. There are often no symptoms prior to the disease being revealed in a complete blood count. When symptoms develop, they usually include fever, night sweats, extreme fatigue, a noticeable swelling of lymph nodes, and weight loss. Prompt assessment by a physician is required. There are five stages of chronic lymphocytic leukemia:

- Stage 0—low risk—lymphocytosis exists
- Stage I—intermediate risk—lymphocytosis plus enlarged lymph nodes
- Stage II—intermediate risk—lymphocytosis plus an enlarged liver or spleen, with or without lymphadenopathy
- Stage III—high risk—lymphocytosis plus anemia
- Stage IV—high risk—lymphocytosis plus thrombocytopenia

Acute Myelogenous Leukemia

Acute myelogenous leukemia is a rapidly progressive neoplasm of myeloid-related cells. In this condition, leukemic cells accumulate in the bone marrow, peripheral blood, and other tissues. It is also known as *acute myeloid*, *granulocytic*, or *myelocytic* leukemia. Rapidly accumulating myeloblasts lead to pancytopenia and anemia. This type of leukemia is the most common adult leukemia and represents about 20% of childhood leukemias.

Chronic Myelogenous Leukemia

Chronic myelogenous leukemia is a slowly progressing neoplasm arising in early progenitor cells or **hematopoietic stem cells**. It results in excessive mature-appearing but hypofunctional neutrophils. Most cases are genetic in origin, identified because of the *Philadelphia chromosome*. This type of leukemia accounts for 15 to 20% of adult leukemias. Nearly one-half of patients are asymptomatic at diagnosis. It is usually diagnosed because of leukocytosis or thrombocytosis found during routine blood tests. The disease usually occurs in adults over the age of 40. The only chance for a complete cure is bone marrow transplantation.

Lymphatic Diseases

Diseases of the lymphatic system include lymphedema, lymphangitis, and various lymphomas.

Lymphedema

Lymphedema is an abnormal collection of **lymph** (usually in the extremities) that results in a painless swelling. It is usually due to an obstruction, but may also be caused by inflammation or the removal of lymph channels. Congenital lymphedema (Milroy's disease) is a hereditary condition characterized by chronic lymphatic obstruction. Secondary lymphedema may follow the surgical removal of lymph channels in **mastectomy**, the obstruction of lymph drainage caused by malignant tumors, or adult filarial parasite infestation of lymph vessels. Lymphedema is most common in the lower limbs. It can also occur in the arms, face, trunk, and external genitalia. Lymphedema may be primary or secondary. There is no cure for lymphedema, but lymph drainage from the extremities can be improved if the patient sleeps with the foot of his or her bed elevated 4 to 8 in. Other helpful measures include the wearing of elastic stockings and regular moderate exercise. Surgery may be performed to remove **hypertrophied** lymph channels and disfiguring tissue.

Lymphangitis

Lymphangitis is an inflammation of the lymph vessels that may be caused by an acute streptococcal infection in one of the extremities. It is characterized by fine red streaks that extend from the infected area to the axilla or groin. Other symptoms include chills, fever, headache, and myalgia. Risk factors include chronic steroid use, diabetes mellitus, long-term placement of a peripheral venous catheter, immunocompromise, bites (from insects, animals, or humans), and any skin trauma.

Lymphomas

Lymphomas are neoplasms of the lymphatic tissue that originate in the lymphatic system. They are usually malignant, but in rare cases may be benign. A lymphoma normally appears initially as a single, painless, enlarged lymph node, usually in the neck. Signs and symptoms progress to include fever, weakness, anemia, and weight loss. The disease may spread to the liver, bones, spleen, and gastrointestinal tract. Lymphomas are usually categorized as Hodgkin's or non-Hodgkin's lymphoma. Hodgkin disease is caused by clonal **proliferation** of transformed B lymphocytes. The presence of **Reed-Sternberg cells** on a pathologic examination is all that is needed to confirm diagnosis of this disease (see **Figure 6–4**). The disease spreads first to continuous lymphoid tissue and then to nonlymphoid tissue.

Transfusion Incompatibility Reaction

It is extremely important that blood components to be transfused be compatible with the individual receiving the transfusion. The correct individual must be identified prior to the transfusion process. Transfusion incompatibility reaction occurs when a transfused blood product has antibodies to the recipient's red blood cells, or when the recipient has antibodies to the donated blood's red blood cells. Individuals must be carefully monitored for a transfusion reaction. The hypersensitivity reaction can range from mild to fatal. Therefore, vital signs should be checked every 5 min during the procedure, and signs and symptoms such as chills, fever, facial flushing, tachycardia, cold or clammy skin, and itching should also be checked. More intensive symptoms may lead to circulatory collapse. This type of reaction produces hemolysis or agglutination of blood cells. Any further transfusion must be quickly stopped, and antihistamines are indicated.

Clotting Disorders

Clotting disorders include hemophilia and disseminated intravascular coagulation. Hemophilia results from a deficiency of

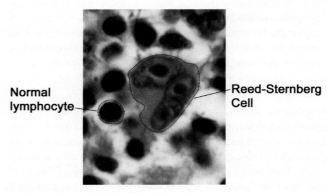

Figure 6–4 Reed-Sternberg cells.

clotting factors, and it is a hereditarily linked disorder. It affects male children and is signified by prolonged bleeding after injury, easy bruising, hematomas, and excessive nosebleeds.

Hemophilia

Hemophilia is a group of hereditary bleeding disorders characterized by a deficiency of one of the factors necessary for blood coagulation. The two most common forms of the disorder are hemophilia A and hemophilia B. **Hemophilia A** is also known as *classic hemophilia*. It is the result of a deficiency or absence of antihemophilic factor VIII. Hemophilia B (Christmas disease) represents a deficiency of plasma thromboplastin component. The greater the deficiency, the more severe the disorder will manifest. Patients with hemophilia experience a greater than normal loss of blood during dental procedures, epistaxis, hematoma, and **hemarthrosis**. Severe nonsurgical internal hemorrhage and hematuria are less common.

The primary treatment for hemophilia is the replacement of deficient factors with recombinant factor products or plasma. Treatment may be prophylactic, or to stop bleeding episodes. Acetaminophen or codeine is used to control pain. Both aspirin and **NSAID** use, as well as intramuscular injections, should be avoided because they may precipitate bleeding. When hemophiliacs need surgery or dental work, extreme care must be exercised. Gene transfer therapy is being experimented with to develop methods of replacing the absent gene.

Disseminated Intravascular Coagulation

Disseminated intravascular coagulation occurs as a complication of diseases and conditions that accelerate clotting. When clotting accelerates, it causes occlusion of small blood vessels and organ necrosis. Clotting in the microcirculation usually affects the lungs, kidneys, extremities, and brain. Disseminated intravascular coagulation is caused by the following:

- Infection (gram-negative septicemia, gram-positive septicemia, or from viruses, fungi, rickettsiae, or protozoans)
- Neoplastic disease (including acute leukemia, aplastic anemia, and metastatic carcinoma)
- Necrotic disorders (including brain tissue destruction, extensive trauma or burns, hepatic necrosis, and transplant rejection)
- Obstetric complications (including **abruptio placentae**, *amniotic fluid embolism*, retained dead fetus, **eclampsia**, and septic abortion)
- Other conditions (including heatstroke, poisonous snakebite, cirrhosis, fat embolism, incompatible blood transfusion, cardiac arrest, shock, severe venous thrombosis, and surgery requiring cardiopulmonary bypass)

Summary

Common disorders related to phlebotomy include those that affect the cardiovascular system, including the blood and blood vessels. Atherosclerosis is the most common type of coronary artery disease. Necrosis of heart tissue results in myocardial infarction. When the coronary arteries are obstructed, this may result in atherosclerosis, a spasm, or a thrombus. A dysrhythmia (arrhythmia) is a disturbance of heart rhythm caused by abnormal electrical conduction or automaticity. Cardiac arrest is a sudden cessation of cardiac output and effective circulation, which is usually precipitated by ventricular fibrillation or ventricular asystole. Common vascular disorders include phlebitis, thrombophlebitis, and varicose veins.

Shock may be caused by anaphylaxis, hemorrhage, respiratory distress, sepsis, heart failure, neurologic failure, emotional catastrophe, or severe metabolic insult. There are many types of anemia, some of which have high fatality rates. Aplastic anemia usually results in fatal bleeding or infection, with the death rate for severe cases being between 80 and 90% of patients. Acute myelogenous leukemia is the most common adult leukemia, while acute lymphocytic leukemia is the most common childhood leukemia.

CRITICAL THINKING

A woman who has been pregnant for 32 weeks has been complaining of weakness, tiredness, and lack of appetite. Her physician orders blood tests to see if she has any type of anemia. The results confirm this.

1. What is the most common type of anemia during pregnancy once iron deficiency anemia is ruled out?
2. Under what form of anemia is this type classified?

WEBSITES

http://digestive.niddk.nih.gov/ddiseases/pubs/hemochromatosis

http://www.americanheart.org/presenter.jhtml?identifier=4440

http://www.heartfailure.org/eng_site/hf.asp

http://www.labtestsonline.org/understanding/conditions/anemia.html

http://www.mayoclinic.com/health/high-blood-pressure/DS00100

http://www.medicinenet.com/heart_attack/article.htm

http://www.merckmanuals.com/professional/sec07.html

http://www.nlm.nih.gov/medlineplus/bloodandblooddisorders.html

http://www.nlm.nih.gov/medlineplus/ency/article/001124.htm

http://www.oncologychannel.com/leukemias/index.shtml

http://www.wrongdiagnosis.com/medical/blood_vessel_disorder.htm

REVIEW QUESTIONS

Multiple Choice

1. An area of dead cells due to lack of oxygen is called
   A. ischemia
   B. infarction
   C. atresia
   D. gangrene

2. The most common type of anemia in the United States is
   A. sickle cell
   B. pernicious
   C. folic acid deficiency
   D. iron deficiency
3. Thrombophlebitis occurs most commonly in the
   A. lower legs
   B. lower arms
   C. lower abdomen
   D. lungs
4. When the heart is pumping inadequately to meet the needs of the body, the condition is called
   A. cor pulmonale
   B. heart failure
   C. arrhythmia
   D. myocardial infarction
5. Which of the following is a sign of shock?
   A. bradycardia
   B. tachycardia
   C. bradypnea
   D. hypertension
6. In which of the following types of anemia may you find hemoglobin S?
   A. hemolytic
   B. aplastic
   C. sickle cell
   D. megaloblastic
7. Stasis of blood flow from immobility, injury to a vessel, or predisposition to clot formation increases the risk of
   A. pulmonary embolism
   B. emphysema
   C. pneumothorax
   D. chronic obstructive pulmonary disease
8. What is the most common type of coronary artery disease?
   A. dysrhythmia
   B. atherosclerosis
   C. anoxia
   D. pancytopenia
9. Aneurysms are often caused by
   A. buildup of atherosclerotic plaque that weakens vessel walls
   B. an inflammation of a vein

C. various cardiac arrhythmias
D. complication of syphilis
10. The presence of Reed-Sternberg cells can confirm diagnosis of
   A. chronic lymphocytic leukemia
   B. acute myelogenous leukemia
   C. Hodgkin's disease
   D. hemophilia
11. Which of the following is a major cause of cardiac disease, renal failure, and stroke?
   A. emphysema
   B. heart failure
   C. hypertension
   D. asthma
12. Which of the following does not cause disseminated intravascular coagulation?
   A. neoplastic diseases such as acute leukemia and metastatic carcinoma
   B. abruptio placentae and septic abortion
   C. severe dehydration and low potassium in the blood
   D. brain tissue destruction and hepatic necrosis
13. Which of the following cardiovascular disorders is the leading cause of death in the United States?
   A. myocardial infarction
   B. hypertension
   C. stroke
   D. angina pectoris
14. Thrombophlebitis results from
   A. inflammation of veins
   B. inflammation of the sac enclosing the heart
   C. hypertension
   D. myocardial infarction
15. The diagnosis of anemia indicates that the patient is experiencing a reduction in
   A. platelets
   B. leukocytes
   C. antibodies or albumin
   D. red blood cells or hemoglobin

Hematology

OUTLINE

Introduction
Hematology
    Red Blood Cells
    White Blood Cells
    Platelets
    Plasma
Hemostasis
    Serum
    Plasma
Appearance of Serum and Plasma
    Blood Clotting
Blood Types and Transfusions
Summary
Critical Thinking
Websites
Review Questions

OBJECTIVES

After studying this chapter, readers should be able to:
1. Distinguish between the formed elements and the liquid portion of the blood.
2. Explain the characteristics of red blood cell counts.
3. Describe *erythropoiesis* and the sites of production of erythropoietin.
4. Distinguish between the five types of white blood cells and discuss their functions.
5. Describe the functions of each of the major components of blood plasma.
6. Describe the characteristics of platelets and their functions.
7. Define *hemostasis* and explain the mechanisms that help achieve it.
8. Explain what prevents the formation of massive clots throughout the cardiovascular system.
9. Explain blood typing and how it is used to avoid adverse reactions to blood transfusions.
10. Distinguish between a thrombus and an embolus.

KEY TERMS

Agglutination: The clumping of red blood cells following a transfusion reaction.

Agranulocytes: Leukocytes without granular cytoplasm.

Albumins: The smallest of plasma proteins; they make up around 60% of these proteins by weight.

Antibodies: Agglutinins; gamma globulin proteins that respond to specific antigens.

Antigens: Agglutinogens; red blood cell surface molecules that react with antibodies from the plasma.

Basophils: Leukocytes that have fewer granules than eosinophils, which become deep blue in basic stain.

B cells: Lymphocytes that are responsible for humoral immunity.

Bilirubin: An orange pigment formed from biliverdin that has potent antioxidant activity; bilirubin is orange and excreted along with biliverdin in the bile.

Biliverdin: A green pigment created from decomposing heme, which is converted to bilirubin.

Coagulation: The formation of a blood clot.

Colony-stimulating factors (CSFs): Glycoproteins that can cause the proliferation and differentiation of leukocytes.

Embolus: A clot that dislodges or fragments, to be carried away in the blood flow.

Eosinophils: Leukocytes with coarse, same-sized granules that appear dark red in acid stain.

Erythropoiesis: The process of developing erythrocytes (red blood cells), which mostly occurs in the red bone marrow (myeloid tissue).

Erythropoietin: A hormone that uses negative feedback to control the rate of red blood cell formation.

Fibrin: Insoluble threads of protein made from the plasma protein fibrinogen.

Fibrinogen: A plasma protein that is important for blood coagulation. It is the largest plasma protein.

Globulins: Antibodies made by the liver or lymphatic tissues that make up around 36% of the plasma proteins.

KEY TERMS CONTINUED

Granulocytes: Leukocytes with granular cytoplasm, including neutrophils, eosinophils, and basophils.

Hematocrit (HCT): The volume percentage of red blood cells in a sample of whole blood.

Hematology: The study of blood and blood disorders.

Hemoglobin: The substance in red blood cells that carries oxygen.

Hemostasis: The stoppage of bleeding.

Interleukins: Hormones upon which many of the effects of leukocytes depend.

Leukocytes: White blood cells; they protect the body against disease and develop from hemocytoblasts in red bone marrow.

Leukocytosis: A condition of white blood cells exceeding 10,000 per cubic millimeter (microliter), indicating an acute infection.

Leukopenia: A condition of the total white blood cell count being below 5,000 per cubic millimeter (microliter); this signifies conditions such as influenza, AIDS, and others.

Lymphocytes: Leukocytes with large, round nuclei inside a thin cytoplasm rim.

Macrophages: Cells that phagocytize and destroy damaged red blood cells, mostly in the liver and spleen.

Mast cells: Connective tissue cells that, during allergic reactions, release histamine and heparin.

Megakaryocytes: Red bone marrow cells that fragment to produce platelets.

Monocytes: Leukocytes that are the largest type of blood cells, with varied nuclei.

Natural killer (NK) cells: Lymphocytes responsible for immune surveillance; they are important in preventing cancer.

Neutrophils: Leukocytes with small granules that appear light purple in neutral stain; older neutrophils are called *segs* while younger neutrophils are called *bands*.

Nonprotein nitrogenous substances: Amino acids, urea, and uric acid in the plasma.

Plasma: The liquid portion of blood.

Plasma cells: Specialized B cells that form and secrete antibodies.

Plasma proteins: The most abundant solutes (dissolved substances) in the plasma.

Platelets: Thrombocytes; platelets are cytoplasm fragments of megakaryocytes that are important in blood clotting.

Polymorphonuclear leukocytes: White blood cells with segmented lobular nuclei, such as neutrophils.

Prothrombin: An alpha globulin made in the liver that is converted to thrombin.

Red blood cells (erythrocytes): Those red blood cells that transport gases, including oxygen.

Serotonin: A substance that contracts smooth muscles in blood vessels, reducing blood loss.

Serum: The clear, yellowish liquid that remains after clot formation; serum is plasma minus fibrinogen and some, but not all, of its clotting factors.

T cells: Lymphocytes that are responsible for cell-mediated immunity.

Thrombin: A substance that causes fibrinogen to be cut into sections of fibrin and then joined into long threads as part of the clotting process.

Thrombocytes: See *platelets*.

Thrombopoietin: A hormone that causes megakaryocytes to develop from hemocytoblasts, resulting in eventual platelet (thrombocyte) formation.

Thrombus: A clot that forms abnormally in a vessel.

Vasospasm: An action of muscle contraction in a small blood vessel that occurs after it is cut or broken; this action can completely close the ends of a severed vessel.

White blood cells: See *leukocytes*.

Introduction

The blood is made up of cells, fragments of cells, and dissolved biochemicals containing nutrients, oxygen, hormones, and wastes. It helps to distribute body heat and maintain stable interstitial fluid. Blood is actually a connective tissue with its cells suspended in a liquid, extracellular matrix. It is heavier and thicker than water. Blood contains erythrocytes (red blood cells), platelets, and leukocytes (white blood cells). Red blood cells (RBCs), white blood cells (WBCs), and platelets are collectively called *formed elements*. The liquid portion of blood is called **plasma**. Blood volume represents about 7% of a person's body weight.

Plasma contains water, amino acids, carbohydrates, lipids, proteins, hormones, electrolytes, vitamins, and cellular wastes (see **Figure 7–1**). An average adult has approximately 4 to 6 L of blood.

Hematology

Hematology is the branch of medicine that is concerned with the study of blood and blood disorders. The blood transports oxygen, nutrients, cellular waste products, and hormones throughout the body. It is involved in heat distribution, protection against infection, and the regulation of acid–base balances. Hematology is a major component of the clinical laboratory. Phlebotomists must be familiar with the composition and normal values of the blood. They must also understand common blood diseases and conditions. This chapter will examine the structure and functions of the blood, which

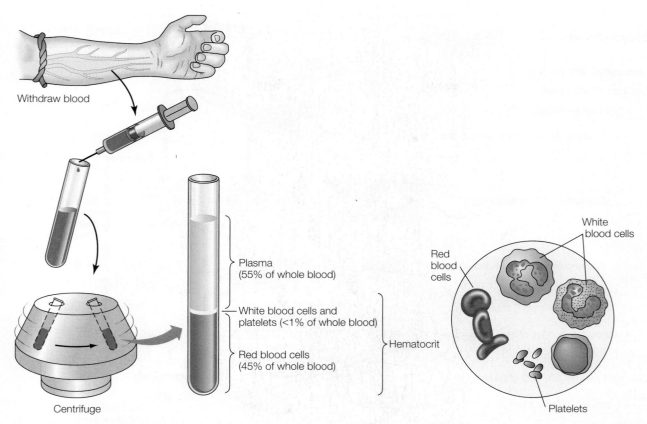

Figure 7–1 The composition of whole blood.

is a specialized fluid connective tissue containing cells suspended in a fluid matrix.

Red Blood Cells

Red blood cells (erythrocytes) have a biconcave shape, meaning that they are basically round, with a center that is depressed in comparison with their edges. They are approximately 7.5 micrometers (μm) in diameter and 2 μm thick at the rim. This shape helps them to transport gases by increasing the surface area of the cell, allowing greater diffusion (see **Figure 7–2**).

The shape of erythrocytes also ensures that the cell membrane is nearer to the **hemoglobin** (which carries oxygen) inside the cell. The cytoplasm of an RBC consists mainly of a 33% solution of hemoglobin. This is the red pigment that gives an RBC its color and name. Erythrocytes make up about 45% of blood volume—this portion is known as the **hematocrit** (HCT). When it binds with oxygen, *oxyhemoglobin* is formed. Oxyhemoglobin is bright red. When oxygen is released, *deoxyhemoglobin* is formed. Deoxyhemoglobin is darker red, and blood rich in deoxyhemoglobin may appear bluish when seen through blood vessels. The cytoplasm of erythrocytes contains an enzyme, *carbonic anhydrase* (CAH), that catalyzes the reaction of carbon dioxide (CO_2) plus water (H_2O) into hydrogen (H_2) and carbon trioxide (CO_3).

Erythrocytes have nuclei that are shed as they mature, allowing more room for hemoglobin. Lacking nuclei, mature RBCs cannot synthesize proteins or divide to form more cells. They produce ATP through glycolysis because they do not have mitochondria, and they use none of the oxygen carried in their hemoglobin.

A *red blood cell count* is the number of RBCs in a microliter of blood. Normal ranges of RBCs are as follows:

- Adult males: 4.6 million to 6.2 million cells per microliter
- Adult females: 4.2 million to 5.4 million cells per microliter

Increased numbers of circulating RBCs increase the blood's *oxygen-carrying capacity*, which can affect health. Red blood cell counts are taken to diagnose many diseases and evaluate their courses. However, the opposite is also true: decreased RBC counts lead to decreased oxygen-carrying capacity, which is more likely to be seen on a regular basis than increased counts.

In humans, RBCs are mostly developed in spaces within bones that are filled with red bone marrow (myeloid tissue). This process is called **erythropoiesis**. Erythrocytes usually live for 120 days, with replacement cells created to maintain a relatively stable RBC count. The rate of red blood cell formation is controlled by negative feedback via the hormone **erythropoietin**. It is released by the kidneys and liver in response to prolonged oxygen deficiency (see **Figure 7–3**).

Production of red blood cells (erythropoiesis) continues at a heightened rate until the amount of them in the blood

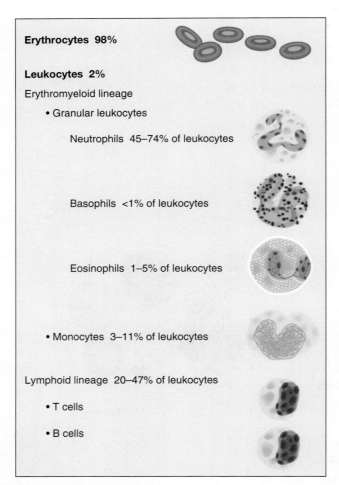

Erythrocytes 98%

Leukocytes 2%

Erythromyeloid lineage

- Granular leukocytes

  Neutrophils 45–74% of leukocytes

  Basophils <1% of leukocytes

  Eosinophils 1–5% of leukocytes

- Monocytes 3–11% of leukocytes

Lymphoid lineage 20–47% of leukocytes

- T cells

- B cells

Figure 7–2 Various blood cells.

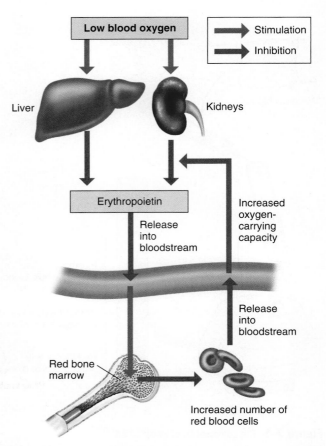

Figure 7–3 Erythropoietin is released by the kidneys and liver is response to prolonged oxygen deficiency.

Source: Adapted from Shier, D. N., Butler, J. L., and Lewis, R. *Hole's Essentials of Human Anatomy & Physiology*, Tenth edition. McGraw-Hill Higher Education, 2009.

circulation is enough to supply oxygen to the body tissues. The stages of formation of RBCs and other blood cells from hemocytoblasts are shown in **Figure 7–4**.

B-complex vitamins such as *vitamin B₁₂* and *folic acid* greatly influence RBC production and are necessary for DNA synthesis. Hematopoietic (blood-cell-forming) tissue is very vulnerable to deficiency of both of these vitamins. Iron is required for normal red blood cell production and for hemoglobin synthesis. Iron is slowly absorbed from the small intestine, and the body reuses much of the iron released by the decomposition of hemoglobin from damaged RBCs. Only small amounts of iron must be taken in via the diet.

Anemia has various causes, but sometimes it is caused by too little hemoglobin, or by too few RBCs. People with anemia may appear pale and lack energy because their blood is not able to carry enough oxygen. Iron-rich foods are important for the pregnant woman especially, in order to supply enough oxygen to her blood supply as well as to the blood supply of the developing fetus. However, not all anemia is due to iron deficiency. Because a pregnant woman's blood volume will increase due to fluid retention that supports the fetus, it decreases her hematocrit levels. *Hemochromatosis* is a condition that involves normal to increased RBCs. It is an iron handling disorder in which the small intestine absorbs

iron at 10 times the normal rate, building up to toxic levels. This is treated by periodic blood removal.

Red blood cells bend as they move through blood vessels, but aging causes them to become more fragile. Cells called **macrophages** phagocytize and destroy damaged red blood cells, mostly in the liver and spleen. Hemoglobin from RBCs is broken down into *heme*, which contains iron, and the protein *globin*. The heme then decomposes into iron and **biliverdin**, a green pigment. The blood may transport the iron to synthesize new hemoglobin. Most of the iron that is removed from degraded hemoglobin is recycled to the bone marrow. Biliverdin is converted into **bilirubin**, an orange pigment, and excreted along with biliverdin in the bile. The life cycle of RBCs is summarized in **Figure 7–5**.

White Blood Cells

Leukocytes, also known as **white blood cells**, protect the body against disease and develop from hemocytoblasts in the red bone marrow in response to hormones. These hormones are either **interleukins** or **colony-stimulating factors (CSFs)**. Interleukins are organized by number, while most of the CSFs are named for the type of cells they stimulate. White blood cells are transported to sites of infection and may then leave the bloodstream.

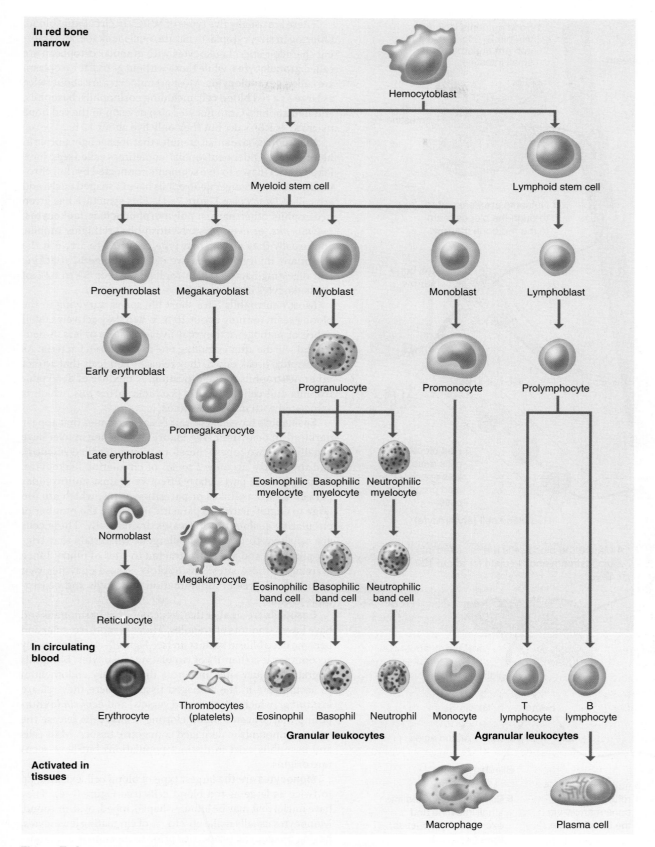

Figure 7–4 The stages of formation of the blood cells from hemocytoblasts.

Source: Adapted from Shier, D. N., Butler, J. L., and Lewis, R. Hole's *Essentials of Human Anatomy & Physiology,* Tenth edition. McGraw-Hill Higher Education, 2009.

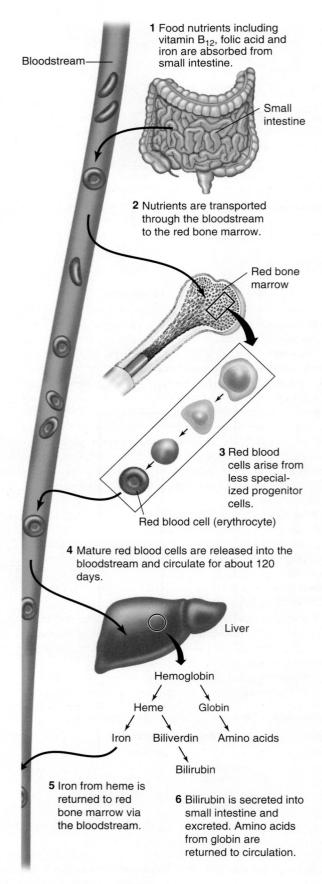

Bloodstream

1 Food nutrients including vitamin B$_{12}$, folic acid and iron are absorbed from small intestine.

Small intestine

2 Nutrients are transported through the bloodstream to the red bone marrow.

Red bone marrow

3 Red blood cells arise from less specialized progenitor cells.

Red blood cell (erythrocyte)

4 Mature red blood cells are released into the bloodstream and circulate for about 120 days.

Liver

Hemoglobin

Heme   Globin

Iron   Biliverdin   Amino acids

Bilirubin

5 Iron from heme is returned to red bone marrow via the bloodstream.

6 Bilirubin is secreted into small intestine and excreted. Amino acids from globin are returned to circulation.

Figure 7–5 The life cycle of RBCs.

There are usually five types of WBCs in circulating blood, differing in size, cytoplasm nature, nucleus shape, and staining characteristics. Leukocytes with granular cytoplasm are called **granulocytes**, while those without granular cytoplasm are called **agranulocytes**. Most granulocytes are about twice as large as a red blood cell, including eosinophils, basophils, and neutrophils. Granulocytes also develop in the red bone marrow, as RBCs do, but they only live about 12 h.

Neutrophils have small granules that appear light purple in neutral stain. Older neutrophils (sometimes called *segs*) have lobed nuclei in two to five segments connected by thin chromatin strands. Younger neutrophils have C-shaped nuclei and are called *bands* (see Figure 7–4). This structure has given neutrophils other names: **polymorphonuclear leukocytes**, *polymorphs*, or even *polys*. Neutrophils are highly mobile, and usually they are the first type of WBCs to arrive at the site of any injury. These active cells specialize in attacking and digesting bacteria. Neutrophils make up 54 to 62% of the leukocytes in most adults.

Most neutrophils have short life spans, surviving in the bloodstream for only about 10 h. When they actively engulf debris or pathogens, they may live for 30 min or less. A neutrophil will die after engulfing one to two dozen bacteria. As neutrophils break down, they release chemicals that attract other neutrophils to their location. A mixture of dead neutrophils and cellular debris products forms *pus*, which is associated with infected wounds.

Eosinophils have coarse, same-sized granules that appear dark red in acid stain (see Figure 7–4). Their nuclei have usually just two lobes (therefore, they are called *bilobed*), and they make up only 2 to 4% of circulating leukocytes. Eosinophils are particularly effective against multicellular parasites such as flukes or parasitic worms, which are too large to engulf. During a parasitic infection, the number of circulating eosinophils increases dramatically. These cells are sensitive to circulating allergens (materials that trigger allergies) and are also attracted to sites of injury. Once arriving at these sites, eosinophils release enzymes that reduce the degree of inflammation **mast cells** and neutrophils produce.

Basophils are smaller than neutrophils or eosinophils and have lower amounts of granules. They are more irregular and become deep blue in basic stain (see Figure 7–4). They usually account for less than 1% of circulating leukocytes. Basophils migrate to injury sites and cross the capillary endothelium to accumulate in the damaged tissues, where they release *histamine* (which dilates blood vessels) and *heparin* (a compound that prevents blood clotting). Mast cells release the same compounds in damaged connective tissues. Mast cells and basophils exist in distinct populations but have separate origins.

Monocytes are the largest type of blood cell, exisiting up to twice as large as red blood cells (see Figure 7–4). They have nuclei that may be kidney-shaped, lobed, oval, or round. Monocytes usually make up 2 to 8% of circulating leukocytes, having phagocytic properties prior to movement to the tissues. An individual monocyte is transported through the bloodstream, remaining in circulation for only about 24 h before entering peripheral tissues. Here, a monocyte becomes a tissue macrophage. Macrophages are aggressive phagocytes that often attempt to engulf items as large as (or larger than) themselves. When phagocytically active, they release chemicals that attract and stimulate neutrophils, monocytes, and other phagocytic cells.

Lymphocytes are usually only a little larger than RBCs, with large, round nuclei inside a thin cytoplasm rim (see Figure 7–4). Lymphocytes make up between 20 and 30% of circulating leukocytes. Lymphocytes continuously migrate from the bloodstream into the peripheral tissues and back into the bloodstream. Circulating lymphocytes constitute only a small fraction of all lymphocytes, and the majority of lymphocytes are in other connective tissues in lymphatic organs. Lymphocytes are vital for immunity. Some of them produce antibodies that attack certain foreign substances.

Circulating blood contains three functional classes of lymphocytes, which cannot be distinguished with a light microscope, as follows:

1. **T cells** are responsible for *cell-mediated immunity*, which is a specific defense mechanism that combats invading foreign cells and tissues. T cells either enter peripheral tissues and attack foreign cells directly or control the activities of other lymphocytes.

2. **B cells** are responsible for *humoral immunity*, which is a specific defense mechanism that involves the production and distribution of antibodies. These antibodies attack foreign antigens throughout the body. Activated B cells differentiate into **plasma cells**, which are specialized to form and secrete antibodies.

3. **Natural killer (NK) cells** are responsible for *immune surveillance*, which involves the detection and subsequent destruction of abnormal tissue cells. NK cells (sometimes known as large granular lymphocytes) are important in preventing cancer.

Normally, there are 4,500 to 10,000 white blood cells in a microliter of human blood. This is called a *white blood cell count* (*WBC count*). White blood cell counts are of interest to determine the clinical conditions of patients. If the WBC count is higher than normal, there may be an infection. If WBCs exceed 10,000 per cubic millimeter (mm^3) (microliter, or μL), the condition is called **leukocytosis**, which may indicate an acute infection. It is important to note that microliters are now being used more than cubic millimeters for this type of measurement, with 1 μL equivalent to 1 mm^3. Also, normal ranges of WBC counts vary slightly from hospital to hospital. Conditions such as leukemia may also be noted as a result of WBC counts.

Appendicitis is an example of an acute infection that an elevated WBC may signify. When the WBC count is greatly elevated, leukemia may exist. **Leukopenia** is defined as a total WBC count below 5,000 per cubic millimeter (microliter). It may be more associated with immune suppression or chemotherapy-related diseases. Leukopenia is associated with diseases such as influenza, measles, mumps, chicken pox, AIDS, poliomyelitis, and typhoid fever.

Percentages of the types of leukocytes in a blood sample are listed in a *differential white blood cell count* (*diff*), which is useful to determine the type of condition that exists with greater accuracy. Bacterial infections usually cause neutrophil counts to increase, while certain parasitic infections cause the number of eosinophils to increase. AIDS causes certain types of lymphocyte counts to drop sharply.

Platelets

Platelets are also known as **thrombocytes**. They are cytoplasm fragments arising from red bone marrow cells (called **megakaryocytes**). Megakaryocytes develop from hemocytoblasts (megakaryoblasts) because of the hormone **thrombopoietin**. Platelets lack nuclei and are not even one-half the size of RBCs. They live for about 10 days and are capable of amoeboid movement. Usually, platelet counts range from 130,000 to 400,000 per microliter. The function of platelets is primarily to block injuries to damaged blood vessels and to start forming blood clots. Therefore, the main event of the platelet phase is the formation of the platelet plug. **Table 7–1** lists the characteristics of RBCs, WBCs, and platelets.

Plasma

Plasma suspends the cells and platelets of the blood. It is a clear, straw-colored liquid made up of 92% water, with organic and inorganic biochemicals. Plasma is close to the same density as water. Plasma makes up 46 to 63% of the volume of whole blood. It helps to transport gases, nutrients, and vitamins while helping to regulate fluid and electrolyte balance as well as pH levels. **Plasma proteins** are the most abundant of the solutes (dissolved substances) in the plasma. They are not usually used as energy sources, remaining in the blood and interstitial fluids. Three primary classes of plasma proteins exist: albumins, globulins, and fibrinogen. These three classes make up more than 99% of the plasma proteins. The remainder consists of circulating enzymes, hormones, and prohormones.

Albumins are the smallest of the plasma proteins, but they make up around 60% of these proteins by weight. They are made in the liver and play an important role in the plasma's *osmotic pressure*. Because plasma proteins are too large to move through capillary walls, they create an osmotic pressure to hold water in the capillaries (known as *colloid osmotic pressure*). This helps regulate water movement between blood and tissues, to aid in controlling blood volume and blood pressure. Albumins are also important in the transport of fatty acids, thyroid hormones, some steroid hormones, and other substances.

Globulins (including *alpha*, *beta*, and *gamma globulins*) make up around 35% of the plasma proteins. Important plasma globulins include antibodies and transport globulins. Antibodies, also called immunoglobulins, attack foreign proteins and pathogens. *Transport globulins* bind small ions and hormones. Alpha and beta globulins are made by the liver to transport lipids and fat-soluble vitamins. Gamma globulins are made by the lymphatic tissues and are a type of antibody. **Fibrinogen** (making up around 4% of the plasma proteins) is important for blood coagulation. It is made in the liver and is the largest (in size) of the plasma proteins. **Table 7–2** summarizes albumin, globulin, and fibrinogen.

Oxygen and carbon dioxide are the most important *blood gases*, with nitrogen also contained in the plasma. *Plasma nutrients* include amino acids, nucleotides, lipids, and simple sugars absorbed from the digestive tract. Glucose is

Table 7-1 Characteristics of Blood Cells and Platelets

Type	Function	Amount	Description
Red blood cells (erythrocytes)	Transport carbon dioxide and oxygen	4.2 million to 6.2 million per microliter	Biconcave discs with no nucleus, about one-third hemoglobin
White blood cells (leukocytes)	Destroy parasites and pathogens and remove worn cells	5,000 to 10,000 per microliter	
Granulocytes			*About twice the size of RBCs, with cytoplasmic granules*
1. Neutrophils	Phagocytize small particles	54 to 62% of WBCs	Nuclei have 2–5 lobes, granules stain light purple
2. Eosinophils	Help control allergic reactions and inflammation and kill parasites	1 to 3% of WBCs	Bilobed nuclei, granules stain dark red
3. Basophils	Release histamine and heparin	Less than 1% of WBCs	Bilobed nuclei, granules stain blue
Agranulocytes			*No cytoplasmic granules*
1. Monocytes	Phagocytize large particles	3 to 9% of WBCs	2–3 times larger than RBCs, varied nuclei shape
2. Lymphocytes	Provide immunity	25 to 33% of WBCs	Only slightly larger than RBCs, with very large nuclei
Platelets (thrombocytes)	Help control blood loss from broken vessels and begin clotting process	130,000 to 360,000 per microliter	Cytoplasmic fragments

transported in the plasma from the small intestine to the liver.

In the liver, glucose is stored as glycogen or converted to fat. The concentration of glucose in the blood is represented in milligrams per deciliter (mg/dL). When the blood concentration of glucose drops, *hypoglycemia* (a potentially dangerous condition) occurs. When glucose is elevated, it is called *hyperglycemia*, which can lead to diabetes (see **Table 7–3**). Plasma carries amino acids to the liver to manufacture proteins or to be used for energy. Plasma lipids include triglycerides, cholesterol, and phospholipids. Lipids are not water-soluble, but plasma is mostly made of water. Hence, lipids join with proteins to form lipoproteins, which the plasma can carry.

Nonprotein nitrogenous substances have nitrogen atoms, but are not proteins. In the plasma, these include amino acids, urea, and uric acid. Blood plasma also contains many *electrolytes*, which include potassium, calcium, sodium, magnesium, chloride, phosphate, bicarbonate, and sulfate ions. The most abundant types are sodium and chloride ions. All plasma constituents are regulated so that their blood concentrations remain mostly stable. **Figure 7–6** summarizes blood composition.

Hemostasis

The stoppage of bleeding is known as **hemostasis**. When blood vessels are damaged, this vital process helps to limit or prevent blood loss. Hemostasis consists of three phases: *vascular phase*, *platelet phase*, and *coagulation phase*. When a smaller blood vessel is cut or broken, smooth muscles in its walls contract (**vasospasm**), and loss of blood slows nearly

Table 7-2 The Plasma Proteins

Protein	Origin	Percentage of Total	Function
Albumins	Liver	60	Help maintain colloid osmotic pressure
Globulins Alpha	Liver	36	Transport lipids and fat-soluble vitamins
¶Beta	Liver		Transport lipids and fat-soluble vitamins
Gamma	Lymphatic tissues		Constitute a type of antibody
Fibrinogen	Liver	4	Plays key role in blood coagulation

Table 7-3 Blood Glucose Levels

Level	Description	Resulting Conditions
Less than 70 mg/dL	Hypoglycemia	Can be potentially fatal; symptoms include lethargy, impaired mental functioning, irritability, and loss of consciousness
Between 70 and 110 mg/dL	Normal	Levels usually lower in the morning and rise after meals
Between 110 and 125 mg/dL	Borderline hyperglycemia	Does not result in diabetes mellitus
126 mg/dL or greater	Hyperglycemia	If persistent, can result in diabetes mellitus, which can cause eye, kidney, and nerve damage

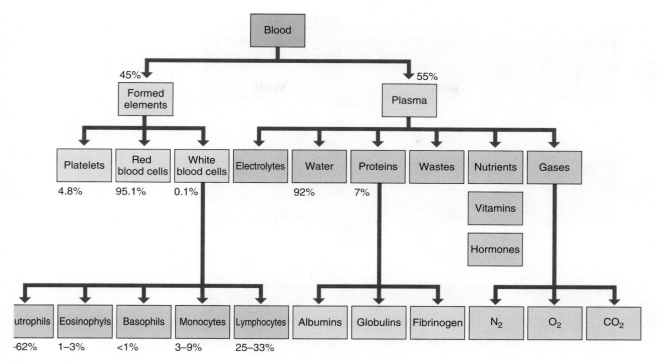

Figure 7–6 Blood composition.

immediately. A vasospasm has the potential to completely close the ends of a severed vessel.

The effects of vasospasm may last for a few minutes up to about 30 min. At that time, a *platelet plug* has formed, and blood begins coagulating. Platelets release **serotonin** to contract smooth muscles in blood vessels, reducing blood loss. Platelets stick to rough surfaces and connective tissue collagen under the endothelial blood vessel lining. They also stick to one another to form a platelet plug in the area of the blood vessel injury. Larger breaks may require a blood clot to stop bleeding (see **Figure 7–7**).

The formation of a *blood clot* is known as **coagulation**. It requires many biochemicals known as *clotting factors*. Some clotting factors promote coagulation while others inhibit it, so a delicate balance between these two types is achieved to address the specific injured tissue. The most important event in coagulation is the conversion of the plasma protein fibrinogen to the insoluble threads of the protein called **fibrin**. The first step is the release of *tissue thromboplastin*, which results in the production of *prothrombin activator*. **Figure 7–8** describes the blood-clotting system. There are two pathways to the activation of the clotting system.

Prothrombin is an alpha globulin made in the liver on a continual basis, and it is always present in the blood plasma. Prothrombin activator converts prothrombin to **thrombin**, which causes fibrinogen to be cut into sections of fibrin. This fibrin then joins to form long threads. The threads stick to the surfaces of damaged blood vessels to create a mesh that traps blood cells and platelets. The result is a blood clot. After the formation of the clot, serum remains.

Serum

Serum is the clear, yellow liquid that remains after a clot forms. It is plasma minus some, but not all, of the clotting factors. Because blood is approximately one-half cells and one-half liquid, any test requiring 1 mL of serum would require 2 mL of blood to be collected.

Following the addition of *clot activator* to most vacuum tubes, serum for testing needs to clot for only 15 to 20 min before it is centrifuged. Plasma fibrinogen traps red blood cells to form a fibrin network. Immunological and chemistry tests are performed on serum. A variety of tests can now be performed on either serum or plasma.

Plasma

Plasma is the fluid portion of blood that remains after all blood cells have been removed. It consists of water and dissolved proteins, amino acids, glucose, fats, fatty acids, electrolytes, gases, and metabolic wastes. It is composed of about 90% water, 9% protein, and other chemical substances that total about 1%. Plasma comprises the liquid portion of whole blood that contains active clotting agents. Plasma is used for "stat" chemistry testing and coagulation studies.

A whole blood specimen is centrifuged to separate the various blood components. Red blood cells will settle in the bottom of the tube, with the white blood cells and platelets forming a thin, white "buffy coat" and the plasma remaining above it. At this point, the plasma contains all of the dissolved components of the blood, including the coagulation factors. Plasma specimens contain an anticoagulant, natural heparin, to prevent clotting.

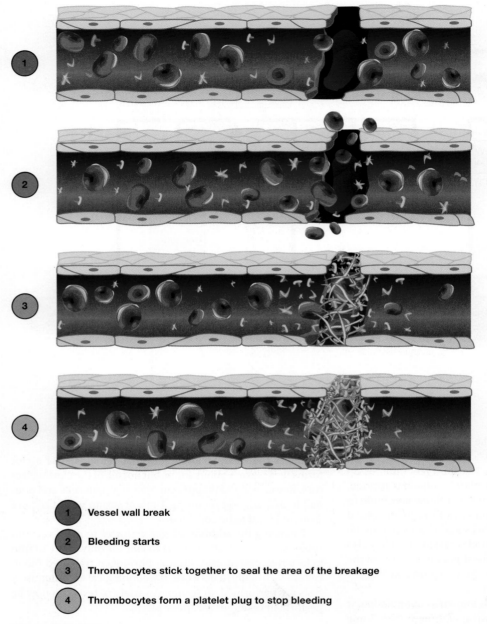

1 Vessel wall break

2 Bleeding starts

3 Thrombocytes stick together to seal the area of the breakage

4 Thrombocytes form a platelet plug to stop bleeding

Figure 7–7 Platelet plug.

Appearance of Serum and Plasma

Blood serum appears as a yellow or straw-colored fluid. It is seen after blood has been allowed to clot, and it does not contain fibrinogen, which is found in the clotted portion of the blood. Blood plasma is the pale yellowish liquid part of whole blood. It contains coagulation factors that help form clots to stop bleeding.

Blood Clotting

More prothrombin activator becomes present if tissue damage is more severe. Continual clotting occurs to stop greater damage. Positive feedback is used to stimulate more clotting action based on the original clotting action. However, this continual process can work only for a short time because it interrupts the stability of the body's internal environment. Excess thrombin is normally carried away to avoid the formation of a massive blood clot. As a result, blood coagulation usually occurs in blood that is not moving or that is only moving slowly. Clotting stops because excess thrombin is absorbed on the clot.

Blood clots in ruptured vessels are invaded by *fibroblasts* to produce fibrous connective tissue that helps seal blood vessel breaks. Clots that form in tissues as a result of blood leakage (*hematomas*) disappear over time. This process requires the plasma protein *plasminogen* to be converted to *plasmin*, an enzyme that digests threads of fibrin and other proteins involved in clotting. While plasmin may dissolve entire clots,

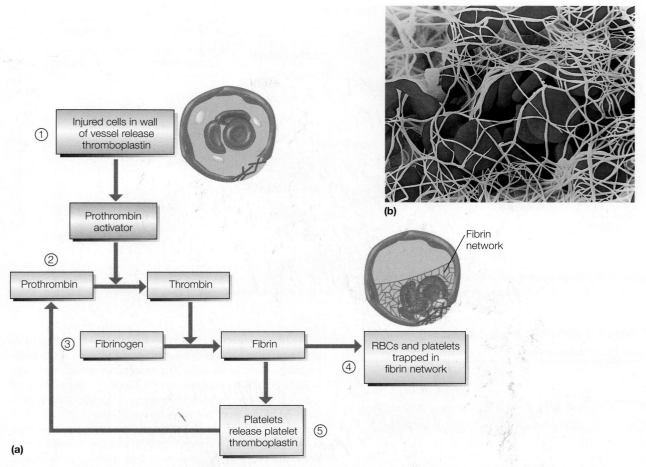

Figure 7–8 Blood Clotting Simplified. (a) Injured cells in the walls of blood vessels release the chemical thromboplastin (1). Thromboplastin stimulates the conversion of prothrombin, found in the plasma, into thrombin (2). Thrombin, in turn, stimulates the conversion of the plasma protein fibrinogen into fibrin (3). The fibrin network captures RBCs and platelets (4). Platelets in the blood clot release platelet thromboplastin (5), which converts additional plasma prothrombin into thrombin. Thrombin, in turn, stimulates the production of additional fibrin. (b) A scanning electron micrograph of a fibrin clot that has already trapped platelets and RBCs, plugging a leak in a vessel. The RBCs are red, and the fibrin network is turquoise.

those that fill large blood vessels are usually not removed naturally.

A **thrombus** is a clot that forms abnormally in a vessel. An **embolus** is a clot that dislodges or fragments to be carried away in the blood flow. Emboli usually move until they reach narrow vessels, which they may block. When a blood clot forms in a vital organ's vessels, it kills the tissues served (*infarction*) by the vessel, a potentially fatal occurrence. If this occurs in the heart, it is known as *coronary thrombosis*. If it occurs in the brain, it is known as *cerebral thrombosis*.

Pulmonary embolism describes a clot blocking a vessel supplying the lungs. In *atherosclerosis*, the endothelial linings of blood vessels change due to fatty deposits that accumulate.

Blood Types and Transfusions

Blood consists of different types, not all of which are compatible. Safe blood transfusions of whole blood depend on matching the blood types of both donors and recipients. The clumping of red blood cells following a transfusion reaction is called **agglutination**. This involves red blood cell surface molecules called **antigens** (*agglutinogens*) that react with **antibodies** (*agglutinins*) from the plasma. There are more than 260 antigens on RBC membranes. A few of them can produce serious transfusion reactions, including antigens of the ABO group and those of the Rh group.

The *ABO blood group* is based on the presence or lack of two major protein antigens (antigen A and antigen B) on RBC membranes. Erythrocytes may have one of the following four antigen combinations:

- Antigen A only—*type A blood*
- Antigen B only—*type B blood*
- Both antigen A and B—*type AB blood* (the least common type)
- Neither antigen A nor antigen B—*type O blood* (the most common type)

Blood types are inherited. Antibodies related to each type of antigen are produced between 2 and 8 months after birth. For example, if antigen A is absent, the antibody called *anti-A* is produced. Therefore, people with type A blood (meaning that antigen A is present but antigen B is absent) have *anti-B*

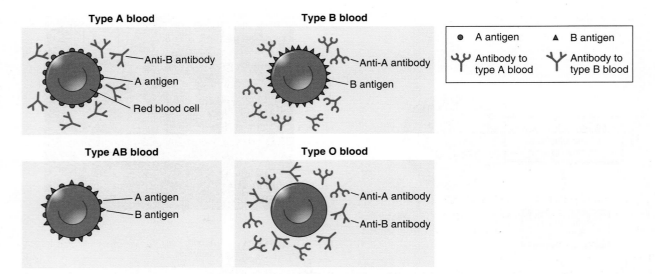

Figure 7–9 Various antigens and antibodies distinguish blood types.

Source: Adapted from Shier, D. N., Butler, J. L., and Lewis, R. Hole's *Essentials of Human Anatomy & Physiology*, Tenth edition. McGraw-Hill Higher Education, 2009.

Table 7–4 ABO Blood Group Antigens and Antibodies

Blood Type	Antigen Present	Antibody Present
A	A	Anti-B
B	B	Anti-A
AB	Both A and B	Neither anti-A nor anti-B
O	Neither A nor B	Both anti-A and anti-B

antibody. The opposite is true for people with type B blood. Those with type AB blood have neither of the two antibodies. People with type O blood have both antibodies (see **Figure 7–9**). Anti-A and anti-B antibodies in blood group O individuals are often IgG class antibodies and *may* cross the placenta, but usually do not. When they do not cross the placenta, a pregnant woman and her fetus may have different blood types, and agglutination in the fetal cells cannot occur. However, when these antibodies do cross the placenta, the result is a mild *hemolytic disease of the newborn (HDN)* because the A- and B-antigens are not fully expressed at birth. **Table 7–4** summarizes blood types, antigens, and antibodies.

Antibodies of a certain type will react with antigens of the same type and cause clumping of RBCs, so these combinations must be avoided. For example, a person with type A (anti-B) blood must not receive blood of either type B or type AB in order to avoid clumping. A person with type B (anti-A) blood must not receive type A or type AB blood. A person with type O (anti-A and anti-B) must not receive type A, B, or AB blood. Because type AB blood lacks both anti-A and anti-B antibodies, those with type AB blood can receive transfusions from any other type. Because of this, type AB individuals are called *universal recipients*. Rapid transfusion must be avoided, however, because agglutination can still occur as a result of certain antibodies in the blood being transfused. It is therefore always best to transfer blood from the same type as the person requiring the transfusion (see **Table 7–5**). Note that the permissible donor types listed in this table should be used only in extreme emergencies. **Figure 7–10** illustrates the concept of agglutination.

Because type O blood lacks antigens A and B, it can be transfused, in extreme emergencies, into people with any other type. Because of this, people with type O blood are

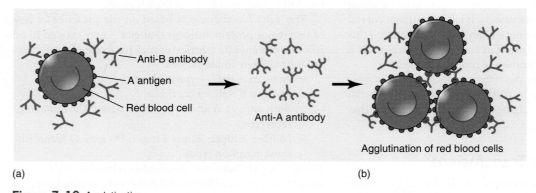

(a)

(b)

Figure 7–10 Agglutination.

Source: Adapted from Shier, D. N., Butler, J. L., and Lewis, R. Hole's *Essentials of Human Anatomy & Physiology*, Tenth edition. McGraw-Hill Higher Education, 2009.

Table 7–5 Blood Transfusion Rules

Recipient's Blood Type	Preferred Donor Type	Permissible Donor Type
A	A	O
B	B	O
AB	AB	A, B, and O
O	O	No alternate types

called *universal donors*. Type O blood still should be given to people of other blood types slowly so that it will be diluted by the recipient's blood volume. This will minimize chances of an adverse reaction.

The *Rh blood group* received its name from the rhesus monkey because it was in this type of monkey that it was first studied. There are several Rh antigens (factors) in humans, the most prevalent of which is *antigen D*. If it is present on the RBC membranes, the blood is called *Rh-positive*. If not, it is called *Rh-negative*. Only 15% of the U.S. population is Rh-negative. The presence or absence of Rh antigen is inherited, but the antibodies that react with it (called *Rh antibodies*) are not spontaneous. They form only in Rh-negative people because of specific stimulation.

An Rh-negative person receiving Rh-positive blood will begin producing anti-Rh antibodies (see **Figure 7–11**). The first transfusion usually causes no serious problems. But after that, the Rh-negative person has become sensitized to Rh-positive blood. A second transfusion, even months later, will usually cause the donated RBCs to agglutinate.

A similar condition can occur when an Rh-negative female is pregnant with an Rh-positive fetus. Although the pregnancy may be normal, at birth (or miscarriage) the placental membranes tear, allowing some of the fetus's Rh-positive RBCs to enter the mother's circulation. This may stimulate her tissues to begin producing anti-Rh antibodies. If she becomes pregnant a second time and the fetus is Rh-positive, these antibodies (*hemolysins*) cross the placental membrane to destroy the fetal RBCs. The fetus develops hemolytic disease of the fetus and newborn, formerly referred to as *erythroblastosis fetalis*. While extremely rare due to the careful management of Rh status, this condition may cause the death of the fetus or infant. Anemia, an enlarged liver or spleen, generalized swelling, and newborn jaundice are signs of this condition.

Summary

Blood is a type of connective tissue. It consists of red blood cells, white blood cells, and platelets suspended in a liquid, plasma, extracellular matrix. Blood transports substances between body cells and the external environment. It helps to maintain a stable internal environment. Blood is separated into formed elements and liquid portions. Red blood cells carry oxygen to the body tissues. White blood cells are important in protecting the body against pathogens and infection. Platelets are vital for blood coagulation.

Blood plasma transports gases and nutrients, helps maintain stable pH, and helps regulate the fluid and electrolyte balance. Hemostasis is the stoppage of bleeding. It involves the steps of blood vessel spasm, platelet plug formation, and blood coagulation. Blood can be typed on the basis of cell surface antigens. The ABO blood group concerns the presence or absence of antigens A and B. The Rh blood group concerns the Rh antigen, which is present on the red blood cell membranes of Rh-positive blood but is not present in Rh-negative blood.

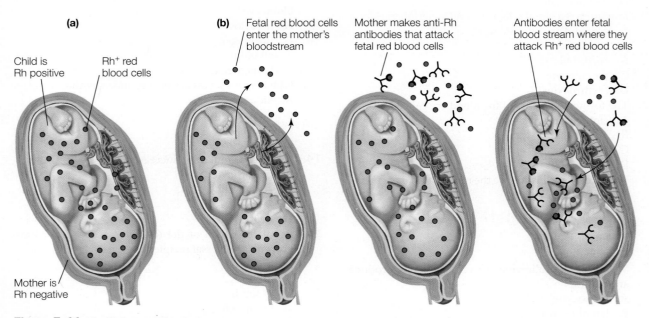

(a) Child is Rh positive — Rh⁺ red blood cells — Mother is Rh negative

(b) Fetal red blood cells enter the mother's bloodstream

Mother makes anti-Rh antibodies that attack fetal red blood cells

Antibodies enter fetal blood stream where they attack Rh⁺ red blood cells

Figure 7–11 The Rh factor and pregnancy.

CRITICAL THINKING

An instructor was conducting an oral examination, and he asked a phlebotomist the following questions. How would you respond to each of these?

1. Why is venipuncture a common technique for obtaining a blood sample?
2. How would the hematocrit change after an individual suffered a significant blood loss?
3. How do basophils respond during inflammation?
4. Which blood type or types can be transfused into a person with type O blood?

WEBSITES

http://surgery.about.com/od/beforesurgery/qt /PTPTTINRtests.htm

http://www.hematology.org/

http://www.mhhe.com/biosci/esp/2002_general/Esp/folder _structure/tr/m1/s7/trm1s7_3.htm

http://www.nhlbi.nih.gov/health/dci/Diseases/bt/bt _whatis.html

http://www.purchon.com/biology/plasma.htm

http://www.redcrossblood.org/learn-about-blood/blood-types

http://www.unomaha.edu/hpa/blood.html

REVIEW QUESTIONS

Multiple Choice

1. Which of the following terms means "the process of red blood cell production"?
   A. erythropoiesis
   B. erythrocytosis
   C. erythropenia
   D. hemocytosis

2. *Immature* red blood cells are found in peripheral blood samples and are referred to as
   A. myeloblasts
   B. erythroblasts
   C. reticulocytes
   D. erythrocytes

3. The formed elements of the blood are called
   A. clotting proteins
   B. lipoproteins
   C. albumins
   D. blood cells

4. Which of the following are the most abundant proteins in blood plasma?
   A. fibrinogens
   B. albumins
   C. lipoproteins
   D. globulins

5. Which of the following white blood cells produce antibodies?
   A. monocytes
   B. lymphocytes
   C. eosinophils
   D. basophils

6. Platelets are formed from cells in the bone marrow known as
   A. megakaryocytes
   B. erythroblasts
   C. lymphoblasts
   D. myeloblasts

7. Which of the following vitamins is needed for the formation of clotting factors?
   A. vitamin A
   B. vitamin D
   C. vitamin K
   D. vitamin E

8. Thrombocytes are
   A. small cells that lack a nucleus
   B. small cells with many-lobed nuclei
   C. fragments of large megakaryocytes
   D. large cells with prominent nuclei

9. Which of the following white blood cells release histamine and heparin?
   A. basophils
   B. monocytes
   C. neutrophils
   D. eosinophils

10. Erythrocytes are formed in
    A. the spleen
    B. red bone marrow
    C. yellow bone marrow
    D. the liver

11. Which of the following hormones regulates production of red blood cells?
    A. erythropoietin
    B. thymosin
    C. epinephrine
    D. somatotropin

12. Which of the following is the major protein in a red blood cell?
    A. myoglobin
    B. fibrinogen
    C. albumin
    D. hemoglobin

13. Older erythrocytes are broken down by the
    A. kidneys
    B. lungs
    C. spleen
    D. pancreas

14. Allergies stimulate an increased _____ count.
    A. erythrocyte
    B. eosinophil
    C. monocyte
    D. neutrophil

15. People of which of the following blood groups are known as universal recipients?
    A. group O
    B. group A
    C. group B
    D. group AB

Clinical Chemistry and Serology Tests

OUTLINE

Introduction
Specimen Requirements
Chemistry Panels or Profiles
    Hepatic Profile
    Renal Profile
    Lipid Profile
    Cardiac Profile
    Thyroid Profile
Glucose Testing
Serology and Immunology Tests
    Rapid Tests
    Common Serology Tests
Drug Testing
Summary
Critical Thinking
Websites
Review Questions

OBJECTIVES

After studying this chapter, readers should be able to:

1. Define *whole blood*.
2. Describe chemistry panels.
3. Describe a hepatic profile, renal profile, and lipid profile.
4. Discuss the common hepatic profile tests.
5. Compare and describe blood urea nitrogen and creatinine.
6. List the two important enzymes that are increased during myocardial infarction.
7. List five common serology tests.
8. List the conditions that a thyroid profile may reveal.
9. Explain what rapid tests are used to determine.
10. What is the anticoagulant of choice for hematology testing?

KEY TERMS

Alanine aminotransferase (ALT): An enzyme normally present in serum and tissues of the body, especially the tissue of the liver; it is released into the serum as a result of tissue injury and increases in persons with acute liver damage.

Albumin (Alb): A water-soluble protein; determination of the levels and types of albumin in urine, blood, and other body tissues is the basis of a number of diagnostic laboratory tests.

Alkaline phosphatase (ALP): An enzyme present in all tissues and in high concentrations in bones, kidneys, intestines, and plasma; it may be elevated in the serum in some diseases of the liver and bones and because of other illnesses.

Aspartate aminotransferase (AST): An enzyme normally present in body serum and in certain body tissues, especially those of the liver and heart.

Blood profile: A complete blood count (CBC).

Blood urea nitrogen: The result of the breakdown of proteins in the body; a blood urea nitrogen (BUN) test is commonly used to measure kidney function.

Creatinine: A breakdown product of creatine phosphate in muscle; creatinine blood levels rise when kidney function is deficient.

Erythrocyte sedimentation rate (ESR): The speed at which red blood cells sediment in a period of 1 h; it is a common hematology test for inflammation.

Graves' disease: An autoimmune disease involving an overactive thyroid, causing hyperthyroidism.

Hypothyroidism: Underactive thyroid; a condition where the thyroid gland lacks adequate amounts of thyroid hormones.

Infantile cretinism: Severely stunted physical and mental growth; untreated congenital deficiency of thyroid hormones due to a maternal nutritional deficiency of iodine.

Lipoproteins: Biochemicals that contain both lipids and proteins; they function to transport fats such as cholesterol throughout the body via the bloodstream.

KEY TERMS CONTINUED

Multiple myeloma: A malignant neoplasm of the bone marrow that is composed of plasma cells and disrupts normal bone marrow functions; it causes abnormal proteins in the plasma and urine as well as anemia, weight loss, and kidney failure.

Syphilis: A sexually transmitted infection caused by the spirochete *Treponema pallidum* and characterized by distinct stages of effects over a period of years.

Systemic lupus erythematosus: A chronic inflammatory disease affecting many body systems; it is an example of a collagen disease.

Treponemal antigen test: Any of various tests detecting specific antitreponemal antibodies in serum in the diagnosis of the *Treponema pallidum* infection of syphilis.

Tularemia: An infectious disease of animals, caused by the bacillus *Francisella tularensis*, that may be transmitted by insect vectors or direct contact.

Introduction

A laboratory examination of blood provides valuable information about many disease processes and body systems. Blood examination is the most common type of diagnostic testing. Results are often obtained quickly. Interventions often occur based upon the findings of blood examinations. The procedures discussed in this chapter correspond to those set forth by the Clinical and Laboratory Standards Institute (CLSI).

Specimen Requirements

Capillary punctures are used for most hematology tests because they require only small amounts of blood. For larger samples, venipuncture is used to collect blood from the veins. For example, a complete blood cell count utilizes venous blood collected into a tube containing an anticoagulant that prevents clotting. The anticoagulant of choice for hematology testing is ethylenediaminetetraacetic acid (EDTA). It is important in this regard that blood not be hemolyzed.

For whole blood testing, an anticoagulant is mixed with the whole blood for a minimum of 2 min, and testing must often occur within 1 h of the blood's being collected. However, whole blood testing is usually good for specimens up to 24 h old. For serology tests, serum should be obtained.

Chemistry Panels or Profiles

Automated blood chemistry analyzers are commonly used to perform blood chemistry testing. When physicians order a **blood profile** (chemistry panel), it means a group of tests that may be performed to help diagnose a pathologic condition. Blood panels include hepatic, renal, lipid, cardiac, and thyroid profiles. **Figure 8–1** shows a panel request form.

Hepatic Profile

Hepatic profile tests include those that test for **alanine aminotransferase (ALT)**, **alkaline phosphatase (ALP)**, **aspartate aminotransferase (AST)**, bilirubin (BILI), **albumin (Alb)**, gamma glutamyl transferase (GGT), total protein (TP), and albumin/globulin ratio (A/G ratio). Each individual test has its own reference ranges that are established by the testing laboratory.

When liver function levels are increased, the test indicates liver disease or damage (such as hepatitis, cirrhosis, gallstones, tumors, inflammation, mononucleosis, obstructive jaundice, and pancreatitis) or genetic defects preventing normal liver function. For example, when newborns have increased bilirubin levels, they may develop jaundice, mental retardation, blindness, and physical abnormalities. When liver function levels are decreased, the hepatic profile may indicate **hypothyroidism**, malnutrition, chronic nephritis, uncontrolled diabetes mellitus, autoimmune diseases, or **multiple myeloma**.

Renal Profile

A renal profile is a diagnostic test designed to collect information about kidney function. It may be performed as part of a full blood panel. In the test, blood levels of **creatinine**, calcium, sodium, chloride, carbon dioxide, albumin, **blood urea nitrogen**, protein, phosphorus, glucose, and potassium are examined. A renal profile may commonly follow a urinalysis after symptoms of a condition are not related to bladder function. Renal profiles are most often utilized for the diagnosis and monitoring of conditions such as gout, kidney failure, and other types of kidney disease and after transplantation surgery.

Lipid Profile

Lipids are fatty substances made up of cholesterol, triglycerides, fatty acids, and phospholipids. **Lipoproteins** are unique plasma proteins that transport otherwise insoluble lipids. Lipids provide energy for metabolism. They are precursors of the steroid hormones (adrenals, ovaries, and testes) and bile acids. Lipids play a part in cell membrane development.

A lipid profile measures three different types of lipids: low-density lipoprotein (LDL), high-density lipoprotein (HDL), and triglycerides. HDL is able to transport cholesterol and remove it from the body via the feces. The lipid profile also measures total cholesterol, or the total of all the types of cholesterol in the blood. High levels of total cholesterol, LDL, and triglycerides as well as low levels of HDL increase the risk of coronary heart disease or atherosclerosis. For lipid profile testing, the client must fast for 12 h prior. During fasting, the patient is allowed to drink only water. The client must avoid alcohol for 24 h and avoid strenuous exercise for 12 to 14 h before the test. The phlebotomist should obtain a 5-mL blood sample. A lipid profile test may reveal hyperlipidemia, which causes atherosclerosis, hypertension, angina pectoris, and even heart attack.

LABORATORY ORDER FORM

Notification to Physicians and Other Persons Legally Authorized to Order Tests for Which Medicare Reimbursement Will Be Sought. Medicare will pay only for tests that meet the Medicare coverage criteria and are reasonable and necessary to treat or diagnose an individual patient. Medicare does not pay for tests which documentation, including the patient record, does not support that the tests were reasonable and necessary. Medicare does not cover routine screening tests even if the physician or other authorized test orderer considers the tests appropriate for the patient.

☐ STAT ☐ ASAP ☐ ROUTINE ☐ CALL _____ ☐ FAX _____

BILLING: ☐ BILL FACILITY ☐ BILL INSURANCE ☐ BILL PATIENT ☐ HMO ☐ PPO ☐ Health First HMO

PATIENT NAME: (LAST) (FIRST) NAME OF INSURANCE: GROUP #: POLICY #:

SEX: SS#: BIRTHDATE: PHONE NUMBER: AUTHORIZATION #: GUARANTOR: GUARANTOR'S SS#: GUARANTOR'S BIRTHDATE:

ADDRESS/ROOM #: ZIP CODE: SPECIMEN COLLECTED BY: DATE/TIME OF COLLECTION: PHYSICAN'S/AUTHORIZED SIGNATURE:

	TESTS	*DX
10080CBC	CBC w/automated differential	
10200HEMGR	Hemogram	
10190HH	Hematocrit & Hemoglobin	
10490RETIC	Reticulocyte	
10500ESR	Sed Rate (ESR)	
10010ATIII	Anti Thrombin III	
10111DIMER	D-DIMER Quant	
10258LUPUS	Lupus Panel	
10440PT	Protime/INR	
10450PTT	PTT (Activated)	
10460PTTTH	PTT Therapeutic	
20120NH3	Ammonia (On ICE)	
20140AMY	Amylase	
20270BILID	Bilirubin, Direct	
20280BILIT	Bilirubin, Total	
21910BUN	BUN	
20360CA	Calcium	
20540CPK	CK	
20500CKMB	CK & MB	
20550CREAT	Creatinine	
20300CRP	CRP	
20640FER	Ferritin	
20700GLU	Glucose	
20870HA1C	Hgb A1C	
20920HBSAB	Hep B Surf Ab (HBsAb)	
20930HBSAG	Heb B Surf Ag (HBsAg)	
20820HCGQ	Preg Test (HCG) Quant.	
20830PREG	Preg Test (HCG) Qual., Serum	
20963HMCYT	Homocysteine (On ICE)	
21060IRONP	Iron Package	
21460K	Potassium	
21090LACID	Lactic Acid (On ICE)	
21150LIPAS	Lipase	
21210MG	Magnesium	
20260PBNP	PBNP	
21410PHOS	Phosphorus	
21615PSASN	PSA Screen	
21614PSA3	Prostate Specific Ag 3rd	
21365PTH	PTH Intact	
21360PTHP	PTH Pkg (Phos, Ca, Mg, Ionized Ca)	
21720T3UP	T$_3$ Uptake	
21750T4	T$_4$, Total	
20670FTIP	FTI, T$_4$, T$_3$ Uptake	
21895TROP	Troponin	
21790TSH	TSH	
21990B12	Vitamin B12	
20650FOLAT	Folate	

	ELECTROPHORESIS	*DX
21540SPEPI	SPEP/Reflex SIFE	
21545SPEP	Serum Electro NO Interp	
21550UPEPI	UPEP/Reflex UIFE	
21555UPEP	Urine Electro NO Interp	
20990SIFEI	Serum IFE/Interp	

	ELECTROPHORESIS (CON'T)	*DX
20995SIFE	Serum IFE/NO Interp	
21000UIFI1	Urine IFE/Interp	
21605UIFE1	Urine IFE/NO Interp	
20880HGBEI	HGB Electro/Interp	
21560OLIGI	CSF Olig/Interp	
	(SERUM Spec Also REQUIRED)	

DRUG LEVELS

LAST DOSE _____ NEXT DOSE _____

20400CRBM	Carbamazepine (Tegretol)	
20600DIG	Digoxin	
20695GENTR	Gentamicin Trough	
20690GENPK	Gentamicin Peak	
21170LITH	Lithium	
21380PHNO	Phenobarbital	
21390PTN	Phenytoin (Dilantin)	
21985VANTR	Vancomycin Trough	
21980VANPK	Vancomycin Peak	
21780THEOP	Theophylline	
21970VALPR	Valproic Acid (Depakene)	

	PROFILES	*DX
20470BMP	Basic Metabolic (Na, K, CL, CO2, Glu, Bun, Creat, Ca)	
21230CMP	Metabolic Panel (Na, K, Cl, CO2, Glu, Bun, Crea, Ca, TP, Alb, ALT, AST, AiP, TBili)	
20885LIVER	Hepatic (Liver) Panel (Alb, AST, ALT, Alk Phos, TBili, DBili, Tot Protein)	
20980HYPOT	Hypothyroid Profile (T3 Uptake, T4 Total, TSH)	
21160LIPID	Lipid Profile (Chol, Trig, HDL, LDL calc, Chol/HDL Ratio)	
21630RENAL	Renal Function Panel (Na, K, Cl, CO2, Glu, Bun, Crea, Ca, Alb, Pho)	
20945HPACU	Acute Hepatitis Panel (Anti-HAV IgM, Anti-HBC IgM, HBS ag, Hepatitis C)	
20950HPPR	Hepatitis Profile (Anti-HBe & HBeAg will be performed if HBsAG Anti-HBc or Anti-HBc-Igm are positive)	

	URINE TESTS	*DX
Source:	☐ Foley Cath ☐ Midstream ☐ Straight Cath ☐ Suprapubic	
20560UCRCL	Creatinine Clearance 24 hr Blood & Urine Ht. Ft____ In ____ Wt. ____ Total Volume	
21600UTP24	Protein, Urine 24 hr. Total Volume _____	
10571UA	Urinalysis	
10581UAMIC	Urinalysis w/Microscopic	
30400CXURN	Culture Urine	
10576UACXI	Urinalysis/Culture if (culture performed if > 5 wbc and/or 2+ Bacteria, Positive Leukocyte Esterase, Positive Nitrite)	
10420UHCG	Preg Test (HCG) Urine	

ADDITIONAL TESTS   **DIAGNOSIS:**

	MICROBIOLOGY CULTURE/VIROLOGY/MISC	*DX
30180CXAEN	Culture & Gram Stain Aerobic & Anaerobic Source	
30120CXBLD	Culture Blood	
30240CXCSF	Culture CSF & Gram Stain	
30220CXFLD	Culture Sterile Body Fluid Source	
30290CXFUN	Culture Fungus/Other Source	
30290CXFNS	Culture Fungus Skin, Hair, Nail Source	
30330CXGAS	Culture Group A Strep	
30820STRA	Strep Group A Antigen	
30340CXGBS	Culture Group B Strep Source	
30360CXLRT	Culture Gram Stain Lower Respiratory (Sputum, etc) Source	
30320CXGOT	Culture Other Source	
30380CXSTO	Culture Stool	
30710OVAP	Ova and Parasites	
30390CXURT	Culture Upper Respiratory (Throat/Nose) Source	
30420CXWND	Culture & Gram Stain Wound Source	
30410CXVIR	Culture Virus Comprehensive Source	
30350CXHSV	Culture Herpes Virus	
30740RSV	RSV Direct Antigen	
30930VRP	Viral Respiratory Direct Panel	
30570FLUAB	Influenza A& B Antigen	
30760ROTA	Rotavirus Antigen	
030650CBLD	Occult Blood - Single Specimen	
30650OCBLM	Occult Blood - Multiple Specimens	
30121CDIF	Clostridium difficile Toxin A & B	
30101CHLGC	Chlamydia & GC Amplification	
30500GIARD	Giardia lamblia Direct Antigen	
30940WETPR	Wet mount	

	IMMUNOLOGY	*DX
30060ANA	ANA	
30755RF	RA Factor	
30020DSDNA	Anti-dsDNA	
30030AMA	Anti-Mitochondrial Antibody	
30050ASMA	Anti-Smooth Muscle Antibody	
30072ENA	ENA Antibodies (Anti-Sm & Sm/RNF)	
30035ANCA	Neutrophil Cytoplasmic Antibodies (ANCA)	
30078SCL70	SCL-70 (Scleroderma) Antibody	
30070SSAB	SSA/RO and SSB/LA Antibodies (Sjogrens)	
30550HIVAB	HIV-1/2 Screening Antibody (Western Blot if positive)	
30630MONO	Mono Screen	
30770RPR	RPR	
20780RUBG	Rubella Antibody, IgG	
30790MEASG	Rubeola (Measles) Antibody, IgG	

	RANDOM URINE TESTS	*DX
21240MABR	Microalbumin Random	
21470UK1	Urine Potassium	
20580UCRE1	Urine Creatinine	
21820TOXIV	Toxi IV Screen	

PLEASE provide narrative diagnostic information for each ordered test. However, if the test is marked as subject to the carrier's Local Medical Review Policy, please provide Medical Necessity.

Figure 8–1 A panel request form.

Cardiac Profile

Cardiac profiles may be utilized to determine disturbed carbohydrate metabolism from various diseases, which can lead to atherosclerotic conditions and heart disease. A lipid profile test is closely related to a cardiac profile. Heart attack and stroke are two commonly diagnosed conditions using these types of tests.

In cases of myocardial infarction, several enzymes increase over time. A cardiac profile is used to determine changes that indicate the development of a heart attack. These enzymes indicate tissue necrosis when their levels are raised. They include troponin T and troponin I, which influence muscle contraction, and creatine kinase (CK), which is present in many other tissues as well as heart tissue. The different isoenzymes (types) of CK are distinguished by specialized tests. The specialized cardiac type of CK is called CK-MB.

Infarcted heart muscle causes these enzymes to leak from necrotic cells into the blood circulation, peaking within a few days. After this, the levels gradually decline. Usually, the larger the infarct, the longer it takes for levels to return to normal. This pattern of rapid rising and gradual decline is characteristic of myocardial infarction. The amount of damage can therefore be assessed based on the amount of rise and decline. Changing levels of the troponins peak at about 24 h and remain elevated for up to 14 days. Changing levels of CK peak in about 24 h and return to normal in a few days.

Also, after about 12 h following necrosis of heart tissue, the **erythrocyte sedimentation rate (ESR)** is increased. White blood cell counts are slightly elevated, and differential WBC counts reveal a progressive infection. Other tests that may accompany a cardiac profile include electrocardiogram, stress tests, CT scan, echocardiogram, and magnetic resonance angiogram.

Thyroid Profile

Thyroid profile tests include those that check the levels of thyroid-stimulating hormone (TSH), thyroxine (T4), triiodothyronine (T3), and thyroid antibodies. The testing laboratory establishes reference ranges for each test. Increased levels of thyroid hormones or antibodies may indicate thyroiditis, hyperthyroidism, or **Graves' disease**. Decreased levels may indicate goiter, congenital hypothyroidism, or **infantile cretinism**.

Glucose Testing

Glucose is used as fuel for body cells, and normal glucose levels are vital in maintaining homeostasis in the human body. Elevated blood glucose levels (hyperglycemia) may signify diabetes mellitus, endocrine disorders, pancreatitis, or chronic renal failure.

Serology and Immunology Tests

The term *serology* is used interchangeably with the term *immunology*. The original tests that involved immune reactions were called serological tests. This is so because the blood serum was tested when these tests were first developed. Today, other body fluids (such as urine), cells, and tissues are tested for immune reactions.

Rapid Tests

Rapid tests include the *rapid plasma regain* (*RPR*) test. A positive result indicates **syphilis**, which must be further confirmed (by a **treponemal antigen test**) due to the possibility of a false-positive result. This test actually works by nonspecific antibodies in the blood that may indicate the organism *Treponema pallidum*. These antibodies oppose substances released by cells when they become damaged by the organism. The RPR test can also be used to track the progress of syphilis.

Common Serology Tests

Serology tests usually diagnose specific antibodies in the serum. They may be performed to determine a specific infection, for rheumatic illnesses, to verify blood type, or for certain autoimmune deficiencies. Common serology tests include the following:

- Anti-HIV—to screen for human immunodeficiency virus
- Antinuclear antibody (ANA)—for autoimmune disorders such as **systemic lupus erythematosus**
- Antistreptolysin O (ASO) titer—for streptococcus infections
- Cold agglutinins—for atypical pneumonia
- C-reactive protein (CRP)—to indicate inflammatory conditions
- Cytomegalovirus antibody (CMV)—to confirm presence of cytomegalovirus
- Epstein-Barr virus (EBV)—to indicate the possibility of infectious mononucleosis
- Febrile agglutinins—for the presence of antibodies to specific organisms (example: **tularemia**)
- FTA-ABS—fluorescent treponemal antibody absorption test, to confirm the presence of syphilis
- Hepatitis B surface antigen (HBsAg)—to demonstrate the presence of hepatitis antigen on red blood cell surfaces
- Human chorionic gonadotropin (HCG)—indicates pregnancy when present in serum and urine
- Rheumatoid factor (RF)—for rheumatoid arthritis

Drug Testing

Many employers today require drug testing of their employees. This requires special protocols and has legal implications. The National Institute on Drug Abuse (NIDA) defines special donor preparation and collection procedures that must be strictly followed. The drugs most commonly tested for include alcohol, amphetamines, barbiturates, benzodiazepines, cocaine, cannabinoids, methadone, opiates, phencyclidine, and propoxyphene.

To prepare the donor for the procedure, he or she must be positively identified using a driver license or other information, and then the test must be explained before it begins. The donor must be advised of all legal rights. All procedures must be followed exactly as outlined in the company's policies and procedures manual. For urine collections, there must be a special area provided. Access to water must be limited so that the donor cannot alter the specimens. The donor must fill in the written information required for the test, and a witness must be present during all specimen collection.

A split sample may be requested, so the contents of the collection cup will need to be poured into two separate containers. The specimens must be packaged correctly, with the donor witnessing all steps, and placed into tamper-proof bags that are sealed. Both the donor and the person handling the collection of samples must complete and sign the collection form. The specimen is delivered to the laboratory for testing, and all people who handle specimens must document their involvement in writing.

Summary

Most clinical chemistry tests utilize capillary or venous blood. Whole blood contains red blood cells, white blood cells, platelets, plasma, and serum. Serum is the clear, yellow liquid left after the clotting factors are removed. Plasma is the fluid portion of blood that remains after all blood cells have been removed. It is the pale, yellowish liquid part of whole blood. Chemistry panels include the hepatic profile, renal profile, lipid profile, cardiac profile, and thyroid profile.

Serology and immunology tests utilize the serum as well as other body fluids to gauge many different types of antibodies, which indicate specific disease states. Blood typing is also accomplished via serological testing. Drug testing commonly involves employer-required tests for alcohol, amphetamines, barbiturates, illegal drugs, and other substances.

CRITICAL THINKING

A 53-year-old man who was overweight went to his physician's office complaining about headaches and dizziness. During the physical examination, his blood pressure was higher than normal. The physician ordered a lipid profile test, which was positive for hyperlipidemia.

1. What are the most common lipoproteins that may indicate hyperlipidemia?
2. Why is hyperlipidemia related to hypertension?

WEBSITES

http://diabetes.webmd.com/blood-glucose

http://health.nytimes.com/health/guides/test/serology/overview.html

http://nobelprize.org/educational/medicine/landsteiner/readmore.html

http://www.bloodindex.com/view_learning_master.php?id=28

http://www.ehow.com/how_2127105_fast-before-blood-cholesterol-test.html

http://www.helium.com/items/1342951-blood-specimens-the-differences-between-serum-and-plasma

http://www.labtestsonline.org/understanding/analytes/lipid/glance.html

http://www.nhlbi.nih.gov/health/dci/Diseases/bdt/bdt_types.html

http://www.nlm.nih.gov/medlineplus/ency/article/003482.htm

http://www.nlm.nih.gov/medlineplus/laboratorytests.html

http://www.webmd.com/baby/oral-glucose-tolerance-test

REVIEW QUESTIONS

Multiple Choice

1. During fasting, the patient is allowed to drink
   A. orange juice
   B. tea with milk
   C. water
   D. soda

2. Which of the following is NOT detected in a liver panel test?
   A. CBC
   B. ALP
   C. ALT
   D. GGT

3. A blood profile is also called a
   A. lipid profile
   B. cardiac profile
   C. hepatic panel
   D. chemistry panel

4. Hepatic profile tests include all of the following EXCEPT
   A. TP
   B. Alb
   C. GTT
   D. GGT

5. The hepatic profile may diagnose all of the following disorders EXCEPT
   A. multiple myeloma
   B. pneumonia
   C. autoimmune diseases
   D. hypothyroidism

6. Creatinine blood levels rise when the function of which of the following is deficient?
   A. kidneys
   B. lungs
   C. bones
   D. spleen

7. HDL
   A. is referred to as the "bad" cholesterol
   B. can result in a greater risk for heart attack if elevated
   C. transports cholesterol
   D. causes inflammation of a gallstone

8. Hormones detected in a thyroid panel include
   A. thyroid antibodies
   B. triiodothyronine
   C. thyroxine
   D. all of the above

9. The buffy coat is
   A. white in color
   B. removed for the differential portion of white blood cells
   C. a layer of thrombocytes between plasma and white blood cells
   D. seen in a centrifuged microhematocrit tube

10. Blood serum
    A. is the pale yellowish liquid part of whole blood
    B. contains coagulation factors
    C. does not contain fibrinogen
    D. none of the above statements is correct

11. The risk of coronary heart disease is increased with high levels of all of the following EXCEPT
    A. LDL
    B. HDL
    C. total cholesterol
    D. triglycerides

12. All of the following tests may be used to determine myocardial infarction EXCEPT
    A. troponin T
    B. creatine kinase-MB
    C. rapid plasma regain
    D. troponin I

13. A treponemal antigen test indicates
    A. syphilis
    B. atypical pneumonia
    C. infectious mononucleosis
    D. tularemia

14. Which of the following tests confirms the presence of syphilis?
    A. FTA-ABS
    B. HBsAg
    C. HCG
    D. ANA

15. All of the following drug tests are commonly used EXCEPT
    A. barbiturates
    B. cocaine
    C. lithium
    D. alcohol

Microbiology

OUTLINE

Introduction
Microorganisms
Classifications of Microorganisms
    Bacteria
    Viruses
    Fungi
    Protozoa
Microbial Growth
Microbes and the Human Body
Microscope
    Structure
    Protection
Summary
Critical Thinking
Websites
Review Questions

OBJECTIVES

After studying this chapter, readers should be able to:

1. Describe the bacterial structures used in identification.
2. Compare bacteria with fungi.
3. Describe various bacterial morphologies.
4. Describe the gram stain.
5. Compare rickettsia with chlamydia.
6. Explain eukaryotes and prokaryotes.
7. Describe the effects of fungal infections on the human body.
8. Explain protozoa and list four protozoal infections.
9. Describe the structure of the microscope.
10. Explain the total magnification of the microscope.

KEY TERMS

Algae: Unicellular or multicellular photosynthetic eukaryotes lacking roots, stems, leaves, conducting vessels, and complex sex organs.

Aperture: The hole in the stage of a microscope through which light is transmitted.

Arthropod: An invertebrate animal with an exoskeleton, such as insects, arachnids, and crustaceans.

Asexual reproduction: The formation of new individual organisms from the cells of a single parent organism.

Bacilli: A generic term that describes the morphology of any rod-shaped bacterium.

Bacteria: A large group of prokaryotic, single-celled microorganisms.

Cocci: Any bacteria that have circular shapes.

Condenser: The microscope structure used to collect and focus light onto the specimen.

Diplococci: Cocci bacteria arranged in two-celled pairs.

Eukaryotes: Organisms whose cells contain complex structures enclosed within membranes.

Fermentation: A metabolic process whereby electrons released from nutrients are ultimately transferred to molecules obtained from the breakdown of the same nutrients.

Microbiology: The study of microorganisms.

Microscopes: Pieces of equipment used to see objects that are too small to be viewed by the naked eye.

Mycology: The study of fungi.

Pathogenic: Able to cause disease or infection.

Periplasm: A metabolic region between the cell membrane and outer membrane of gram-negative cells.

Physiochemical: Relating to both physiology and chemistry.

Prokaryotes: A group of organisms that lack a cell nucleus and any other membrane-bound organelles.

Protozoa: Microorganisms generally classified as unicellular, eukaryotic organisms lacking cell walls.

Resolution: The capability of a microscope to visualize certain objects.

Rheostat: A variable resistor that controls electric current in a circuit.

Spirilla: Bacteria with spiral shapes.

Spores: Reproductive structures adapted for surviving over longer periods in unfavorable conditions.

KEY TERMS CONTINUED

Staphylococci: Gram-positive bacteria that form grapelike clusters.

Streptococci: Gram-positive bacteria that form chains or pairs of round structures.

Symptomatology: The study of the symptoms of diseases.

Teichoic acid: A negatively charged polysaccharide in the cell wall of gram-positive bacteria.

Virions: Complete viral particles, making up the infective forms of viruses.

Viruses: The smallest infectious agents; they can replicate only within living host cells.

Working distance: The distance between the front lens of a microscope and the specimen when the microscope is correctly focused.

Introduction

Microbiology is the study of very small living organisms. These include bacteria, **algae**, fungi, protozoa, and viruses. Microorganisms are often called *microbes, germs,* or *single-celled organisms.* **Pathogenic** microorganisms cause a wide spectrum of illnesses. These include meningitis, pneumonia, tuberculosis, upper respiratory tract infections, and urinary tract infections. Phlebotomists must understand how infectious diseases are transmitted and how they may be prevented. A simple way to reduce the risk of transmission of disease is by proper hand washing. This chapter focuses on microorganisms and microbial growth.

Microorganisms

Microorganisms are organisms that are not visible to the naked eye and that are able to carry out all life processes, including metabolism, reproduction, and motility. Less than 1% of microorganisms are pathogenic. The majority of microorganisms are either beneficial or permanent in their relationship to human beings and are called *normal flora.*

Microorganisms are responsible for the decomposition of waste and natural recycling. The organisms that are normally present on and inside our bodies ensure that food is digested, that blood clots properly (resulting from vitamin K production by the organs that inhabit the intestines), and that pathogens are kept from invading our skin, mucous membranes, gastrointestinal tract, and genitourinary tract. When these *normal microbiota* are disrupted by the use of antibiotics, hormonal changes, or other causes, certain organisms that are normally present in low numbers proliferate, causing a *superinfection.* There are two main types of microorganisms: **eukaryotes** and **prokaryotes.**

Classifications of Microorganisms

Microorganisms are classified as bacteria, viruses, fungi, and protozoa.

Bacteria

Bacteria are single-celled prokaryote microorganisms that reproduce by binary fission. This process involves duplication of the chromosome and subsequent fission (splitting in half) of the cell. This is a process of asexual reproduction that results in large numbers of bacteria developing from a single cell. It explains why bacterial infections can quickly overwhelm a patient's immune system and cause a superinfection. Bacteria are often classified according to their shape,

staining characteristics, and the environmental conditions in which they thrive. Pathogenic bacteria assume these three different *morphologic* shapes:

- **Bacilli**—rod-shaped bacteria, which include *coccobacilli* and *streptobacilli*
- **Cocci**—in general, spherical bacteria, which include the following:
  - **Diplococci**—either spherical or coffee-bean-shaped bacteria usually found in pairs
  - **Staphylococci**—spherical bacteria that appear in grapelike clusters
  - **Streptococci**—spherical bacteria that appear in chains
- **Spirilla**—spiral-shaped bacteria

Figure 9–1 shows various shapes of bacteria.

Bacteria may also be classified by staining, according to their cell wall composition. In pathogenic bacteria, three types of cell wall structures exist: gram-positive, gram-negative, and acid-fast. These types are based on reactions to specialized stains used to view the bacteria under a microscope.

The bacterial cell wall is composed of *peptidoglycan*, a molecule that is composed of carbohydrate and protein. Most gram-positive bacterial cells have a thick layer of rigid peptidoglycan cell wall without a surrounding lipid layer. The gram-positive cell wall also contains a sugar-alcohol called **teichoic acid**. A gram-negative cell has a thin layer of peptidoglycan surrounded by a lipid layer. It lacks teichoic acid. The unique feature of the gram-negative cell wall is the presence of an outer membrane, which is separated from the cell membrane by a gap (called **periplasm**). The peptidoglycan layer is

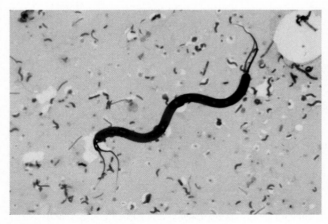

Figure 9–1 Various shapes of bacteria.

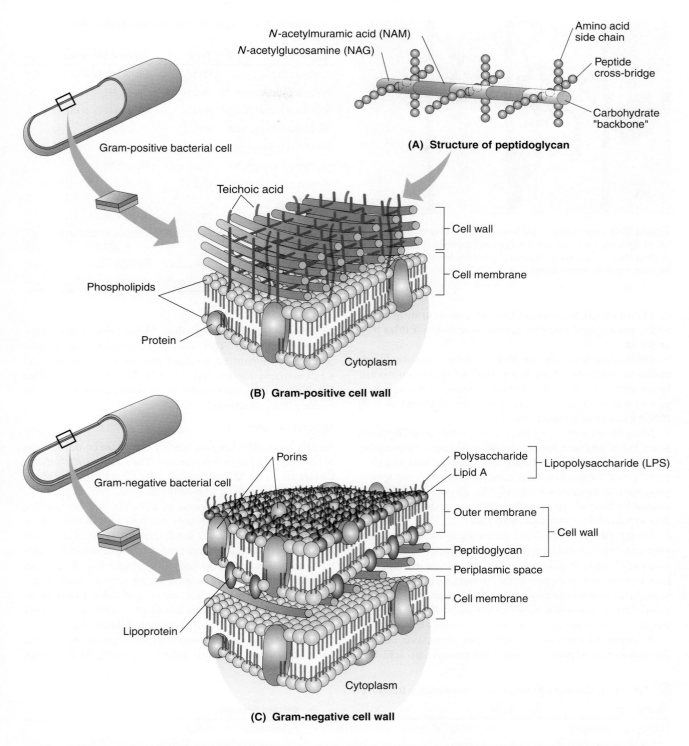

N-acetylmuramic acid (NAM)

N-acetylglucosamine (NAG)

Amino acid side chain

Peptide cross-bridge

Carbohydrate "backbone"

(A) Structure of peptidoglycan

Gram-positive bacterial cell

Teichoic acid

Cell wall

Cell membrane

Phospholipids

Protein

Cytoplasm

(B) Gram-positive cell wall

Gram-negative bacterial cell

Porins

Polysaccharide

Lipid A

Lipopolysaccharide (LPS)

Outer membrane

Cell wall

Peptidoglycan

Periplasmic space

Cell membrane

Lipoprotein

Cytoplasm

(C) Gram-negative cell wall

Figure 9–2 A comparison of the cell walls of gram-positive and gram-negative bacterial cells. (A) The structure of peptidoglycan is shown as units of NAG and NAM joined laterally by amino acid cross-bridges and vertically by side chains of four amino acids. (B) The cell wall of a gram-positive bacterial cell is composed of peptidoglycan layers combined with teichoic acid molecules. (C) In the gram-negative cell wall, the peptidoglycan layer is much thinner, and there is no teichoic acid. Moreover, an outer membrane overlies the peptidoglycan layer such that both comprise the cell wall. Note the structure of the outer membrane in this figure. The outer half is unique in containing primarily lipopolysaccharide and porin proteins.

located in the periplasm and attached to lipoproteins in the cell membrane. An acid-fast bacterium will not stain well in gram stain, while both gram-positive and gram-negative bacteria stain negative in an acid-fast stain (see **Figure 9–2**).

Gram stains are used to classify bacteria. They utilize crystal violet and iodine solutions, followed by alcohol. Gram-negative microorganisms stain red or rose-pink, while gram-positive microorganisms stain blue or purple

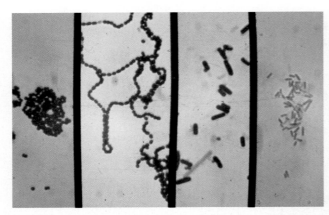

Figure 9–3 Appearance of bacteria as seen in Gram stains. From left to right: gram-positive cocci in clusters (staphylococci), gram-positive cocci in chains (streptococci), gram-positive bacilli, gram-negative bacilli (original magnification × 1,000).

Table 9–2 Common Pathogenic Gram-Negative Bacteria

Bacterium	Type	Related Diseases
Escherichia coli	Rod	Urinary infections
Haemophilus ducreyi	Rod	Chancroid
Haemophilus influenzae	Rod	Meningitis or pneumonia
Klebsiella pneumoniae	Rod	Pneumonia
Neisseria gonorrheae	Diplococci	Gonorrhea
Neisseria meningitides	Diplococci	Meningitis
Rickettsia rickettsii	Rod	Rocky Mountain spotted fever
Salmonella typhi	Rod	Typhoid fever
Shigella species	Rod	Shigellosis (bacillary dysentery)
Treponema pallidum	Spirochete	Syphilis
Vibrio cholerae	Curved rod	Cholera

(see **Figure 9–3**). Some important pathogenic gram-positive and gram-negative bacteria are summarized in **Tables 9–1** and **9–2**.

Gram stain tests require 24 to 48 h to complete. Gram stains are performed on every type of specimen except blood cultures. Once it is known whether a bacterium is gram-positive or gram-negative, the correct choice of drug therapy is able to be determined.

Most bacteria multiply by simple cell division. However, some types produce **spores**, which withstand unfavorable environments such as extreme heat, drying, and disinfectants. Once the environment returns to normal, the spores germinate to form new bacteria cells. Examples of diseases caused by bacteria include diarrhea, pneumonia, sinusitis, gonorrhea, and urinary tract infections.

Bacteria are also classified according to oxygen requirements. *Aerobes* are bacteria that require oxygen to live. *Anaerobes* are bacteria that do not require oxygen to live and that may even die in its presence. Some bacteria are more "flexible" regarding oxygen requirements, and although they are considered to be anaerobes, they can survive in the presence of oxygen. These organisms are called *facultative* anaerobes.

Examples of various different types of bacteria include the following: *Mycobacterium tuberculosis*, an acid-fast aerobic bacteria affecting white blood cells in the lungs, causes tuberculosis. The gram-negative *Bacteroides fragilis* is the predominant bacterium found in the intestines, and it is anaerobic. *Escherichia coli*, a facultative anaerobe, also inhabits the intestines, and it is the most common cause of urinary tract infections.

Specific Bacteria

Specific types of bacteria are smaller than more common types of bacteria, but larger than viruses. They include *Rickettsiae*, *Chlamydiae*, and *Mycoplasmae*. The classification of these organisms has proved to be difficult to microbiologists.

Rickettsiae are tiny forms of bacteria that cannot live without a host. They can only multiply within the cells of an infected person. Many small animals, such as dogs, are infected by rickettsiae. They are gram-negative *intracellular* bacteria that require host cells for reproduction. Rickettsial infections are spread through a vector such as insect bites, including those of fleas, lice, mites, and ticks. Examples of rickettsial infections include Rocky Mountain spotted fever and typhus, two of the most common rickettsial diseases.

Chlamydiae are very small, gram-negative, nonmotile bacteria that require host cells for growth. At one time,

Table 9–1 Common Pathogenic Gram-Positive Bacteria

Bacterium	Type	Related Diseases
Clostridium botulinum	Spore-forming rod, motile, noncapsulate	Botulism (food poisoning)
Clostridium perfringens	Spore-forming rod, nonmotile, noncapsulate	Gas gangrene, wound infections
Clostridium tetani	Sporing, motile, noncapsulate	Tetanus
Corynebacterium diphtheriae	Rod, nonmotile	Diphtheria
Mycobacterium leprae	Rod	Leprosy
Mycobacterium tuberculosis	Rod	Tuberculosis
Staphylococcus aureus	Cocci in clusters	Boils, carbuncles, pneumonia, septicemia
Streptococcus pneumoniae	Diplococcus	Pneumonia
Streptococcus pyogenes	Cocci in chains	Rheumatic fever, scarlet fever, septicemia, strep throat

chlamydiae were considered to be viruses. Chlamydiae, unlike rickettsiae, are not transmitted by **arthropod** vectors. Examples of chlamydiae infections include inclusion conjunctivitis and pneumonia. Tissue culture or serologic testing is required to identify rickettsiae and chlamydiae.

Mycoplasmae are very small bacteria that are extremely fragile because they lack a cell wall. They are not obligate parasites like rickettsiae and chlamydiae, which cannot grow on artificial media in the laboratory. Most types of mycoplasmae can easily be identified in standard agar cultures. One member of this group causes a type of pneumonia known as *primary atypical pneumonia*.

Viruses

Viruses are microorganisms that can only exist and reproduce inside host cells. They are the smallest of all microorganisms and are visible only with an electron microscope. Not considered cellular, viruses are simpler than bacteria (prokaryotes). They consist of a nucleic acid core, containing either deoxyribonucleic acid (DNA) or ribonucleic acid (RNA) that is surrounded by a coat of antigenic protein (see **Figure 9–4**), sometimes surrounded by an *envelope* of lipoprotein. A *capsid* is a layer of protein enveloping the genome of a virion. A capsid is composed of structural units called *capsomeres*.

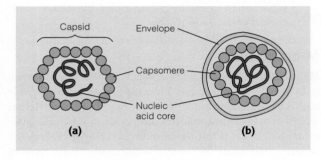

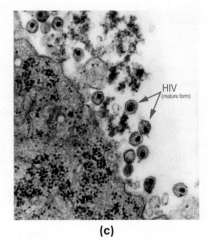

Figure 9–4 General structure of a virus. (a) The virus consists of a nucleic acid core of either RNA or DNA. Surrounding the viral core is a layer of protein known as the capsid. Each protein molecule in the capsid is known as a capsomere. (b) Some viruses have an additional protective coat known as the envelope. (c) Electron micrograph of the human immunodeficiency virus (HIV).

The envelope is structurally similar to the plasma membranes of eukaryotic cells. Once inside a host cell, viruses block its normal protein synthesis and utilize its metabolism so that they can reproduce.

A *bacteriophage* is a type of virus that uses bacteria for part of its life cycle. Typically, bacteriophages enter bacteria using bacterial enzymes and proteins to reproduce themselves, and then they escape the bacteria. Depending upon the specific type of bacteriophage, the host bacteria may or may not be harmed.

Viruses are classified based on **physiochemical** characteristics of **virions**, mode of transmission, **symptomatology**, host range, and other factors. Some trigger an immediate disease response, while others remain latent for years. Viruses usually enter the body through the digestive and respiratory systems, although other routes of entry are also possible. For example, viruses may also enter through the skin during sexual contact. A specific viral infection may cause symptoms in one person that are different from the symptoms caused in another person.

Fungi

Mycology is the study of *fungi* and the diseases they cause. They are important sources of food and are essential for the **fermentation** of various substances such as alcohol, antibiotics, antitoxins, and other drugs. Fungi are eukaryotes, larger than bacteria, and include unicellular yeasts and multicellular molds.

Fungi are present in soil, air, and water. However, only a few species cause disease. Fungal infections may be superficial (affecting the hair, nails, or skin). Examples of superficial fungal infections include *tinea* (ringworm), *tinea pedis* (athlete's foot), and *tinea barbae* (which affects the facial hair follicles). The term *ringworm* is used because the infected area is often circular and appears wrinkled at the center, which is a result of the healing process.

Certain types of fungi can penetrate internal body tissues to produce serious diseases that affect the heart, lungs, mucous membranes, and other organs. An example of a yeast infection affecting the mucous membranes is *Candida albicans*, which commonly affects the reproductive system or mouth. Because fungal infections are resistant to antibiotics (which are used to treat bacterial infections), fungal infections must be treated with drugs that are active against the unusual cell walls of fungi.

Protozoa

Protozoa are single-celled parasitic eukaryotes ranging in size from microscopic to macroscopic (able to be seen by the naked eye). They are the lowest forms of animal life. Protozoa are found in both water and soil, and they have the ability to move. Protozoa usually obtain their food from organic matter that is dead or decaying. Most protozoa are saprophytes. Protozoal infections are spread through the ingestion of contaminated food or water as well as through insect bites. Examples of protozoal infections include gastroenteritis, malaria, amebic dysentery, and the vaginal infection known as *Trichomonas vaginalis*.

Microbial Growth

Microbes increase in number via **asexual reproduction**, which is a process that maintains genetic constancy while increasing the numbers of cells. *Microbial growth* requires an energy source, specific nutrients, adequate temperature, adequate pH (acidity), and adequate moisture. Microbial growth occurs via the processes of fermentation, respiration, and photosynthesis. *Fermentation* is the decomposition of complex substances through the action of enzymes. *Respiration* is the interchange of gases between an organism and its environment. Microbes that may grow either with or without oxygen are called facultative anaerobes. *Photosynthesis* is the process by which light energy produces organic molecules (usually used by plants, although certain bacteria are also capable of photosynthesis).

Microorganisms require various types of nutrients to grow and replicate. These include *macronutrients*, such as oxygen, carbon, hydrogen, nitrogen, phosphorus, sulfur, calcium, potassium, iron, and magnesium, as well as minor amounts of other nutrients (*micronutrients* or *trace elements*). Micronutrients include manganese, zinc, cobalt, molybdenum, copper, and nickel. Each different microorganism may have additional particular requirements, but overall every microorganism requires a balanced mixture of nutrients.

Certain microorganisms have all of the enzymes and biochemical pathways required to synthesize their needed cell components. Others need to extract enzymes from their environment to be able to live and grow. There are three major classes of *growth factors*:

- Amino acids—needed for protein synthesis
- Purines and pyrimidines—needed for nucleic acid synthesis
- Vitamins—usually make up all or some of the enzyme cofactors; vitamins are needed only in very small amounts to sustain growth

It is important to understand the growth factor requirements of microbes. Microbes with certain growth factor requirements can be used in *bioassays* such as *growth-response assays*, which allow the amount of growth factor in a solution to be determined. Ideally, the amount of growth factor is directly related to the amount of growth. Some microorganisms can synthesize large quantities of vitamins to manufacture certain compounds for human use. Certain water-soluble and fat-soluble vitamins are partly or completely produced using *industrial fermentations* via organisms that include *Clostridium*, *Candida*, and *Streptomyces*.

Microbes and the Human Body

The study of pathogens and disease processes is known as *medical microbiology*. Disease processes, due to microbes in the human body, involve *epidemiology, diagnosis, treatment, infection control,* and *immunology*. Other terms used in the discussion of microbes and the human body include the following:

- *Symbiosis*—any close relationship that exists between two different species
- *Mutualism*—a relationship in which both organisms benefit; for example, certain normal flora living in the human intestine synthesize vitamin K, biotin, riboflavin, pantothenate, and pyridoxine
- *Commensalism*—a one-sided relationship in which only one member benefits, but neither organism is harmed; yeast, *Candida albicans*, is one of the normal flora that has a commensural relationship with the skin (meaning that it benefits from contact with the skin and does not harm it)
- *Parasitism*—a one-sided relationship between a host and a parasite (an organism that lives on, in, or at the expense of another)
- *Opportunism*—a relationship in which a usually harmless organism becomes pathogenic when the host's resistance is impaired
- *Pathogenicity*—the ability of a pathogenic agent to cause a disease
- *Virulence*—the degree of pathogenicity or relative power of an organism to produce a disease
- *Infective dose*—the number of organisms required to cause a disease in a susceptible host
- *Vector*—a carrier of pathogenic organisms (such as insects and other creatures)
- *Resistance*—the body mechanisms that oppose infection; the host's state of health and other factors (race, age, sex, occupation) affect the ability of a pathogen to cause disease. Resistance is also the ability of a microorganism to live in the presence of antibiotics, antimicrobial agents, and phages.

Microscope

Microscopes are used to view structures that are too small to be seen by the naked eye. The magnification they provide allows us to see abnormalities of the blood and body tissues as well as many pathogenic microorganisms. When the laboratory technician is testing the blood, microscopes allow her or him to recognize the stage of maturation of cells, types of bacteria that may be present, and their characteristic shapes, sizes, growth, and staining.

Structure

A microscope consists of eyepiece lenses (*oculars*) at the top, a revolving *nosepiece* that holds several different magnifying lenses known as *objectives*, slide clips to hold slides in place, a *stage* where slides are placed for viewing, a *condenser, iris*, and a light source. The *arm* of the microscope serves as the unit's "backbone," to which most of the pieces previously listed are mounted. On the arm are fine and coarse focus controls. The entire structure has a *base* upon which it stands (see **Figure 9–5**).

The Lenses of the Microscope

A microscope's ability to magnify extremely small objects works because of multiple lenses, known as the oculars and objectives. *Monocular* microscopes have one ocular, while *binocular* microscopes have two. Most oculars magnify objects by 10 times. The objective lenses, usually consisting of three or four different magnifications, commonly range from 4 to 10 to 40 to 100 times ($4\times$ to $10\times$ to $40\times$ to $100\times$)

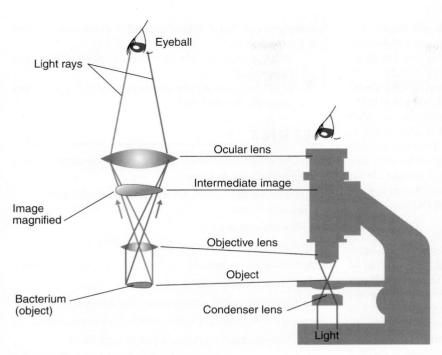

Figure 9–5 The parts of a microscope.

in magnification size. Only one objective is used at a time. The objective lenses are rotated on the revolving nosepiece so that the desired magnification can be easily obtained.

Primarily, the following information describes the major uses of each magnification of the objective lenses:

- 4×—used to scan a slide for areas to examine under high magnification
- 10×—"low power," used in initial focusing, to count cells, and to scan urine sediment
- 40× (may be 43× or 45× on some microscopes)—"high power," used to count blood cells, scan differential smears, and view urine sediment
- 100× (may be 95× or 97× on some microscopes)—"oil-immersion objective" uses an oil layer between the specimen and objective to refract light and is employed to identify different types of bacteria and white blood cells; the oil should be wiped from the objective after each slide to prevent it from damaging the cement around the lens

The 4×, 10×, and 40× objectives are called "dry lenses" because they do not require oil to assist in magnification. Oil should not contact these lenses, or it may damage the cement that holds them in place.

A microscope's total magnification is calculated by multiplying the magnification of the oculars (10×) by the objective used. This means that a standard microscope is capable of 10× multiplied by 100×, achieving 1000× the magnification. The **resolution** of a microscope is its ability to view fine details. This depends on the quality of the microscope and its components. A better quality of microscope will have higher resolution.

The Stage of the Microscope

The stage is a platform that holds the slide to be viewed. The slide is placed over a circular or oval hole in the center of the stage that allows light to enter from below.

The Light of the Microscope

The light source is usually located in the base of the microscope, and it has a filter to change wavelengths. Blue daylight is usually used because it allows the most comfortable viewing. Other filters are available, however. Light intensity is controlled with a **rheostat**. A substage called the **condenser** is located just below the opening in the mechanical stage and above the light source. The condenser controls the stream of light and may be raised or lowered. Its **aperture** narrows and widens to control how much light passes through to the specimen on the slide. The aperture is also called the *iris diaphragm* because it looks like the iris of a human eye.

Because the light shines up through the specimen, the specimen must be thin enough to allow light to pass through it without diffusion. Glass slides help in this capacity. There also must be enough dark and light contrast for a structure to be viewed clearly.

The Focusing of the Microscope

Focusing a microscope requires either moving the objective up or down relative to the stage or moving the stage itself. Round knobs usually located on both sides of the microscope allow for these movements, and they are labeled as fine or coarse focus controls. The *coarse adjustment* knob moves the objective a greater distance quickly, while the *fine adjustment* knob moves it only a slight amount. At high power magnification, only the fine adjustment knob should be used to focus, moving at tiny increments.

The **working distance** is the distance between the specimen on the stage and the objective lens. It is longest at lower magnification and shorter as magnification increases. With the 100× objective, the working distance is only about as thick as a heavy piece of paper. The oil on the oil immersion lens actually touches the glass slide as well as the objective. Because of the short working distance, you should always examine the microscope from the side when changing from 40× to 100× to avoid grinding the slide into the lens.

Protection

Microscopes must be protected from excess dust, oil, light, and vibrations, and, of course from falling. They should be stored in a safe place and cleaned carefully after each use. Maintenance records should be kept to make sure that every component is being properly and regularly maintained. Only recommended brands of immersion oil may be used. Ideally, microscopes should be kept in cabinets or under plastic covers when not in use. Whenever the microscope is carried, you should support it underneath with one hand while fully grasping the arm of the microscope with the other hand.

Dust should be blown from the microscope's glass surfaces without touching the lenses. Only the outer surfaces of lenses should be cleaned, using a circular motion from the center outward. For this purpose, lens paper that is slightly moistened with 70% isopropyl alcohol should be used. If the 100× objective has been used, the oil should be carefully cleaned from the objective and all other parts of the microscope.

Summary

Microorganisms require a microscope to view them. The smallest of all microorganisms are viruses, which require an electron microscope to see. Bacteria are found in a variety of different shapes, and they may also be identified by their response to staining with different types of solutions, which include gram stains. Other microorganisms that are related to disease include rickettsiae, chlamydiae, mycoplasmae, fungi, and protozoa. For microbes to grow, energy sources and nutrients, along with other substances, are required. The study of microorganisms and disease processes is known as medical microbiology. Integral to this field is the use of various types of microscopes, which utilize different types of lenses and magnifications to view objects of all sizes. Common magnifications used in nonelectron microscopes include 4×, 10×, 40×, and 100×. By using these lenses in conjunction with ocular lenses in the eyepiece portion of a microscope, magnifications of up to 1000× may be achieved.

CRITICAL THINKING

Amanda, who has been a phlebotomist for a few months, was trying to focus on a blood smear specimen to view specific white blood cells. She was utilizing the fine and coarse adjustments on her microscope and accidentally crushed the lens and slide.

1. What could Amanda have done to prevent this from happening?
2. If the lens was indeed crushed, what is the next step Amanda should take?

WEBSITES

http://health.howstuffworks.com/diseases-conditions/infectious/virus-human.htm

http://micrographia.com/tutoria/micbasic/micbpt01/micb0100.htm

http://www.asm.org/

http://www.livescience.com/bacteria/

http://www.merck.com/mmhe/sec17/ch195/ch195a.html

http://www.microbes.info/

http://www.opticsplanet.net/using-microscope-guide.html

http://www.sciencedaily.com/articles/p/protozoa.htm

http://www.ucmp.berkeley.edu/fungi/fungi.html

REVIEW QUESTIONS

Multiple Choice

1. Which of the following microorganisms appears in grapelike clusters?
   A. streptococci
   B. spirochetes
   C. staphylococci
   D. vibrio cholerae
2. Which of the following organisms requires a vector?
   A. diplococcus
   B. mycoplasma
   C. rickettsia
   D. chlamydia
3. Microbes that can grow either with or without oxygen are called
   A. obligate anaerobes
   B. facultative anaerobes
   C. anaerobes
   D. aerobes
4. The smallest microorganisms are called
   A. viruses
   B. chlamydia
   C. rickettsia
   D. bacteria
5. Bacteria that are permanent and beneficial residents in the human body are called
   A. pathogens
   B. hosts
   C. normal flora
   D. parasites
6. Viruses are
   A. visible to the naked eye
   B. simpler than prokaryotes
   C. the same as fungi
   D. the same as bacteria

7. Spiral-shaped bacteria are called
   A. cocci
   B. diplococci
   C. bacilli
   D. spirilla

8. Streptococci appear in
   A. clusters of cocci
   B. chains of cocci
   C. spirilla
   D. pairs of cocci

9. Both bacteria and fungi can be
   A. unicellular
   B. multicellular
   C. prokaryotes
   D. eukaryotes

10. Which of the following can be seen only with an electron microscope?
    A. fungi
    B. viruses
    C. bacteria
    D. rickettsia

11. When the high-power objective (40×) is used, which of the following parts of the compound microscope is used to focus the image?
    A. revolving nosepiece
    B. coarse adjustment
    C. fine adjustment
    D. eyepiece

12. Organisms that cause disease are called
    A. inflammative
    B. fulminative
    C. pathogens
    D. chronic

13. Which of the following items should be used to clean the lenses of a microscope?
    A. cotton cloth
    B. lens paper
    C. soft facial tissue
    D. paper towels

14. The degree to which an organism is pathogenic is known as
    A. resistance
    B. pathogen
    C. infective dose
    D. virulence

15. A part of a microscope used to collect and focus light onto the specimen is referred to as a(n)
    A. resolution
    B. condenser
    C. aperture
    D. binocular

CHAPTER 10

Safety, Infection Control, and Standard Precautions

OUTLINE

Introduction
Physical Hazards
    Fire Hazards
    Electrical Hazards
    Mechanical Hazards
    Chemical Hazards
    Disposal of Chemicals
    Chemical Spill Cleanup
Patient Safety Related to Latex Products
Infection Control
    Pathogens and Infections
    Nosocomial Infections
Chain of Infection
    Infectious Agent
    Reservoir Host
    Portal of Exit
    Mode of Transmission
    Portal of Entry
    Susceptible Host
Standard Precautions
    Biologic Hazards
    Blood-borne Pathogens Standard
    Disposal of Hazardous Wastes
    Safety Showers and the Eyewash Station
    Sharps/Needlestick Injury Prevention
    Exposure Control
Prevention of Disease Transmission
    Hand Washing
    Sanitization
    Disinfection
    Sterilization
    Decontamination
Cardiopulmonary Resuscitation
Summary
Critical Thinking
Websites
Review Questions

OBJECTIVES

After studying this chapter, readers should be able to:
1. Describe the classifications of fires.
2. List techniques that may minimize physical, chemical, and biologic risks in the clinical laboratory.
3. Explain electrical safety in the clinical laboratory.
4. Describe chemical identification.
5. Discuss chemical spill cleanup.
6. Explain the major areas included in the OSHA Compliance Guideline.
7. Specify potentially infectious bodily fluids.
8. Explain the chain of infection.
9. Describe various precautions used to stop the spread of disease.
10. Differentiate disinfectants and antiseptics.

KEY TERMS

Airborne precautions: Formerly called *respiratory isolation*, these additional safety precautions are applied to certain diseases such as tuberculosis.

Anoxia: Partial or complete absence of oxygen from inspired gases, arterial blood, or tissue.

Antiseptics: Substances that inhibit the growth of microorganisms in living tissue.

Asepsis: The state of being free of pathogenic microorganisms.

Aseptic techniques: Procedures that are performed under sterile conditions.

Blood-borne pathogen (BBP): Any microorganism in the blood (or other body fluids) that can cause illness and disease.

Carcinogenic: Able to cause cancer or make it more likely to develop.

Cardiopulmonary resuscitation (CPR): An emergency procedure commonly performed on patients who are in cardiac or respiratory arrest.

KEY TERMS CONTINUED

Carrier: An individual (host) with no overt disease who harbors infectious organisms.

Caustic: Capable of burning, corroding, or destroying living tissue.

Centrifuge: A piece of laboratory equipment used to "spin" substances such as blood samples to separate out various elements that they contain.

Chain of infection: The method of infection proliferation; it includes an infectious agent, a reservoir, a portal of exit, a mode of transmission, a portal of entry, and a susceptible host.

Communicable disease: An infectious disease that is able to be transmitted between individuals because of a replicating agent (rather than a toxin).

Contact precautions: Procedures that reduce the risk of transmission of serious diseases through direct or indirect physical contact.

Disinfectants: Substances that can destroy microorganisms from nonliving objects.

Double bagging: The use of two trash bags for disposing of waste from patient rooms (usually from patients who are in isolation).

Droplet precautions: Procedures used to reduce the transmission of diseases via droplets that are expelled during sneezing, coughing, or talking; these diseases include meningitis, pertussis, pneumonia, and rubella.

Fomites: Inanimate objects that may transmit infectious organisms or infectious agents (such as sinks, toilets, doorknobs, linens, glasses, and phlebotomy supplies).

HazCom: The OSHA Hazard Communication Standard, which requires chemical manufacturers to supply Material Safety Data Sheets (MSDSs) for their chemicals.

Infection control programs: Guidelines that address community-acquired and health care-associated infections, including their monitoring, reporting, required isolation procedures, education, and management.

Intensive care unit (ICU): A specialized treatment area for critically ill patients, those needing additional monitoring, and those who are more susceptible to infections.

Isolation procedures: Methods used to protect healthcare workers from patients with certain infectious diseases; usually divided into category-specific and disease-specific types.

Material Safety Data Sheets (MSDSs): Required paperwork about all chemicals used in a workplace that lists chemical, precautionary, and emergency exposure information.

Mode of transmission: The method by which pathogenic agents are transmitted.

Nosocomial infections: Health care-acquired infections; those acquired after being admitted into a health facility.

Protective (reverse) isolation: Precautionary methods designed to protect patients who may be highly susceptible to infections.

RACE: Rescue Alert Confine Extinguish: A system designed to help healthcare workers remember how to respond when a fire emergency occurs.

Source: The origin of an infection.

Standard precautions: Safeguards to reduce the risk of transmission of microorganisms. These precautions are more comprehensive than universal precautions, applying to patients, body fluids, nonintact skin, and mucous membranes, and they include barrier protection, hand hygiene, and proper use and disposal of needles and other sharps.

Susceptible host: A person who lacks resistance to an agent and is vulnerable to contracting a disease.

Teratogenic: Able to cause birth defects in an embryo or fetus.

Transmission-based precautions: A set of procedures designed to prevent the communication of infectious diseases.

Universal precautions: Approaches to infection control designed to prevent the transmission of blood-borne diseases.

Introduction

Safety in the laboratory is of the utmost importance. Most laboratory accidents are prevented by exercising proper techniques and by using common sense. Safe laboratory practices require a personal commitment to and concern for others. It is important to know the proper safety factors and precautions to take to prevent accidents and injuries while on the job. Hazards include fire, explosives, laboratory hazards, electrical hazards, radioactivity, chemical spills, mechanical hazards, and allergies. All patients and healthcare workers must be protected from hazardous events on a daily basis.

For infection control, healthcare facilities must provide biologically safe working environments as set forth by the Occupational Safety and Health Administration (OSHA), the Centers for Disease Control and Prevention (CDC), accrediting agencies, and state regulatory agencies. Every healthcare worker must assist in protecting patients from hazardous events each time they enter the healthcare facility.

Besides OSHA and the CDC, there are other governing agencies that deal with safe laboratory practices. These include a nonprofit educational organization known as the Clinical and Laboratory Standards Institute (CLSI), which provides a forum for the development, promotion, and use of national and international standards. The College of American Pathologists (CAP) is a leading organization in the provision of laboratory quality improvement programs, and the Environmental Protection Agency (EPA) is a government organization that strives to protect human health while safeguarding the natural environment.

Physical Hazards

Physical hazards in the laboratory can be classified as fire, electrical, and mechanical hazards.

Fire Hazards

It is the responsibility of every healthcare employee to practice good fire safety because fire or explosions can result from stored chemicals and other substances in the workplace. Employees should be familiar with the locations and uses of all fire safety equipment, such as fire extinguishers and fire blankets (see **Figure 10–1**). Fire extinguishers are available in several types, and employees should be familiar with all types used in their facilities. Fire blankets should be available wherever there is any risk of flames or explosions. Fire blankets are used to extinguish flames before serious injury can occur.

Regular fire safety education and fire drills should be conducted to keep employees knowledgeable and practiced in fire safety procedures. It is also important to be familiar with the escape routes from each facility, and fire escape routes and evacuation plans must be posted conspicuously (see **Figure 10–2**).

Classification of Fires

Fires are caused by the combination of fuel, oxygen, heat, and a specific chain reaction. There are five general classifications of fires, according to the National Fire Protection Association (NFPA) (see **Figure 10–3**). This figure explains what each classification means.

Emergency Response to Possible Fire

When a fire or explosion occurs, healthcare workers should practice the RACE system of steps. **RACE: Rescue Alert Confine Extinguish** is a system that provides the best and quickest correct reactions to a fire or explosion (see **Figure 10–4**).

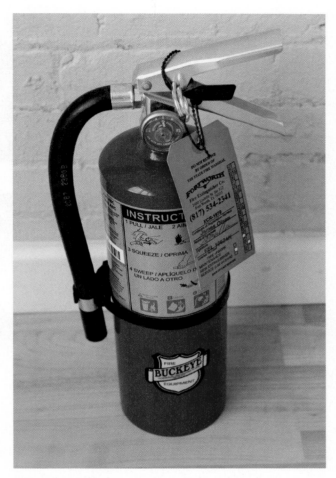

Figure 10–1 Fire extinguisher.

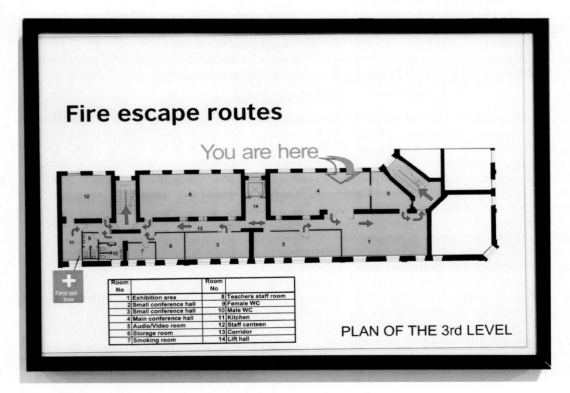

Figure 10–2 A posted fire escape route/evacuation plan mounted on a wall.

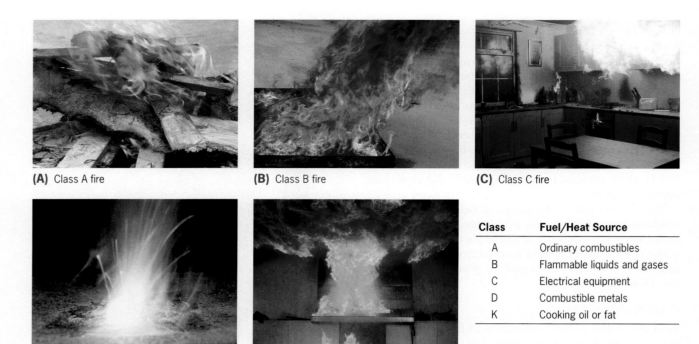

(A) Class A fire

(B) Class B fire

(C) Class C fire

(D) Class D fire

(E) Class K fire

Class	Fuel/Heat Source
A	Ordinary combustibles
B	Flammable liquids and gases
C	Electrical equipment
D	Combustible metals
K	Cooking oil or fat

Figure 10–3 Classification of fires.

It is important in these situations to NOT do the following:

- Block entrances
- Reenter the building
- Panic
- Run

When a fire is likely to block exits or is very large, you should leave the area immediately by taking the stairs, not the elevator. When clothing catches on fire, you should drop to the ground and roll (preferably in a fire blanket) to smother the flames. When there is a lot of smoke, you may have to crawl to an exit because breathing will be easier at floor level. Breathing through a wet towel also helps to avoid smoke inhalation.

Electrical Hazards

Electrical equipment can cause shocks as well as electrical fires. Employees should know where circuit breaker boxes are located in the facility. Steps that can be taken to practice good electrical safety include the following:

- Do not use frayed power cords.
- Avoid using poorly working switches and thermostats.
- Unplug all equipment prior to performing any maintenance.
- Unplug and then dry any equipment that has come into contact with any liquids.
- Avoid opening any equipment with an electrical caution warning.
- Avoid the use of extension cords.
- Avoid contacting any electrical equipment while collecting blood.
- Make sure to use *three-prong* (grounded) plugs for all equipment.

When an electrical accident or shock occurs, you should do the following:

- Shut off the electrical power source.

- If you cannot do this, use a nonconductive substance or fabric to carefully remove the electrical contact from the victim.
- Never touch the victim while he or she is in contact with an electrical source, or else you will also be electrocuted.
- Call for medical assistance.
- After checking reveals that the victim's pulse and respirations are absent, begin **cardiopulmonary resuscitation (CPR)** immediately.
- Do not move the victim.
- Place a fire blanket or warm clothing over the victim until medical help arrives.

Mechanical Hazards

Mechanical hazards may occur because of the use of laboratory equipment. Special care should be used when you are working with equipment that has moving parts, such as a **centrifuge** (see **Figure 10–5**), or those pieces of equipment that rely on high pressure (such as an *autoclave*). Those working in the clinical laboratory must become very proficient in working with centrifuges and the parts that they contain. The "carriers" for blood specimens must be correctly in place prior to use so that they do not swing out of the holding disks. Correctly sized heads and cups must be used, and tubes must be balanced correctly. Incorrect use of a centrifuge may result in the breaking of blood specimen tubes and potential exposure to blood-borne pathogens. Centrifuges must be checked on a regular preventive maintenance schedule.

Chemical Hazards

The clinical laboratory is home to chemicals that are **caustic**, flammable, **carcinogenic**, poisonous, and **teratogenic**. Exposure to any of these chemicals may be through inhalation, direct absorption through the skin, entry through a

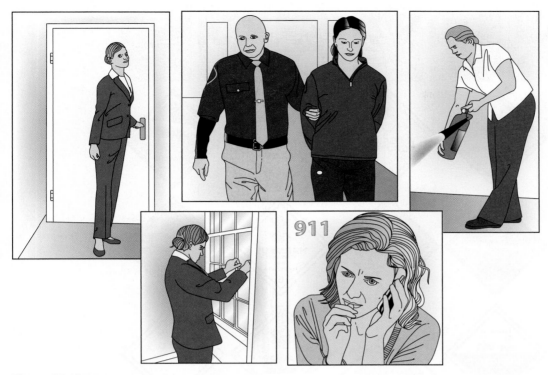

Figure 10–4 RACE: Rescue Alert Confine Extinguish.

mucous membrane, ingestion, or entry through a break in the skin. OSHA maintains regulatory standards directed at minimizing occupational exposure to hazardous chemicals in laboratories. Chemical safety labels are vital in providing employees with information about the potential hazards of every chemical in the workplace (see **Figure 10–6**). Proper labeling indicates the contents of containers as well as amounts and specific qualities of chemicals.

Employees must always carefully read labels before using any reagents. Labels for hazardous chemicals must give the following information:

- Warnings about corrosive qualities, potential explosions, poisons, flammability, gases, oxidation, radioactivity, and other hazards
- Explanations of these hazards
- Special precautions that can eliminate risks

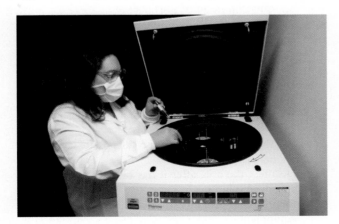

Figure 10–5 Centrifuge.

- Explanations of types of first aid treatment in the event of leaks, spills, or other exposure

Chemical Identification

The Occupational Safety and Health Administration regulates workplace safety, and it has amended the *Hazard Communication Standard* to include healthcare facilities. OSHA is a part of the Department of Labor. Its "Right to Know Law" is also known as the **HazCom** standard. This standard requires chemical manufacturers to supply **Material Safety Data Sheets (MSDSs)** for their chemicals. An MSDS is required for each chemical that bears a hazard warning label and lists general information (such as the chemical name, trade name, synonyms, manufacturer's name, address, and telephone number for emergencies). Each MSDS also contains information about protective measures that should be taken when working with a chemical (see **Figure 10–7**).

The National Fire Protection Association (NFPA) has developed a labeling system for hazardous chemicals, which uses a diamond-shaped symbol; quadrants colored red, yellow, white, and blue; and a hard rating scale (from 0 to 4) (see **Figure 10–8**). Red indicates a flammability hazard, yellow indicates an instability hazard, white indicates a specific hazard, and blue indicates a health hazard. Common laboratory chemicals stored in "squirt" bottles must be labeled using this system.

Important protective measures for chemical use include the following:

- Personal protective equipment (PPE) (see **Figure 10–9**)
- Protective clothing, including laboratory coats, safety glasses, face shields, gloves, and aprons
- Acid carriers (to transport acids or alkalis)

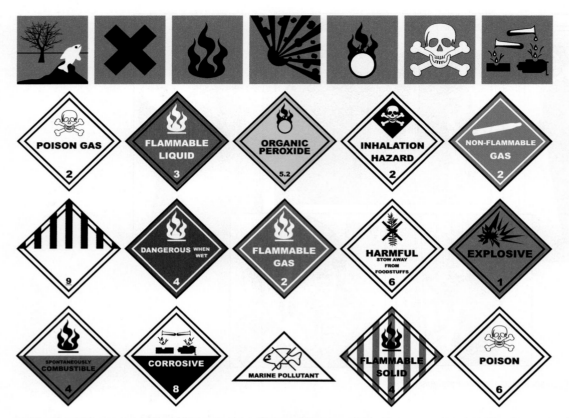

Figure 10–6 Hazardous Materials Warning Signs List Provided by the Department of Transportation (DOT).

- Chemical caution signs posted on entrance doors
- Storage of chemicals below eye level to reduce risks of danger or breakage due to reaching for them
- Proper labeling of all storage containers
- Avoiding the pouring of chemicals into previously used or dirty containers
- Storage of all explosive materials in explosion-proof or fireproof rooms away from other flammable materials

Disposal of Chemicals

Local and state regulations apply to all chemical disposal procedures. Healthcare workers must be familiar with which chemicals may be flushed into sanitary sewer systems and which must be disposed of otherwise. Policies and procedures for proper chemical disposal must always be followed.

Chemical Spill Cleanup

Spill cleanup kits should be readily available to begin prompt cleanup of spilled materials. These kits contain absorbents and neutralizers to clean up acids, alkalis, mercury, and other substances (see **Figure 10–10**). The safety department of a facility should be contacted immediately if there is a chemical spill.

For biohazard spills (such as blood), 10% bleach, made daily, is recommended to be used for cleanup because it will kill all pathogens. Approved disinfectants may also be used.

When a blood specimen is spilled, a phlebotomist must cover the spill with paper towels, pour 10% bleach solution on the towels, and wait for 15 min. Then, while wearing gloves, he or she should wipe up the spill, discarding the paper towels in an infectious waste container.

For extremely toxic spills, a specially trained hazardous cleanup team should be called in. When hazardous materials are spilled, take these general steps:

- Put on gloves and personal protective equipment. The CDC publishes guidelines in various formats demonstrating the correct methods of donning and removing PPE (for example, see www.cdc.gov/ncidod/dhqp/pdf/ppe/PPEslides6-29-04.ppt).
- Bring needed cleanup supplies and a hazardous waste container to the spill area.
- Use tongs or other equipment to pick up any broken glass.
- Dispose of broken glass in the approved fashion (following the policies and procedures manual).
- Wipe up the spill with the cleanup supplies from the spill kit.
- Use the biohazard container to dispose of used cleaning materials.
- Disinfect the area after it has been cleaned with an approved solution.
- Remove and discard gloves and personal protective equipment.
- Wash your hands thoroughly.

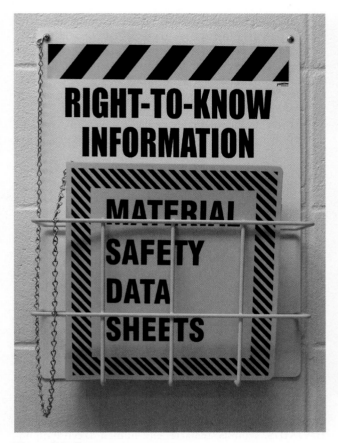

Figure 10-7 Material safety data sheet.

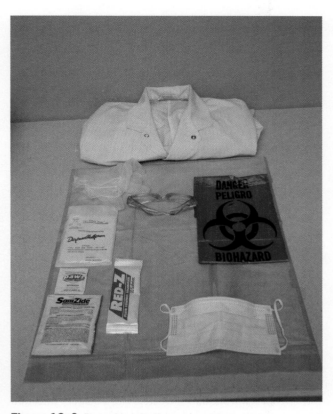

Figure 10-9 Personal protective equipment.

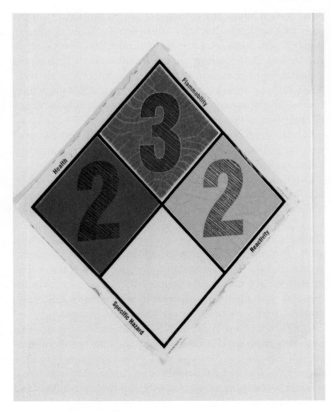

Figure 10-8 NFPA hazard identification symbol.

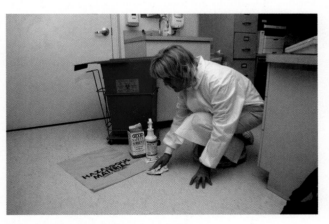

Figure 10-10 A common spill cleanup kit.

Patient Safety Related to Latex Products

Certain individuals are allergic to latex products, including latex gloves. Latex allergies may cause hives; skin rashes; irritation to the nose, eyes, or sinuses; and occasionally shock. If a phlebotomist is sensitive to latex gloves, he or she should ask for nonlatex gloves. Latex-free alternative products are widely available for those who have latex allergies. **Table 10-1** lists items often used in healthcare facilities that contain latex, although today many facilities are changing to latex-free.

Infection Control

Infection control is based on the policies and procedures of a hospital or other health facility. It is aimed at minimizing the risk of spreading nosocomial or community-acquired infections to patients or staff members. Laboratory specimens may contain *pathogens* (disease-causing microorganisms), to which phlebotomists and other personnel must not be exposed. To decrease the risk of disease transmission, general principles of hygiene and safety must be maintained. Infection control requires a variety of procedures, which include sanitization, ultrasonic cleaning, disinfection, autoclaving, and sterilization (which may be via chemicals, dry heat, gases, or microwaving). Hand washing also plays a very large role in infection control because it minimizes the transfer of pathogens between individuals as well as onto inanimate objects such as medical equipment.

Pathogens and Infections

An *infection* occurs when the body is invaded by pathogens. Pathogens may be bacteria, fungi, viruses, and parasites. *Normal flora* is a term used to describe naturally occurring nonpathogenic microorganisms on the skin and inside the body. It is possible for normal flora to sometimes enter parts of the body where they do not normally occur, causing a disease state to develop. An example of this occurs when *Escherichia coli* from the GI tract causes a bladder infection because of poor hygiene. A **communicable disease** may be caused when an infectious microorganism is transmitted via direct or indirect contact, or because of an airborne infection. Various precautions are used to stop the spread of disease, including the following:

- **Airborne precautions** were formerly called *respiratory isolation*. These are additional safety precautions applied to certain diseases such as tuberculosis. Phle-

botomists must wear appropriate personal protective equipment that relates to the patient's condition.
- **Contact precautions** are procedures that reduce the risk of transmission of serious disease through direct or indirect contact. Phlebotomists must wear appropriate personal protective equipment that relates to the patient's condition.
- **Droplet precautions** are procedures used to reduce the transmission of diseases via droplets that are expelled during sneezing, coughing, or talking; these diseases include meningitis, pertussis, pneumonia, and rubella. Phlebotomists must wear appropriate personal protective equipment that relates to the patient's condition.
- **Transmission-based precautions** are a set of procedures designed to prevent the communication of infectious diseases.
- **Universal precautions** are approaches to infection control designed to prevent the transmission of blood-borne diseases.
- **Protective (reverse) isolation** is a precautionary method designed to protect patients who may be highly susceptible to infections.

Patients in healthcare facilities are usually ill due to injuries or infections. These settings are havens for microorganisms of all types carried in by patients, healthcare providers, and visitors. A **blood-borne pathogen (BBP)** is any infectious microorganism present in blood or other body fluids and tissues. BBPs commonly cause various forms of hepatitis, HIV/AIDS, syphilis, malaria, and human T-cell lymphotrophic virus (HTLV).

Nosocomial Infections

Nosocomial infections are acquired by patients after admission to healthcare facilities. Between 1.75 and 3 million patients will contract a nosocomial infection every year in the United States, out of about 35 million institutionalized patients. Approximately 80,000 of these infections are fatal. The CDC and other organizations have mandated guidelines for the development of **infection control programs** to reduce the numbers of these infections. Approximately 5% of all hospitalized patients in the United States develop some type of nosocomial infection. The most common type of nosocomial infection is a urinary tract infection.

An infection that a healthcare worker catches would not be considered a nosocomial infection. However, it may become a source of nosocomial infection in patients. Nosocomial infections are usually symptomatic. Managers of healthcare facilities are encouraged to develop these programs, which stress the concepts of **asepsis**, education, **isolation procedures**, and the management of all types of infections. The **intensive care unit (ICU)** is a specialized treatment area for critically ill patients, those needing additional monitoring, and those who are more susceptible to infections.

The CDC is a part of the U.S. Public Health Service and primarily oversees the investigation and control of communicable diseases. It provides guidelines that protect healthcare workers as well as patients from contracting infections. **Aseptic techniques** are the mainstays of these guidelines and include the following:

Table 10–1 Products Containing Latex

Medical Equipment	Medical Supplies	Personal Protective Equipment	Office Supplies
Blood pressure cuffs	Condom-style urinary collection devices	Gloves	Adhesive tape
Breathing circuits	Enema tubing tips	Goggles	Erasers
Disposable gloves	Injection ports	Rubber aprons	Rubber bands
IV tubing	Rubber tops of stoppers on multi-dose vials	Surgical masks	
Oral and nasal airways	Urinary catheters		
Stethoscopes	Wound drains		
Syringes			
Tourniquets			

- Following **standard precautions**
- Frequent hand washing and the use of alcohol-based hand rubs
- Using barrier garments and protective personal equipment
- Using proper cleaning solutions
- Using sterile procedures whenever necessary
- Utilizing proper waste management for contaminated materials

Aseptic techniques must be made part of the facility's standards of practice, and all workers should be familiar with all of these standards. Home healthcare workers have an even more complex set of standards due to the variables that may exist in every patient's home.

Chain of Infection

Infectious diseases are spread when certain specific factors occur. These factors, or "links," make up the **chain of infection**. Breaking the chain results in stopping the infectious process (see **Figure 10–11**).

Infectious Agent

The chain of infection begins with an infectious agent. There are five groups of potentially pathogenic microorganisms. These include bacteria, viruses, protozoa, fungi, and rickettsia. Infections cannot occur without the presence of an infectious microorganism. Therefore, the most important way to prevent the spread of disease is to use adequate infection control procedures. These include consistent hand washing, the proper use of **antiseptics**, and effective disinfection and sterilization methods.

Reservoir Host

A reservoir host is the second link in the chain of infection. Reservoirs may actually be people, animals, insects, food, water, or contaminated equipment. A reservoir host supplies nutrition for a pathogenic microorganism, which allows it to multiply. The pathogen will either cause infection in the host or exit from the host (via a vector, such as an insect) in numbers that are great enough to cause disease in another host. A **carrier** is an individual (host) with no overt disease who harbors infectious organisms.

Portal of Exit

A pathogen escapes a reservoir host via a portal of exit. This may include the mouth, nose, eyes, ears, intestines, urinary tract, open wounds, or the reproductive tract. The use of standard precautions helps to control the pathogen's ability to spread from one host to another. Standard precautions that help to control the spread of infection include latex gloves, masks, the correct disposal of contaminated items, proper wound care, and hand washing.

Mode of Transmission

After they exit a reservoir host via a portal of exit, pathogens spread by either direct or indirect transmission. Direct transmission occurs from contact with an infected person or with his or her bodily fluids. Indirect transmission occurs from droplets expelled into the air by coughing, sneezing, speaking, various vectors, contaminated food or drinks, and contact with **fomites** (objects that harbor infectious agents and can transmit infection). The transmission of pathogens may be

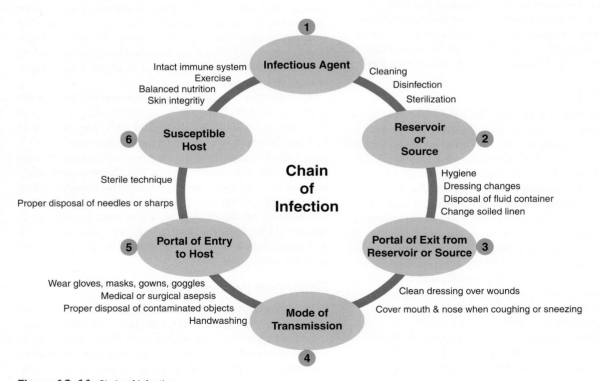

Figure 10–11 Chain of Infection.

decreased by proper sanitation, disinfection, and germicidal and sterilization procedures.

Invasive medical instruments may easily become contaminated, and they should be discarded (if "single-use") or sterilized after each use. Examples of such instruments include catheters, safety needles, and needle holders. Other types of medical supplies that also may become easily contaminated include tourniquets and linens. To reduce transmission via this mode, isolation procedures should be followed, sterile techniques utilized, gloves worn during equipment handling, and the use of common facilities or toys restricted.

Other vectors that may transmit infection include insects and rodents. Diseases transmitted via this mode include malaria, rabies, and plague. These vectors can transmit infectious microorganisms via the saliva and broken skin due to a bite.

Portal of Entry

The portal of entry is the method with which a pathogen gains entry into a new host. A portal of entry may be any of the same methods as the previously listed portals of exit. The first line of body defense against infection is an intact integumentary system (skin and related structures), which are mechanical barriers. Other body defenses against infection include cilia, tears, mucous membranes, and body fluid pH. The second line of body defense is the inflammatory reaction, which is a nonspecific response to any harmful agent. It includes phagocytosis of the material by neutrophils and macrophages. *Phagocytosis* (the ingestion and destruction of pathogens) occurs when *macrophages* engulf these microorganisms.

The third line, which depends on the immune system, consists of the development of an acquired immunity. The immune system produces *antibodies* to combat specific foreign substances (*antigens*) in a process known as *humoral immunity*. At the cellular level, *cell-mediated immunity* causes the destruction of pathogenic cells at the site of invasion.

Susceptible Host

A **susceptible host** is a person who lacks resistance to an agent and is vulnerable to contracting a disease. A microorganism may establish an infection after first overcoming surface barriers that include the skin, enzymes, and mucus. These barriers may be either antimicrobial or able to stop attachment of the microorganism to the host. Pathogens that succeed in penetrating these barriers may reach underlying tissues, but then may encounter both nonspecific resistance mechanisms and the specific immune response.

A *compromised host* is a person with impaired defense mechanisms, making susceptibility to infection more likely. The following characteristics influence a person's susceptibility to infections while also increasing the likelihood of more severe infections developing:

- Aging, which causes decreased immunity
- Concurrent disease, which increases susceptibility
- Heredity, which may predetermine susceptibility
- Immunization status, when people have not been fully vaccinated
- Lifestyle practices, such as smoking, drug use, multiple sex partners, and sharing needles
- Nutritional status, because those who are of normal weight for their height are less prone to infections
- Occupation, because some jobs expose workers to pathogens
- Stress, which lowers defense mechanisms against infection

Standard Precautions

The CDC mandates that standard precautions be followed regarding all specimen handling. This organization recommends that the workplace have an infection control plan in place, with specific work practice controls, the use of personal protective clothing and equipment, adequate training and education, readily available hepatitis B vaccinations, and medical intervention when an exposure occurs. Additional guidelines from the CLSI and CAP must also be followed, with the labeling of potential biohazards being extremely important.

Biologic Hazards

Biologic hazards are also known as biohazards. They may be either materials or situations that present an actual or potential risk of infection. Biohazards may cause infection during the collection, handling, transportation, or testing of specimens. Blood, body tissue biopsies, other body fluids, *exudates*, cultures, and smears may all be potentially infective. However, the CDC does not recommend standard precautions for urine unless it contains visible blood. Most clinical laboratories do, however, observe standard precautions for urine specimens. Pathogens can cause infection via aspiration, needlesticks, the uncapping of specimen tubes, accidents concerning centrifuges and other equipment, and the entry of pathogens through skin wounds. OSHA strictly regulates exposure to biologic hazards. Workplaces are required to have the Occupational Exposure to Blood-borne Pathogens program in place.

Biologic agents include human immunodeficiency virus (HIV), hepatitis B virus (HBV), hepatitis C virus (HCV), and the tubercle bacillus. HIV, HBV, and HCV are transmitted by blood infected with these viruses. Tuberculosis (TB) is transmitted by contact with respiratory secretions infected with *Mycobacterium tuberculosis*. The Occupational Safety and Health Administration requires that healthcare workers be tested in varying time periods for tuberculosis because it is such an infectious disease. These time periods are as follows: (1) for high-risk facilities, every 3 months; (2) for intermediate-risk facilites, every 6 months; (3) for low-risk facilities, every year.

Blood-borne Pathogens Standard

Clinical laboratory personnel must be aware of the constant threat of exposure to HIV, HBV, and HCV, which are all transmitted via exposure to blood and body fluids. According to OSHA, thousands of healthcare workers contract hepatitis B every year, and approximately 200 die as a result. Therefore, HBV is the most commonly occurring laboratory-acquired infection. Studies have indicated that HBV may survive up to 7 days in dried blood on work surfaces, equipment, and other objects. According to the CDC, hepatitis C (HCV) infection is the most widespread chronic blood-borne illness in the United States. The symptoms of HCV are similar to those of HBV infection. There is no vaccine currently available for HCV.

OSHA's Blood-borne Pathogens (BBP) Standard covers all employees who may be reasonably anticipated to come into contact with blood and other potentially infectious materials during their regular job duties. The BBP Standard was revised in 2001 to conform to the Needlestick Safety and Prevention Act that was passed by Congress and became law in 2000. The BBP Standard requires employers to have a written exposure control plan.

Federal law mandates enforcement of the BBP Standard, which requires implementation of work practice and engineering controls to prevent exposure incidents, special training, the availability and use of personal protective equipment, medical surveillance, and the availability of the HBV vaccination for all "at-risk" employees. The 2001 revision focused on the following four key areas:

- Modification of definitions that relate to engineering controls
- New requirements for record keeping
- Revision and updating of the exposure control plan
- Solicitation of input from employees about the selection of work practice and engineering controls

The most effective means of preventing infection is proper hand washing. You should always wash your hands when you enter a work area, when you leave a work area, before and after patient procedures, after contact with any body fluid (even if gloves are worn), before and after eating, and before and after using the lavatory.

The workplace should have a safety manual that details all safety practices and precautions, with clear explanations of procedures to be followed when a mishap occurs. Emergency numbers for the local hospitals, police, fire, and security personnel should be included, along with evacuation plans. This information should also be clearly posted near telephones and in strategic locations on the walls of the facility. There should be documentation for accidents, an accident log, and instructions on how to correctly document accidents.

Disposal of Hazardous Wastes

Hazardous wastes include all materials that have come into contact with blood or body fluids. Hazardous material is collected in various containers labeled with the *biohazard symbol* so that all employees are aware of the contents within (see **Figure 10–12**).

Soft materials such as gloves, dressings, and paper towels are deposited into red plastic bags that have been placed inside cardboard boxes bearing the biohazard symbol. They are leakproof and puncture-resistant. Sharps (including needles, scalpel blades, disposable syringes, and glass slides) are deposited into rigid containers that bear the biohazard symbol. These rigid containers are also usually red. **Figure 10–13** shows both types of biohazard containers.

Hazardous wastes are usually removed from the medical facility by companies that specialize in the removal and disposal of these wastes. Janitorial staff members should not empty hazardous waste containers. The changing of plastic hazardous waste bags, when needed, requires healthcare staff members to wear gloves, protective eyewear, and masks. These bags must be closed securely. If there is any chance that they may leak, they must be placed inside a second hazardous waste bag (a technique known as **double bagging**).

Safety Showers and the Eyewash Station

To protect against accidental chemical spills, safety showers should be in close proximity to areas where chemicals are used. Any body area that comes into contact with potentially harmful chemicals should be rinsed for at least 15 min after contaminated clothing is removed. If a chemical comes into contact with the eyes, the victim should use an eyewash station to rinse the eyes for at least 15 min, after removing any contact lenses (see **Figure 10–14**). The victim should avoid rubbing the eyes, which can cause further damage. In most cases, the victim should be taken to a nearby emergency room for treatment after the eyes have been rinsed properly.

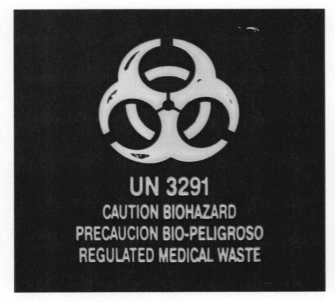

Figure 10–12 Biohazard symbol.

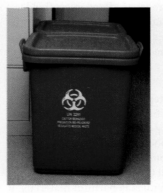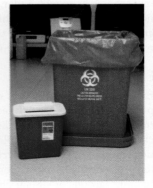

Figure 10–13 Biohazard containers.

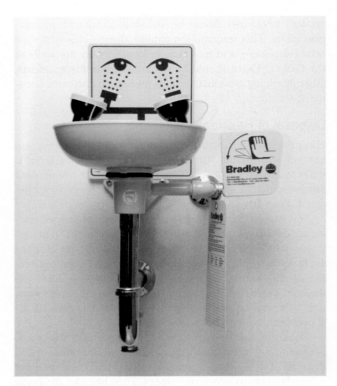

Figure 10–14 Eyewash station.

Sharps/Needlestick Injury Prevention

Sharps are defined as needles, scalpels, scissors, and other objects that may cause wounds or punctures while being handled. *Needlestick injuries* are accidental skin punctures that result from handling or accidentally coming into contact with needles. Steps to prevent needlestick injuries should always be taken because these injuries can be very dangerous. For example, if a needle has been used in a patient with a severe blood-borne infection and another person is stuck by the same needle, the possibility of contracting the infection is very real.

To minimize needlesticks, needles should never be recapped or broken. They should be discarded immediately into a leakproof, puncture-resistant biohazard container. When an injury does occur, the first step in controlling infection is to wash the hands and cover the injury. The injury should be documented and reported, and immediate treatment should be sought. Today, most needle adapters (holders) now have a safety cap attachment that encloses the needle after the draw. Proper use of these types of engineering control devices helps to prevent needlesticks.

Exposure Control

Exposure control consists of steps designed to minimize the potential for exposure to infectious agents. *Exposure potential* is defined as the possibility of contact with a hazardous chemical, safety hazard, or blood (or other potentially infectious material). An *exposure control plan* is defined as a written procedure for the treatment of any person who is exposed to biohazardous or similar chemically harmful materials. It is designed to minimize exposure risks to both infectious

materials and blood-borne diseases, and it must be written and updated as necessary. OSHA has regulations concerning hazards, including radioactive materials.

Prevention of Disease Transmission

The goal of medical asepsis is to prevent the reinfection of a specific patient, or cross-infection of other patients, healthcare workers, and other people who may be in close proximity to a patient. *Medical asepsis* is defined as the destruction of disease-causing organisms after they leave the body. OSHA's Blood-borne Pathogens Standard is designed to eliminate or minimize pathogens and involves disinfecting objects as soon as possible after they become contaminated.

Surgical asepsis is the destruction of disease-causing organisms before they enter the body. Any time the body's skin or tissues are invaded (including during surgery and via injections), surgical aseptic techniques are practiced. All drapes, gowns, gloves, and instruments must be *sterile*. Minor surgeries, injections, urinary catheterizations, and certain types of blood collection and biopsies are performed with surgical aseptic techniques.

Hand washing reduces skin bacteria via antimicrobial soaps, mechanical friction, and warm, running water. *Transient bacteria* on the skin are introduced by fomites and remain present for only a short time. *Resident bacteria* are found under fingernails, in hair follicles, in sebaceous gland openings, and in deeper skin layers. Thorough hand washing aids in reducing the numbers of transient bacteria and helps to prevent them from becoming resident bacteria.

As long as the skin and mucous membranes are intact, medical asepsis can be practiced for most noninvasive procedures. Instruments and objects used during medical aseptic procedures must always be decontaminated or sterilized before being used on a different patient. Medical aseptic procedures (including the wearing of gowns and masks) are not actually sterile, but they help to protect first the healthcare worker and then the patient.

Hand Washing

Correct hand washing technique is critical in minimizing disease transmission. Hands should be washed *before* and *after* each patient is examined or treated. An extended scrub is not required each time, but the first period of hand washing in the morning should always last for at least 20 s to 2 min, and each time a good antimicrobial soap with chlorhexidine should be used. Also, a water-soluble solution may be rubbed into the hands after washing and drying are completed, to reduce any cracking or chapping of the skin, which interrupts skin integrity and greatly increases the potential for disease transmission.

During hand washing, the water should be warm—not hot or cold. Warm water is less likely to cause chapping of the skin. Proper friction should be used, with all surfaces of the hands and wrists being scrubbed (see **Figure 10–15A through D**). Both upper and lower portions of each fingernail should also be scrubbed. Always remember to remove all jewelry before hand washing. The hands should be positioned with the fingertips downward during hand washing

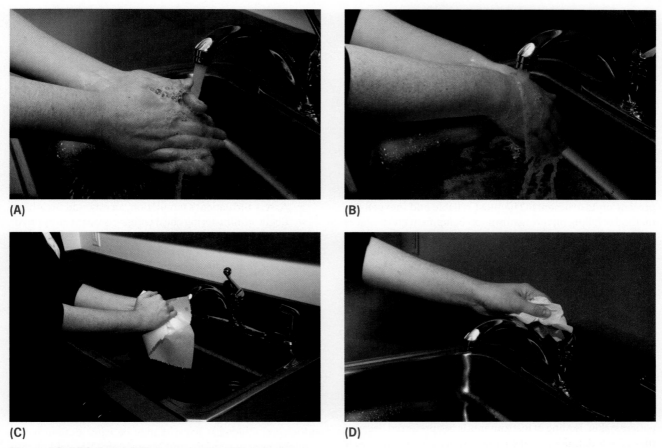

(A)   **(B)**

(C)   **(D)**

Figure 10–15A through D Proper hand washing procedure.

so that the water washes away debris from the wrists down toward the fingertips.

Antiseptic hand washing protects the healthcare worker from infection and prevents cross-contamination of microorganisms from one patient to another. The hands should also be washed *in between* handling different specimens, *before and after* going to the restroom, *after* any contact with potentially contaminated objects, *before* beginning work, *after* finishing work, as well as *before and after* eating. Alcohol handrubs may also help to cleanse the hands, but should not be the preferred method above antiseptic hand washing. Antimicrobial wipes such as towelettes are also not preferred over antiseptic hand washing. Note that hand washing should occur *after* removing the gloves, even if the hands were not in contact with visible body fluids.

Sanitization

Sanitization decreases the amount of microorganisms on instruments and other items to safe levels. It removes debris such as blood and other body fluids, which means that later disinfection methods can penetrate all surfaces of each instrument fully and completely. When performing sanitization, individuals should wear appropriately protective gloves to prevent possible personal contamination. Sanitization should be completed immediately after using instruments in a separate area designed for the process, in order to minimize

potential cross-contamination. If complete sanitization cannot be performed immediately, used items should be rinsed under cold water and then placed in a special detergent solution that has low levels of suds, is rust-inhibiting, and contains enzymes that attack microorganisms.

Blood and other substances should never be allowed to coagulate or dry on instruments. When sanitization may be completed, first drain off the soaking solution and rinse each instrument again in cold, running water, separating the sharper instruments from others. Thicker gloves should be worn when cleaning sharper instruments. All hinges should be opened, and small scrub brushes should be used to scrub ratchets and serrations. The instruments should then be rinsed in hot water and examined for proper functioning before being disinfected or sterilized. Towels should be used to hand-dry them to prevent spotting. Sanitization should never be done carelessly or overlooked. New, disposable instruments are becoming more popular because they minimize the need for sanitization, disinfection, and sterilization.

Ultrasonic sanitization utilizes sound waves and an ultrasonic bath of cleaner and water. The sound waves vibrate the solution, loosening attached materials. Ultrasonic cleaners do not damage any instruments, regardless of how delicate they are, and they minimize potential sharps injuries because there is little handling required. Current phlebotomy practice utilizes nearly completely disposable equipment—therefore, sanitization and other methods of cleaning equipment apply only to nondisposable equipment. Most phlebotomists do not deal with sanitization processes unless they are specially trained in a facility-specific protocol.

Disinfection

Disinfection is the process of killing or inactivating pathogenic microorganisms. However, it is not always effective against certain viruses, spores, and the bacilli that cause tuberculosis. **Disinfectants** may kill microorganisms very quickly, but often are harmful to instruments and should not be used on human skin. Antiseptics are designed for cleansing the skin. There are certain less damaging chemicals available, but they require many hours of immersion to kill all microorganisms present on instruments. The most reliable and inexpensive method of killing microorganisms on equipment and surfaces is 1:10 bleach, made daily, which also can be used for soaking reusable items before sanitizing them. Bleach solution is effective for the disinfection of surfaces that have come into contact with viruses (including HIV).

Disinfection is difficult to verify even when manufacturers' directions are followed. It may be inaccurate due to incomplete sanitization, poor drying of sanitized instruments, changes in concentrations of solutions due to evaporation, expiration of solutions' effectiveness, improper preparation or mixing of solutions, and improper storage techniques. Although alcohol is the most widely used antiseptic solution, it is not the most effective. Povidone-iodine solution is an example of an effective antiseptic that is safe to use on patients' skin. Boiling of instruments is not preferred because many bacterial spores and viruses can survive the process. It also takes at least 15 min of full boiling to achieve adequate disinfection.

Sterilization

Sterilization is the destruction of all microorganisms. It is essential for surgical asepsis, and it should be done in a specific area designed for this process. One part of the sterilization area should be used for receiving contaminated materials, and it should have a sink along with receiving basins, brushes, cleaning agents, autoclave wrapping paper, sterilizer envelopes and tape, disposable gloves, sterilizer indicators, and biohazard waste containers. The other part of the sterilization area should be used for receiving sterile items after they have been removed from the autoclave. Sterile packs should be stored inside clear plastic bags. Both parts of the sterilization area should be totally clean and organized.

Decontamination

OSHA uses the term *decontamination* to describe the use of physical or chemical means of removing, inactivating, or destroying blood-borne pathogens. Decontamination frees a person or object of contaminating substances. It is also sometimes referred to as the *neutralization* of contaminants. It may not eliminate microorganisms, but it is a necessary step that precedes disinfection or sterilization.

Cardiopulmonary Resuscitation

Cardiopulmonary resuscitation, or CPR, must be a skill of all allied health professionals, including phlebotomists. For example, if a patient were to have a heart attack, or experience another emergency situation, and the phlebotomist was the only person closeby, he or she must be able to perform CPR, at least until other healthcare practitioners can arrive.

To be effective, CPR must be correctly administered quickly. Tissue **anoxia** for more than 4 to 6 min can cause irreversible brain damage or death. The steps involved in CPR are as follows:

- Ascertain that the patient is unresponsive.
- Call for help.
- Note the exact time of collapse.
- Position the patient horizontally on the floor or a hard surface.
- Assess the patient's circulation, airway, and breathing.
- Begin administering chest compressions at an approximate rate of 100 per minute; each compression should be at least 1½ to 2 in deep.
- After 1 min, check the vital signs of the patient; if there are no vital signs, continue chest compressions until help arrives.

Summary

Safety may be compromised by physical hazards, which include fire, electrical, and mechanical hazards. Fires are caused by fuel, oxygen, heat, and a specific chain reaction. Electrical equipment can cause shocks as well as electrical fires. To avoid mechanical hazards, special care should be taken when working with equipment such as centrifuges or autoclaves. Chemical hazards may be caustic, flammable, carcinogenic, poisonous, and teratogenic. To avoid chemical hazards, employees should always carefully read chemical labels prior to use. OSHA's Hazard Communication Standard requires the use of Material Safety Data Sheets (MSDSs) to protect employees from the effects of chemicals and provide information about what to do if exposure occurs.

Biologic hazards are also known as biohazards. They may cause infection during the collection, handling, transportation, or testing of specimens. Standard precautions should be followed to limit risk of exposure to potentially infectious materials. Proper hand washing is the most effective means of preventing infection. Safety showers and eyewash stations should be in close proximity to areas where employees work with hazardous chemicals. When a chemical spill occurs, spill cleanup kits are used to begin prompt cleanup, although for extremely large or hazardous spills, specially trained cleanup firms should be called in.

Infections occur when the body is invaded by pathogens. A blood-borne pathogen is any infectious microorganism present in blood or other body fluids and tissues. Patients acquire nosocomial infections after admission to healthcare facilities. The chain of infection includes a **source, mode of transmission,** and susceptible host. Sharp instruments such as needles may transmit infection because they can come into direct contact with the skin of healthcare workers and other people. The transmission of infectious diseases may be reduced by both medical and surgical asepsis. Correct hand washing is critical as the basis for asepsis. Sanitization decreases the amounts of microorganisms on equipment and other objects to safe levels. Disinfection is the process of killing or inactivating pathogens. Sterilization is the destruction of all microorganisms.

CRITICAL THINKING

While a phlebotomist was carrying some blood sample collection tubes, one dropped on the floor and broke. She put on heavy-duty work gloves to clean up the spill.

1. What is the first step she should take to clean up this spill?
2. Which chemical substance is recommended for cleaning up blood spills? Why?

WEBSITES

http://esfi.org/

http://health.mo.gov/training/epi/Mod2StudentOutline.pdf

http://www.cdc.gov/ncidod/dhqp/

http://www.cdc.gov/ncidod/dhqp/pdf/ppe/PPEslides6-29-04.ppt

http://www.cdc.gov/niosh/topics/chemical-safety/
http://www.healthline.com/galecontent/nosocomial-infections

http://www.infectioncontroltoday.com/articles/2002/07/breaking-the-chain-of-infection.aspx

http://www.isips.org/

http://www.osha.gov/SLTC/firesafety/index.html

http://web.princeton.edu/sites/ehs/emergency/spills.htm

REVIEW QUESTIONS

Multiple Choice

1. The CDC does not recommend standard precautions for which of the following body fluids if the fluid does not contain visible blood?
   A. cerebrospinal fluid
   B. urine
   C. synovial fluid
   D. pleural fluid
2. When blood spills on a laboratory table, the most appropriate procedure for cleaning up the spill is to
   A. wipe up the spill with soapy cloth towels and rinse the table thoroughly with warm water
   B. spray the spill with a strong detergent and allow the table to dry
   C. wipe up the spill with paper towels, then spray disinfectant on the table for 10 min
   D. cover the spill with paper towels, wait 15 min, then wipe up the spill while wearing gloves
3. The most important step in achieving asepsis is
   A. wearing gloves
   B. removing jewelry
   C. using surgical soap
   D. washing hands
4. Which of the following microorganisms is the main blood-borne hazard for a phlebotomist?

A. hepatitis B virus
B. human immunodeficiency virus
C. hepatitis E virus
D. cytomegaolvirus

5. Which of the following terms is used by OSHA to describe the use of physical or chemical means to remove, inactivate, or destroy blood-borne pathogens?
   A. sterilization
   B. disinfection
   C. decontamination
   D. sanitization
6. The destruction of pathogens by physical or chemical means is called
   A. disinfection
   B. sterilization
   C. sanitization
   D. asepsis
7. Which of the following is NOT classified as a physical hazard?
   A. fire
   B. a mechanical hazard
   C. body tissue biopsy
   D. an electrical hazard
8. OSHA is a part of which of the following departments?
   A. Department of Health
   B. Department of Justice
   C. Department of Labor
   D. Department of Safety
9. Universal precautions should be followed if the phlebotomist is exposed to which of the following?
   A. human body fluids
   B. chemical substances
   C. radioactive substances
   D. chemotherapy agents
10. A person who lacks resistance to an agent and is vulnerable to contracting a disease is referred to as a
    A. source of infection
    B. mode of transmission
    C. standard precaution
    D. susceptible host
11. Which of the following is an example of normal flora?
    A. *Tubercle bacilli*
    B. *Escherichia coli*
    C. *Bacillus anthracis*
    D. *Chlamydia trachomatis*
12. Which of the following is NOT included in the chain of infection?
    A. mode of transmission
    B. susceptible host
    C. portal of vein
    D. reservoir host
13. Which of the following is NOT an element needed for a fire to occur?
    A. oxygen
    B. carbon monoxide
    C. an ignition source
    D. sufficient heat to ignite a fire

14. The Blood-borne Pathogens Standard is primarily concerned with
    A. regulating the use of personal protective equipment
    B. mailing blood samples to the state laboratory
    C. taking blood samples from patients
    D. reducing the transmission of HIV, HBV, and HCV

15. An example of a mechanical hazard is
    A. a frayed wire
    B. a centrifuge
    C. wet electrical equipment
    D. a carcinogen

Phlebotomy Equipment

OUTLINE

Introduction
Types of Equipment
    Gloves
    Other Personal Protective Equipment
    Tourniquets
    Venoscopes
    Antiseptics
    Evacuated Tubes
    Needle Holders
    Additive and Nonadditive Tubes
    Anticoagulants
    Syringes
    Needles
    Butterfly Collection Systems
    Lancets
    Micropipettes
    Microcollection Tubes
    Gauze Pads
    Bandages
    Centrifuge
    Blood-Drawing Chair
    Infant Phlebotomy Station
    Specimen Collection Trays
    Sharps Containers
Needle Safety
Summary
Critical Thinking
Websites
Review Questions

OBJECTIVES

After studying this chapter, readers should be able to:

1. List the equipment needed for venipuncture.
2. Explain the purpose of a tourniquet.
3. Describe the various tube additives.
4. Compare a syringe and an evacuated tube.
5. Explain why OSHA requires needle holders to be "single-use."
6. Describe butterfly needles and the reasoning behind choosing them over an evacuated tube.
7. Describe containers that may be used to collect capillary blood.
8. Explain venoscopes.
9. Describe infant phlebotomy stations.
10. Explain specimen collection trays.

KEY TERMS

Additive: Any substance added intentionally or indirectly that becomes a part of the product.

Anticoagulants: Substances added to blood collection tubes to slow or stop coagulation of specimens.

Antiglycolytic agent: A substance that prevents glycolysis (the breakdown of glucose, which yields pyruvic acid and ATP); the most common antiglycolytic agent is sodium fluoride.

Benzalkonium chloride: A disinfectant and fungicide prepared in an aqueous solution in various strengths.

Blood-drawing chair: A special seat designed for phlebotomy procedures.

Butterfly needles: "Winged infusion sets," often used in phlebotomy for people who have either spasticity or thin "rolling" blood vessels that are difficult to access.

Chlorhexidine: An antimicrobial agent used as a surgical scrub, hand rinse, and topical antiseptic.

Clot activators: Substances added to blood collection tubes to speed coagulation of specimens.

Coagulation cascade: The series of steps beginning with activation of coagulation.

Evacuated tubes: Blood tubes that discharge or remove blood from blood vessels.

Gauge: The size of a needle's lumen.

Glycolysis: The breakdown of glucose into pyruvic acid and ATP.

KEY TERMS CONTINUED

Glycolytic inhibitor: A substance that stops the breakdown of glucose, such as bromopyruvic acid and dichloroacetic acid.

Hemolyze: To rupture the red blood cells.

Lancets: Small, extremely sharp-bladed instruments used for puncturing the skin, as used in capillary puncture.

Microhematocrit capillary tubes: Collection tubes used to measure the hematocrit (the proportion of blood volume occupied by red blood cells) in very small quantities.

Micropipettes: Very small, thin pipettes used to measure samples that range from less than 1 μL up to 1 mL.

Multiple-sample needles: Double-pointed needles that allow the drawing of multiple blood samples.

Needle holder: A translucent cylinder that is used to hold double-pointed needles and evacuated tubes.

Povidone-iodine: An antiseptic microbicide.

Sodium fluoride: An inorganic chemical compound commonly used as an antiglycolytic agent.

Thixotropic gel: A material that appears to be a solid until subjected to a disturbance such as centrifugation, whereupon it becomes a liquid.

Velcro: A brand name of fabric "hook and loop" fasteners; usually made of nylon and polyester; the hook side of the fabric presses onto the loop side to make a firm bond.

Venoscopes: Devices for locating veins for blood collection.

Introduction

Phlebotomy is primarily performed for diagnoses and to monitor patients' conditions. It requires highly developed procedures and equipment to keep patients as safe and comfortable as possible. The most common method of obtaining blood is by venipuncture, utilizing a needle to puncture a vein. Blood is collected into either a stoppered tube or a syringe. Equipment commonly used to collect blood includes double-pointed safety needles, evacuated tubes with stoppers, needle holders, sharps containers, syringes, *winged infusion sets* (**butterfly needles**), marking pens, tourniquets, alcohol swabs, *sterile gauze pads*, bandages, and gloves.

Types of Equipment

For the collection of blood for testing, there are several varieties of equipment. These include venipuncture, skin puncture, and arterial puncture equipment. *Venipuncture* is defined as "blood collection from a vein." Skin punctures are usually done from the fingers or from the heels. Related equipment includes vacuum tubes, safety-needle collection devices, lancets, tourniquets, cleansing supplies, labels, gloves, and special transport trays for blood specimens.

Gloves

Gloves for phlebotomy must be supplied by the employer and should include several types: hypoallergenic gloves, powderless gloves, and glove liners. Nitrile or vinyl gloves are now standard in most hospitals. The Occupational Safety and Health Administration (OSHA) requires that gloves always be worn during venipuncture procedures. It is permissible to palpate the arms to detect the locations of veins with the fingertips and then put on gloves for the cleansing of the site and the actual venipuncture. Note any distinguishing marks on the skin that will help to remember the exact venipuncture location. Never touch the prepared site except with the venipuncture needle device because the gloves themselves carry contaminants.

Other Personal Protective Equipment

Besides gloves, other types of personal protective equipment are used to create a barrier between blood or bodily fluids and employees. These types of equipment are sometimes called *barrier precautions*. They minimize the risk of exposure to blood and body fluids. Personal protective equipment helps to protect the skin and the mucous membranes. Examples of other personal equipment include gowns, laboratory coats, eye protection, face shields, and masks (see **Figure 11–1**). Eye protection, face shields, and masks protect against the splashing or splattering of blood, body fluids, and chemicals.

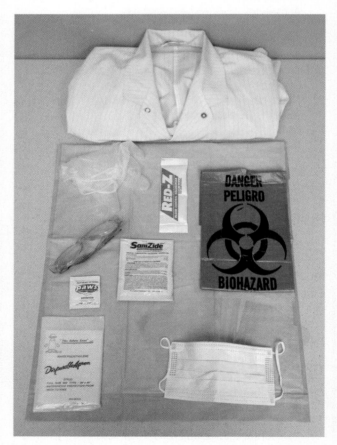

Figure 11–1 Examples of other personal equipment include gowns, laboratory coats, eye protection, face shields, and masks.

Eye wash stations are required by law in all facilities for emergencies, enabling employees to flush out their eyes or mucous membranes with water after exposures.

Tourniquets

Tourniquets are constricting bands applied to one or more limbs to restrict blood flow. Application of a tourniquet helps in locating the vein needed for venipuncture. A tourniquet prevents venous blood flow out of the site, causing the veins to bulge. Tourniquets are most commonly strips made of various materials that are tied around the upper arm tightly but not uncomfortably. When patients are allergic to latex, other types should be used, such as those with **Velcro** closures or nonlatex tourniquets.

Venoscopes

Venoscopes are devices for locating veins for blood collection. However, they are not commonly used. The most popular type of venoscope is the Venoscope II transilluminator, which allows a noninvasive procedure to visualize veins that may be difficult to find. It also prevents "vein rolling," which occurs when a vein moves or rolls away from the point of the needle.

Antiseptics

Antiseptics are used to clean venipuncture sites prior to the procedure. They usually contain rubbing alcohol (70% isopropyl alcohol). The most commonly used type is the prepackaged alcohol "prep pad," which is rubbed on the skin in a circular motion, and then the skin is allowed to dry. Alcohol simply inhibits the reproduction of bacteria that could possibly contaminate the blood sample. The alcohol should remain on the skin for between 30 and 60 s. For certain tests, instead of isopropyl alcohol, the following may be used: **benzalkonium chloride**, **povidone-iodine**, or sterile soap pads. For blood cultures, **chlorhexidine** gluconate is the preferred antibacterial. Blood cultures must be drawn into a specifically designed bottle or a sterile tube (see **Figure 11–2**).

Evacuated Tubes

Evacuated tubes are also known as Vacutainer® systems. They consist of evacuated tubes of various sizes that have color-coded tops, which indicate the tubes' contents (see **Table 11–1**). Tubes are available in regular glass, shatter-resistant glass, and plastic (which is preferred for safety reasons). The

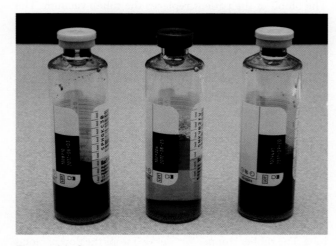

Figure 11–2 Blood cultures must be drawn into a specifically designed bottle or a sterile tube.

Table 11–1 Additive and Nonadditive Tubes

Stopper Color	Additives	Uses
Red (glass)	None	Blood bank, chemistry, serology/immunology
Red (plastic)	Clot activator	Chemistry
Yellow	Acid citrate dextrose (ACD)	Blood culture in blood bank/ immunohematology
Yellow	Sodium polyanethol sulfonate (SPS)	Blood culture in Microbiology
Light blue	Sodium citrate	Coagulation
Red/light gray (plastic)	Nonadditive	NA (discard tube only)
Red/black (tiger), gold, red/gold	Clot activator and gel separator	Chemistry
Green/gray, light green	Lithium heparin and gel separator	Chemistry
Green	Lithium heparin, sodium heparin	Chemistry
Lavender, pink	EDTA	Hematology, blood bank
Gray	Sodium fluoride and potassium oxalate, sodium fluoride and EDTA, sodium fluoride	Glucose determinations
Orange, gray/yellow	Thrombin	Trace element chemistry
Royal blue	None (red label), EDTA (lavender label), sodium heparin (green label)	Trace element chemistry
Tan (glass tube)	Sodium heparin	Chemistry
Tan (plastic)	EDTA	Chemistry

tube contents may include anticoagulants, **clot activators**, and/or **thixotropic gel**. The vacuum in the tube draws a measured amount of blood into it. Tube volumes range from 2 to 15 mL. The needle **gauge** must be matched to the size of the blood vessel. The larger the tube, the greater the vacuum and the more likely it is that the blood will **hemolyze** if a high-gauge needle with a small lumen is used.

Evacuated collection tubes may be any type of evacuated blood collection system that is similar to the patented Vacutainer brand. Tubes are selected based on the age of the patient, the amount of blood required, the test being performed, and the condition of the patient's veins. Evacuated systems consist of a collection tube that already has a vacuum inside, which is attached to a double-pointed needle. The blood of the patient replaces the tube's vacuum. The needles used in evacuated systems may include a safety device that is attached to the needle holder or needle itself (see **Figure 11–3**), or they may lack this device. One end of the double-pointed needle is longer than the other. The shorter end is covered by a protective rubber sheath to prevent blood leakage when the evacuated tubes are changed or removed.

The double-pointed needles used in these systems consist of a needle on each end with a screw hub close to the center (see **Figure 11–4**). One end of the needle pierces the patient's skin to enter the vein, while the other end pierces the rubber stopper on the evacuated tube, allowing the vacuum within to cause the blood to move from the vein into the tube.

When the tube is pushed into the holder, the rubber sleeve is compressed, exposing the needle so that it can enter the tube. The rubber stopper (or "sleeve") stops the flow of blood when the tube is removed from the **needle holder**. The needles used in evacuated systems are between 1 and 1½ in long, with gauge sizes usually being 21 to 23 in. The needles are coated with silicon to make puncture into the skin smoother. New types of these needles have a thinner steel wall, reducing the outside diameter and thus being less painful while still allowing the same flow rate of blood. All needles are

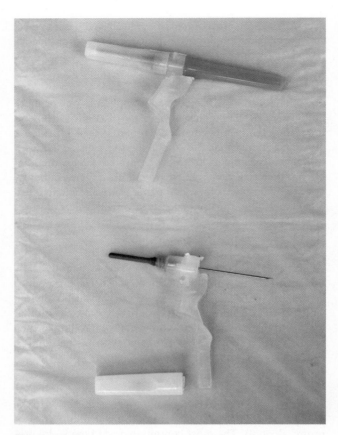

Figure 11–4 The double-pointed needle (removed from the syringe assembly) used in an evacuated system, with a rubber stopper on one end.

required to have some sort of safety engineering (usually a sheath to cover the needle after venipuncture). The needle holders used in evacuated systems are available in a large size for adults (see **Figure 11–5**) and a smaller size for children.

Needle Holders

When a double-pointed needle is used, it must be placed firmly into a needle holder (adapter) or tube holder. These are commonly translucent cylinders, with a ring that shows how far the tube may be pushed onto the needle without reducing the vacuum (see **Figure 11–6**). To reduce potential accidental needlesticks, OSHA requires that needle holders be disposed after a single use. In most cases, the entire needle and the holder are discarded simultaneously.

Additive and Nonadditive Tubes

Most evacuated tubes contain some type of **additive**, which is a substance placed inside the tube besides the tube stopper or coating. The type of additive determines whether the blood inside the tube will clot or not. Whole blood specimens are examples of unclotted blood specimens. When a tube contains a clot activator, the blood will clot, and the specimen requires centrifuging to separate the serum from the remainder of the specimen. The amount of additive placed in a tube is adjusted so that it will interact optimally with a specific amount of blood—the tube must not be underfilled

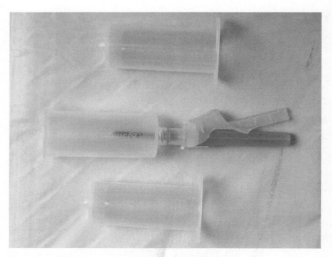

Figure 11–3 The needles used in evacuated systems may include a safety device that is attached to the needle holder or needle itself.

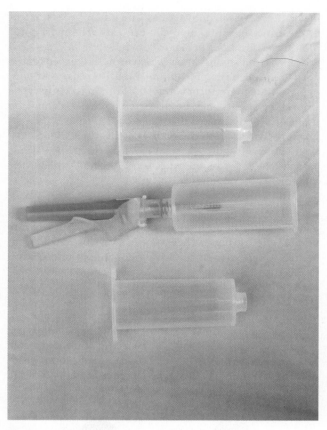

Figure 11–5 An adult evacuated system holder.

or overfilled. This is easily accomplished by allowing additive tubes to fill with blood until the vacuum is exhausted.

Almost all collection tubes contain some form of additive. If made of plastic, even serum tubes need an additive to promote clotting. Any nonadditive plastic tubes are used for clearing or discard purposes only. A few glass nonadditive tubes are available, but are generally being discontinued. Because collected blood will clot in a tube that does not have an additive, nonadditive tubes are used for serum samples. Some examples of nonadditive tubes include those used for serology/immunology, chemistry, and blood banks.

Expiration dates printed on the labels of tubes guarantee how long additives and evacuated tube vacuums are allowed to be used. This is based on proper tube handling and storage between 4 and 25°C. If a tube's integrity is compromised, test results may be compromised, or the tube may not fill properly.

Anticoagulants

When a blood sample is taken, blood clotting may be stopped by the presence of **anticoagulants** inside the sample tube. Common anticoagulants include citrates, ethylenediaminetetraacetic acid (EDTA), fluoride/oxalates, and heparin. Commonly used *citrates* include 3.2% or 3.8% *sodium citrate*, which is indicated as being present when the collection tube has a light blue stopper. Sodium citrate prevents coagulation by binding calcium in a nonionized form. The ratio of drawn blood in these

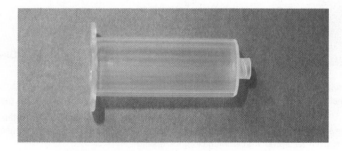

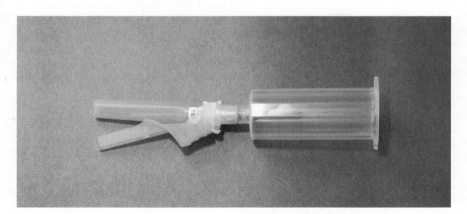

Figure 11–6 These are commonly used translucent cylinders, with a ring that shows how far the tube may be pushed onto the needle without reducing the vacuum.

tubes must be 9 parts blood to 1 part sodium citrate. Citrates are also found in yellow-stoppered tubes, which contain an additive called acid citrate dextrose (ACD).

EDTA is an anticoagulant present in lavender-stoppered tubes. It also acts by binding calcium to prevent coagulation. *Tripotassium EDTA* is used in glass tubes in a liquid form, while *Dipotassium EDTA* is used in plastic tubes in a dried powder form. Dipotassium EDTA is the recommended type because it preserves cell morphology for complete blood counts (CBCs) and differential blood smears and also provides stable microhematocrit results. It does not distort cell size or shape as other anticoagulants do.

Fluoride/oxalates such as *potassium oxalate*/**sodium fluoride** are present in gray-stoppered tubes. This combination of anticoagulants works by precipitating calcium in the blood to stop the **coagulation cascade**. In this mixture, sodium fluoride acts as a **glycolytic inhibitor** to preserve blood glucose. Any substance that prevents glycolysis (the breakdown of glucose, which yields pyruvic acid and ATP) is called an **antiglycolytic agent**. Sodium fluoride is an inorganic chemical compound commonly used as an antiglycolytic agent.

Heparin works in a different manner than most other anticoagulants. It is present in green-stoppered tubes. Heparin stops coagulation by neutralizing thrombin and the resultant stages that form a clot. Heparin occurs naturally

in very low levels in body tissues, and it has the least effect of the anticoagulants upon clinical tests. The most common forms are *lithium heparin* and *sodium heparin*, and the phlebotomist must know which form is required for the needed sample. The phlebotomist must not use a lithium heparin tube to perform a draw for lithium levels because laboratory results may be distorted. Heparin cannot be used for blood samples that are stored for more than 48 h before they are tested, because by this time, blood clotting will have begun. **Figure 11–7** lists the many various stopper colors for blood collection tubes and explains the ingredients they contain.

Syringes

Syringes come in both nondisposable glass types and disposable one-use types. They come in a variety of sizes, from 60 mL, to insulin syringes, to some that hold only 0.5 mL (see **Figure 11–8**). Some syringes are packaged with a needle attached (see **Figure 11–9**). The most commonly used syringes in phlebotomy are 10 mL.

The component parts of a syringe consist of a plunger, barrel, flange, and tip (see **Figure 11–10**). The *plunger* is a movable cylinder designed for insertion within the barrel. The *barrel* is the part that holds blood or medication, which is calibrated on its surface. The *flange* is at the end of the

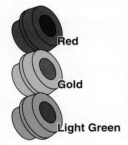 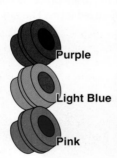 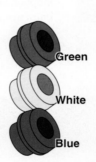 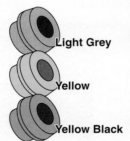 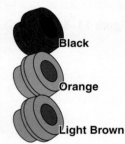

RED: No additive, blood clots, centrifugation is used to separate the serum; used for blood bank crossmatching, serology and immunology, and chemistries.

GOLD: No additive, this is a serum separator tube (SST) containing a gel on the bottom, which separates blood from serum during centrifugation, used for serology and immunology, and chemistries.

LIGHT GREEN: Is a plasma separating tube (PST) containing lithium heparin, which causes anticoagulation; the PST gel at the bottom separates the plasma, used for chemistries.

PURPLE: Contains EDTA, which removes calcium by forming calcium salts, used for blood bank crossmatching and hematology (CBC); This requires a full draw, and the tube must be inverted 8 times to prevent platelet clumping and clotting.

LIGHT BLUE: Contains sodium citrate, which removes calcium by forming calcium salts, used for protime and prothrombin time, which are coagulation tests; a full draw is required.

PINK: Contains potassium EDTA, which forms calcium salts, used for immunohematology.

GREEN: Contains lithium heparin or sodium heparin, which inactivates thromboplastin and thrombin; sodium heparin should be used for lithium level, and either sodium or lithium heparin can be used for ammonia level.

WHITE: Contains potassium EDTA, which forms calcium salts, and is used for molecular/PCF and bCNA testing.

DARK BLUE: Contains EDTA, and the tube is designed so that it does not contain any conatminating metals, used for toxicology and trace element testing.

LIGHT GRAY: Contains potassium oxalate and sodium fluoride; an antiglycolytic agents preserves glucose for up to 5 days, used for glucoses. It requires a full draw since a short draw may cause hemolysis.

YELLOW: Contains acid-citrate-dextrose (ACD), which inactivates complement, used for DNA studies, paternity tests, and HLA tissue typing.

YELLOW-BLACK: Contains a broth mixture, which preserves the viability of microorganisms, used for microbiology.

BLACK: Contains buffered sodium citrate, which removes calcium by forming calcium salts, used for Westergren Sedimentation Rate. It requires a full draw.

ORANGE: Contains thrombin, which quickly clots blood, used for STAT serum chemistries.

LIGHT BROWN: Contains sodium heparin, which inactivates thromboplastin and thrombin, and contains almost no lead; used for serum lead determination.

Figure 11–7 Illustrations and text showing various stopper colors for blood collection tubes and the ingredients they contain.

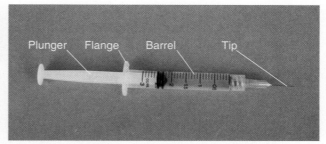

Figure 11–10 The component parts of a syringe.

barrel where the plunger is inserted. The *tip* is at the end of the barrel where the needle is attached.

Larger syringes have greater vacuum than smaller syringes. The correct size of syringe must be used because too large a size will cause greater vacuum than the vein can withstand, causing it to collapse. This occurs more often in patients with thinner, more fragile veins, such as the elderly and children. In general, syringes larger than 10 mL are not recommended. If more blood is required for sampling, a butterfly collection set should be used instead.

Needles

Needles are made in many lengths and widths (diameters), or gauges. The needle is actually a hollow metal tube with a sharp point that pierces the skin to draw blood or to deliver medications. Needles may be purchased separately, or the needle may be already attached to the syringe. Other options include syringes and needles that are separate but packaged together as a needle-syringe unit for specific use. **Multiple-sample needles** are double-pointed needles that allow the drawing of multiple blood samples.

The parts of a needle include the hub (where it attaches to the syringe), cannula (shaft), and bevel (the angled tip that allows for easy puncture into the vein) (see **Figure 11–11**). The lumen of the needle is the opening at its bevel end. The bevel should be extremely sharp, which allows it to puncture the vein with less pain. Silicon coating on the needle also helps it to be inserted more easily. The needle is attached by sliding the hub onto the syringe or screwing it into a threaded insert such as a *Luer lock*. The common lengths of needles remain between 1 and 1½ in. Needle gauges range from size 14, which has the largest lumen or opening, to size 31, which has the smallest lumen.

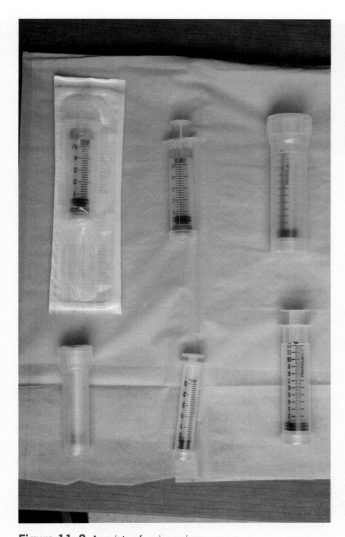

Figure 11–8 A variety of syringe sizes.

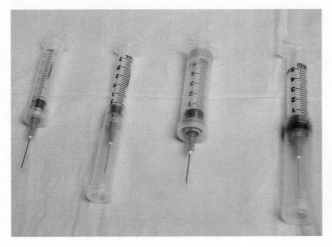

Figure 11–9 Syringes that are packaged with needles attached.

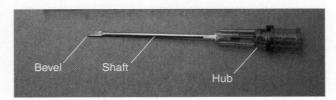

Figure 11–11 The component parts of a needle.

Most commonly, 21- to 23-gauge needles are used for venipuncture, with 22-gauge needles being used for children or adults with small blood vessels. When butterfly collection sets are required, 23-gauge needles are commonly used. However, 25-gauge needles are not used for venipuncture because of the potential of destruction of red blood cells. Large 16- or 18-gauge needles are used in blood banks to collect pints of blood for transfusion. This is done because the lumens of these needles are wide, which reduces the chance of hemolysis. **Table 11–2** summarizes common needle gauges and their uses.

The use of syringes now requires safety shields that cover the needles immediately after they are withdrawn from the body. These devices may be either additional syringe barrels that slide over the needle or devices that slide over the needle after it is used (see **Figure 11–12**).

An *activating safety device* is one that slides over the needle by pushing it forward with the thumb (see **Figure 11–13**).

Butterfly Collection Systems

For small veins, butterfly needles (winged infusion sets) are used (see **Figure 11–14**). These needles are usually 23 gauge in size, with needles ranging between ½ and ¾ in long, featuring a flexible plastic butterfly-shaped grip that is attached to a short amount of tubing. One end of the tubing is fitted into the syringe or the vacuum tube adapter. Syringes are often used because they allow the vacuum to be better controlled. These, or smaller evacuated tubes with less powerful vacuums, are preferred while using butterfly needles.

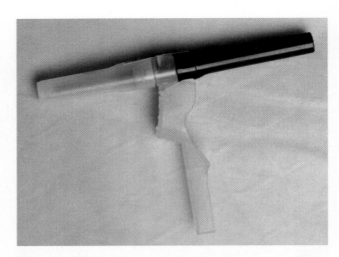

Figure 11–13 An activating safety device.

The needles used in these systems should also have safety devices that work after the procedure is complete. The tubing used is between 3 and 12 in long. The entire assembly should be discarded into a sharps container after the venipuncture is completed. The assembly should be held by the needle end, which is inserted into the sharps container first, as the remainder is allowed to drop into the container.

Butterfly collection systems are used for small veins, such as those on the back of the hand, the arm, or the foot. The plastic wings of the butterfly portion allow easy access, with the winged needle being inserted at only a 5° angle instead of the normal 15° angle used for other venipunctures. The

Table 11–2 Needle Gauges and Common Uses

Gauge	Use
25	Intramuscular injections
23	Butterfly or syringe collection
22	Syringe or evacuated system collection; preferred for small-veined patients such as children
21	Syringe or evacuated system collection
20	Syringe or evacuated system collection (not commonly used)
16–18	Blood collection or transfusion

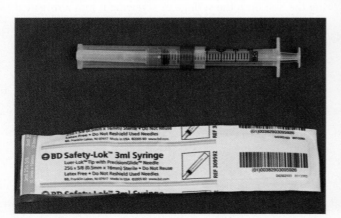

Figure 11–12 Two needles—one with the safety syringe unengaged, and one with it engaged.

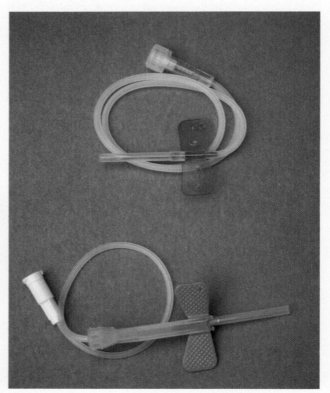

Figure 11–14 A winged infusion set attached to an evacuated tube holder with a Luer needle holder.

flexible tubing of these systems may move, but the needle can stay anchored into the vein. Vein collapse usually does not occur when these systems are used. They also allow the ability to begin drawing blood with a syringe and then follow up with an evacuated tube system.

Lancets

Lancets are microcollection devices used to make a puncture or cut into the skin through a capillary bed. The lancet must be sterile, and it should also have a controllable puncture depth. OSHA requires that lancets have retractable blades and/or locks that prevent their reuse, and therefore potential accidental punctures. When lancets are used, usually the fingers or heels of the feet are utilized. Many different skin *puncture lancets* are used in microcollection, with specific designs that allow a controllable depth of puncture. Lancets may consist of a blade or needle that may be used manually (see **Figure 11–15A**) or via a spring-loaded device. The spring-loaded type is preferred today (see **Figure 11–15B**). Lancets must be discarded in a sharps container.

A *laser lancet* is a reusable device that vaporizes water in the skin to make a small hole in the capillary bed. Because no sharp instrument is involved, there is no risk of accidental injury, and there is no "sharp" to discard. Although the device is reusable, single-use disposable inserts are utilized with it to prevent cross-contamination between patients. Spring-loaded microcollection devices quickly and easily puncture the capillary bed of the patient and then automatically withdraw the lancet up into the plastic body of the device. They are designed specifically for certain areas of the body and for certain ages of patients. Most microcollection equipment is intended for one-time use. They differ from home-use devices that are made for blood glucose monitoring because they are designed to draw more blood. The home use or "personal" laser lancets offer patients such as diabetics the ability to access capillary blood for regular self-testing without pain. **Table 11–3** lists recommendations for the types of lancet blades that should be used in specific applications.

Micropipettes

Disposable, calibrated **micropipettes** draw between 1 and 200 μL of blood so that it can be transferred to containers or certain solutions. Plastic or plastic-coated glass micropipettes are preferred over regular glass micropipettes. However, microcollection tubes are now replacing micropipettes in most facilities.

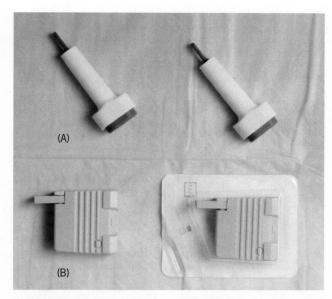

(A)

(B)

Figure 11–15 (A) Non-spring-loaded lancets and (B) spring-loaded lancets.

Microcollection Tubes

Microhematocrit capillary tubes are similar to calibrated micropipettes, but are designed for determining packed red blood cell volume. **Figure 11–16** shows various microcollection tubes.

For children and the elderly, smaller collection containers are commonly used. *Microtainer* tubes hold less than 1 mL (0.75 mL) of blood, and they may contain a variety of anticoagulants and additives. A microcollection container is sometimes called a *bullet* because of its size and shape. They are color-coded the same way as standard adult collection tubes.

Gauze Pads

Gauze pads are made with a transparent fabric of open weave and differing degrees of fineness. They are used for absorbent sponges, bandages, and dressings. Gauze pads may be sterilized and permeated by an antiseptic or lotion. There are three kinds of gauzes: absorbable gauze, absorbent gauze, and petrolatum gauze. In the clinical laboratory, absorbable gauzes are usually used, which may be sterile or nonsterile. For holding pressure over a venipuncture site, gauze or gauzelike pads are preferred rather than cotton balls. This is so because the

Table 11–3 Various Types of Lancets

Sizes	Uses	Blood Volume
28-gauge needle, 2.25-mm depth	Finger sticks	Single drop
23-gauge needle, 2.25-mm depth	Finger sticks, glucose test	Single drop
1- × 1.5-mm blade	Finger sticks, microhematocrit tube, or drop of blood for glucose or cholesterol test	Low blood flow
1.5- × 1.5-mm blade	Finger sticks, to fill a single Microtainer tube	Medium blood flow
2- × 1.5-mm blade	Finger sticks, to fill multiple Microtainer tubes	High blood flow

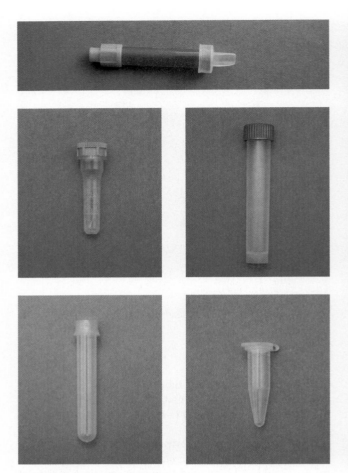

Figure 11–16 Various microcollection tubes.

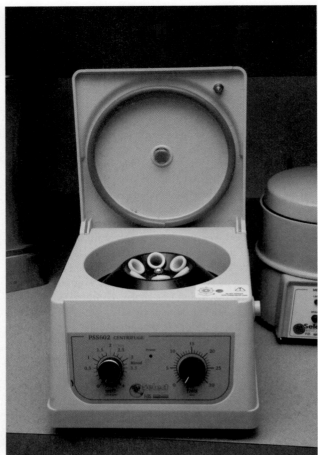

Figure 11–17 A centrifuge.

fibers from cotton, Dacron, or rayon balls tend to stick to the site and reinitiate bleeding when removed.

Bandages

After venipuncture, gauze pads are used to cover the puncture site. Cotton balls are not preferred because they tend to stick to wounds and can cause further bleeding when they are removed. After the patient has stopped bleeding, surgical tape is placed over the gauze. Although latex tape adheres better than other types, it may damage the skin of older patients or those with latex allergies. Bandages and tape should not be used on patients under 2 years of age, as they may be removed and are potential choking hazards. Bandage alternatives include such items as:

- Coflex® self-adherent bandaging tape
- Foam compression dressings
- Absorbent foam dressings
- Collagen wound dressings

Centrifuge

A type of equipment that is essential for processing specimens is a *centrifuge*. A centrifuge is a device for separating components of different densities contained in liquid by spinning them at high speeds. *Centrifugal force*, which is created by the spinning motion, causes the heavier components to move to one part of the container, leaving the lighter substances in another part. A centrifuge is shown in **Figure 11–17**.

For serum specimens, blood in an evacuated tube must be allowed to clot for 15 to 30 min before being loaded into a centrifuge (see **Figure 11–18**). Serum is then extracted from the specimen so that it can be sent for testing in a correctly labeled tube with a laboratory requisition form. Plasma specimens result due to the anticoagulant present in the vacuum tube, and care must be taken when removing the specimen from the centrifuge to prevent mixing the blood cells and the plasma. Centrifuges are also used to separate solid materials, such as crystals, casts, and cells from urine.

Centrifuges may be either bench-top or floor models, and some may be refrigerated. Centrifuges must be loaded correctly because they must be properly balanced to function. When it is not balanced, the centrifuge can vibrate to such a degree that it moves across a countertop, and it may even fall off. A centrifuge should never be used by anyone who has not been properly trained. Various sizes of tubes are used in centrifuges.

Blood-Drawing Chair

A variety of **blood-drawing chairs** are available that make phlebotomy safer and easier (see **Figure 11–19A** and **Figure 11–19B**). Some of these chairs recline and have adjustable armrests and/or leg extensions, neck pillows or supports, mounts for scales, hydraulic lifts, storage cabinets, and foot covers. When no blood-drawing chair is available, patients

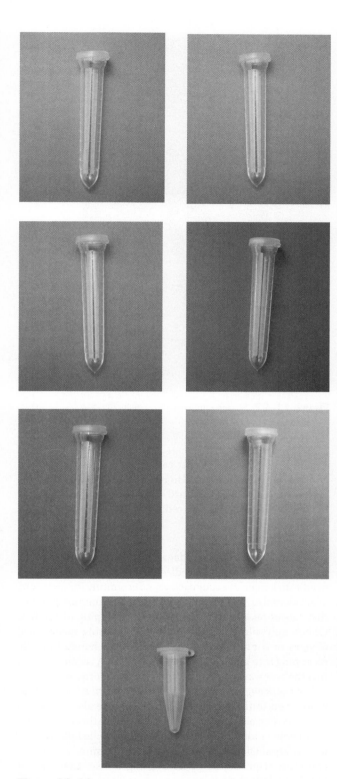

Figure 11–18 Various sizes of tubes used in centrifuges.

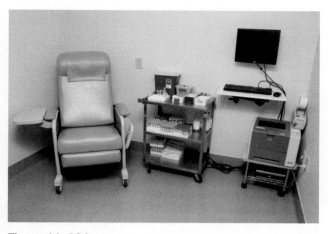

Figure 11–19A Blood-drawing chair.

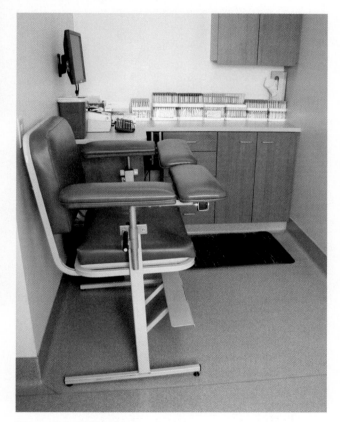

Figure 11–19B Blood-drawing chair.

can simply lie on examination tables, or sit in chairs without arms and wheels, while blood is collected. This is always a good idea to prevent the patient from fainting and falling because of the stress of the procedure.

Infant Phlebotomy Station

Infant phlebotomy stations are used to safely collect infant blood. These stations are wheeled so that they can be maneuvered into various areas at on- and off-site locations. Newborns and infants should be placed in a supine position on the infant phlebotomy station table to have their blood drawn. Older children (ages 3 to 8) should lie supine on a pediatric table in order to have their blood drawn (see **Figure 11–20**).

Specimen Collection Trays

Specimen collection trays are used for the collection of blood specimens (see **Figure 11–21**). Usually made of plastic that can be sterilized, these trays should include the types of equipment needed for the specific procedures to be performed in the facilities where they are kept. These trays

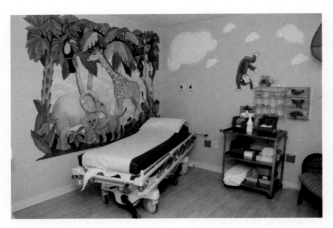

Figure 11–20 Pediatric table.

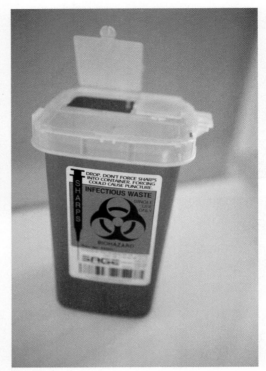

Figure 11–22 Sharps container.

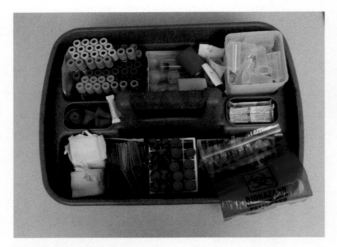

Figure 11–21 Specimen collection tray.

should be lockable, have tight seals to reduce blood-borne pathogen transference, and include the following:

- Antimicrobial hand gel or foam
- Biohazardous waste containers
- Chemicals such as iodine and isopropyl alcohol
- Disposable gloves
- Marking pens or pencils
- Microcollection blood serum and plasma separator tubes
- Microcollection capillary whole blood collectors
- Nonlatex tourniquets
- Pads or swabs with chlorhexidine
- Safety blood collection sets (with butterfly needles)
- Safety lancets for skin puncture
- Safety needles for vacuum tubes and syringes
- Safety syringes
- Sterile gauze pads and bandages
- Vacuum tubes with needed anticoagulants
- Vacuum tube safety holders
- Warming devices appropriate to the facility

Sharps Containers

OSHA requires that sharps containers be rigid, leakproof, puncture-resistant, and disposable (see **Figure 11–22**). They

should have locking lids that can be easily sealed when the containers are full. OSHA also requires that sharps containers be marked with a biohazard symbol, but does not require that all of the containers be red.

Needle Safety

Needle safety is required because it is relatively easy for phlebotomists to receive needlestick injuries. Nearly 800,000 needlestick injuries occur each year, accounting for up to 80% of accidental exposures to blood. The most common practice that causes needlestick injuries is the recapping of needles. OSHA only allows needle recapping by using mechanical devices or a one-handed technique—two-handed needle recapping is to be avoided at all costs. OSHA recently stated that the best way to prevent these types of injuries is to utilize a *sharp with engineered sharps injury protection* (SESIP) that is attached to the needle holder. SESIPs are also known as *safety needles*, eliminating the need to remove the needle from the needle holder, and to help shield the needle following its use. Safety shields used for needles must be simply designed and must require little or no training to use. Examples of SESIPs include the following:

- Self-sheathing safety devices with sliding needle shields attached to disposable syringes and vacuum tube holders (see **Figure 11–23**)
- Retractable safety devices that retract the needles after use into the syringe or needle holder (see **Figure 11–24**)
- Needle-blunting safety mechanisms, wherein a blunt tube is moved through the needle to cover its sharp point after use

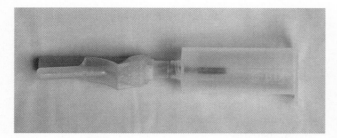

Figure 11–23 A self-sheathing device.

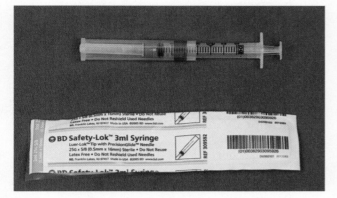

Figure 11–24 A retractable safety device.

- Hinged (sliding safety) mechanisms, which are manually engaged after use (see **Figure 11–25**)

The following steps are designed to protect phlebotomists and other personnel from needlestick injuries:

- Dispose of used needles immediately in appropriate sharps disposal containers.
- Follow recommended infection prevention practices (including hepatitis B vaccinations).
- Plan for safe handling and disposal before starting any procedure requiring the use of needles.
- Do not recap needles.
- Report all needlestick and sharps-related injuries immediately to ensure that appropriate follow-up care is given.
- Help your employer to evaluate and select devices with safety features.
- Tell your employer about hazards that you observe in your work environment.
- Participate in blood-borne pathogen training.
- Use devices that have safety features, as provided by your employer.
- Avoid using needles when safe and effective alternatives are available.

OSHA requires employers to maintain sharps injury logs to record injuries from contaminated sharps. These logs must contain complete information about the device involved, the location where the injuries occurred, and a full explanation of the incident, keeping employee confidentiality in mind.

Summary

Phlebotomists must be familiar with all types of laboratory equipment, not just the equipment that they will utilize for venipuncture. Venipuncture equipment includes double-

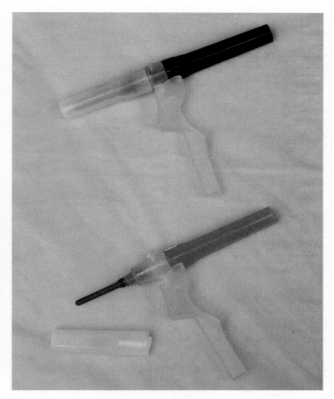

Figure 11–25 A hinged (sliding safety) device.

pointed safety needles, evacuated collection tubes, needle holders or syringes that are fitted with safety needles, tourniquets, alcohol prep pads, gauze or cotton, sterile bandages, gloves, and biohazard disposal containers. Needles used for venipuncture consist of a bevel, shaft, and a hub that is attached to a syringe. The gauge of a needle to be used for various types of blood collection is very important.

Syringes are used more often for blood collection from elderly patients and children because their veins tend to be more fragile. Collection tubes are color-coded based on the anticoagulants they contain. Different sizes of collection tubes exist for adults and for children. Microcollection equipment is used to collect capillary blood instead of venal blood. There are four common types of anticoagulants: citrates, EDTA, fluoride/oxalates, and heparin. Needle safety is designed to minimize accidental exposure to sharps and potential needlestick injuries.

CRITICAL THINKING

Greg is a phlebotomist who must draw blood from an elderly patient, and the physician has ordered that three separate tubes be filled. The patient's veins in her arms are sclerotic.

1. How should Greg draw blood from this patient?
2. What equipment will help him prevent her veins from rolling during the procedure?

WEBSITES

http://www.austincc.edu/mlt/phb_tubes

http://www.bd.com/vacutainer/pdfs/plus_plastic_tubes_wallchart_tubeguide_VS5229.pdf

http://www.clsi.org

http://www.medscape.com/viewarticle/509098

http://www.ncbi.nlm.nih.gov/pmc/articles/PMC130950/

http://www.osha.gov/SLTC/bloodbornepathogens/index
.html

http://www.phlebotomy.com

http://www.phlebotomycert.com/traing_components
.htm

http://www.science.smith.edu/departments/Biology/Bio231/
glycolysis.html

http://www.tpub.com/content/armymedical/MD0853/
MD08530077.htm

REVIEW QUESTIONS

Multiple Choice

1. Which device might be used to collect blood from fragile veins?
   A. a finger stick lancet
   B. a butterfly needle
   C. a Vacutainer system
   D. an automatic puncturing device

2. The color code for an evacuation tube that does not contain an additive is
   A. red
   B. gray
   C. lavender
   D. yellow

3. Which of the following instruments is used to examine the vein for a venipuncture?
   A. gloves
   B. a tourniquet
   C. a blood-drawing chair
   D. a specimen collection tray

4. Which of the following is the most common gauge of needle used for phlebotomy in adults?
   A. 25
   B. 23
   C. 19
   D. 16

5. A light blue stopper indicates that a collection tube
   A. is to be used only for capillary puncture
   B. contains the additive EDTA
   C. contains an antiseptic
   D. contains sodium citrate

6. The color code for an evacuation tube that does not contain an additive is
   A. gray
   B. red
   C. lavender
   D. red and black

7. Which vacuum tube stopper color is used to test for septicemia?
   A. yellow
   B. red
   C. black
   D. blue

8. The hollow channel inside the hypodermic needle is called the
   A. shaft
   B. hub
   C. lumen
   D. bevel

9. Which anticoagulants inhibit the conversion of pro-thrombin to thrombin?
   A. heparin
   B. oxalate
   C. sodium citrate
   D. EDTA

10. Which of the following needles has the smallest "bore"?
    A. 18
    B. 21
    C. 23
    D. 25

11. Which anticoagulant cannot be used for blood samples that are stored for more than 48 h before they are tested?
    A. potassium oxalate
    B. EDTA
    C. heparin
    D. citrates

12. Which part of the needle is attached onto the syringe?
    A. bevel
    B. hub
    C. shaft
    D. lumen

13. Which of the following is used to locate veins for blood collection?
    A. needle holder
    B. venoscope
    C. telescope
    D. sharps container

14. Double-pointed needles are used for
    A. multiple evacuated tubes
    B. only adults and the elderly
    C. only newborns and young infants
    D. collecting blood with syringes

15. Which of the following parts of a needle describes the lumen size?
    A. bevel
    B. shaft
    C. gauge
    D. hub

CHAPTER 12

Phlebotomy Procedures

Outline

Introduction
Requisitions
Patient Preparation
Preparing for the Venipuncture
Performing the Venipuncture
    The Order of the Draw
    Venipuncture with the Evacuated Tube Method
    Venipuncture with the Syringe Method
    Venipuncture with the Butterfly Set (Winged Infusion Set)
Performing Capillary Puncture
Routine Capillary Puncture
    Heel Puncture in Infants
    Finger Punctures
Postcollection Specimen Handling
Routine Blood Film (Smear)
Specimen Recollection
Summary
Critical Thinking
Websites
Review Questions

OBJECTIVES

After studying this chapter, readers should be able to:
1. State the importance of correct patient identification, complete specimen labeling, and proper handling.
2. List the equipment needed for venipuncture.
3. Explain the requisition form for blood collection.
4. Explain the purpose of a tourniquet.
5. List the correct order of draw for blood specimens.
6. Describe cross-contamination.
7. Describe why a phlebotomist may choose a syringe for blood collection rather than an evacuated tube.
8. Explain why a butterfly set may be chosen instead of an evacuated tube.
9. Name and describe the veins that may be used for blood collection.
10. Explain the major cause of specimen rejection and the signs that it has occurred.

KEY TERMS

Antecubital: Relating to the region of the arm in front of the elbow.

Basilic vein: One of the four superficial veins of the arm, beginning in the ulnar part of the dorsal venous network and running proximally on the posterior surface of the ulnar side of the forearm.

Bifurcation: The splitting of a structure into two parts.

Capillary puncture: Dermal puncture; the puncturing of the capillaries of usually the fingers or heels to withdraw blood for testing.

Cephalic vein: One of the four superficial veins of the upper limb. It receives deoxygenated blood from the dorsal and palmar surfaces of the forearm.

Ethylenediaminetetraacetic acid (EDTA): An anticoagulant used extensively for analysis of blood, such as in complete blood counts.

g Force: The unit of measure of gravitational force in the International System of Units.

Heel stick: A method of blood collection in very young children; the heel of the foot is punctured and capillary blood is collected for testing.

Hemoconcentration: An increase in the concentration of blood cells resulting in loss of plasma or water from the bloodstream.

Hemolysis: The breaking open of red blood cells and the release of hemoglobin into the blood plasma.

Lateral: Farther from the middle or center.

Microcollection: Blood collection from a finger or heel into microcontainers; it requires smaller amounts of blood than from venipuncture.

Microtainer: A patented type of capillary tube that holds less than 1 mL of blood and often contains varieties of anticoagulants and additives.

Plantar: Related to the sole or bottom of the foot.

Syncope: Fainting.

Thixotropic gel: A substance that changes from a gel to a liquid when stirred or shaken; after centrifugation, the gel forms a barrier over red blood cells in the tube, keeping them separate from the blood serum.

Introduction

Phlebotomy is critical in determining various types of diseases and infections. Nearly 80% of physicians' decisions are based on laboratory tests, and the majority of these are blood tests. Phlebotomy involves highly developed procedures and equipment. Phlebotomists must be adequately trained in skillful procedures to ensure accuracy and patient comfort as well as safety. Venipuncture is the most common method of obtaining blood, and it requires a lot of practice to achieve skill and confidence.

Requisitions

Test requisitions are the legal beginnings of blood collection procedures. They are usually made by a physician or other qualified healthcare professional and involve laboratory testing. Law enforcement officials may also request certain tests to be used for evidence. Certain states allow *direct access testing* (DAT) so that patients can order some of their own blood tests.

A *requisition* is a form on which test orders are entered. They become part of the patient's medical record. Requisitions require specific information to ensure that the physician's orders are fulfilled, the correct patient is tested, the correct tests are performed, the testing time and conditions are appropriate, and the patient is correctly billed. A sample required manual requisition form is shown in **Figure 12–1**.

Manual requisitions are available in various forms, including three-part forms that have requesting, reporting, and billing functions. Computer requisitions are becoming more common than manual requisitions today, although manual forms are still used as backups when computer systems fail.

Computer requisitions (see **Figure 12–2**) usually contain the actual labels that will be adhered onto the specimen tubes immediately after blood collection. They identify the patient, test information, and type of tube needed for the specimen, and they may indicate additional patient information, if required. Required information for a requisition includes the following:

- Name of the ordering physician
- Full name of the patient
- Inpatient medical record number, if applicable
- Date of birth or age of the patient
- Inpatient room number and bed, if applicable
- The type of test ordered
- The date on which the test is to be performed
- Outpatient billing information and ICD-9 codes, if applicable
- Timed, fasting, priority test status, etc.
- Latex sensitivity or other special precautions

Both manual and computer requisitions may contain a *bar code*. On a manual requisition, a copy of a bar code (or codes) is usually printed on a removable label so that it can be placed on a specimen container. On a computer requisition, the bar code is usually printed on each label. Bar codes are easy to use and can be scanned into a printer by using a special light or laser. This speeds up processing and ensures accuracy. Bar codes have been proved to decrease laboratory and clerical errors.

Special computer terminals at a phlebotomist station in the laboratory are used to print out computer requisitions for inpatients (see **Figure 12–3**).

Outpatients are usually given laboratory requisitions or prescription slips with test orders written on them by their physicians. Patients are then instructed to take them to a blood collection site. The personnel at the site either ascertain whether adequate information is provided on the requisition or fill out a requisition from the physician's prescription slip.

Test requisitions must be thoroughly reviewed to avoid duplication of orders, ensure specimen collection at correct times and under correct conditions, and identify required equipment. The phlebotomist must make sure to do the following:

- Check that all required information is complete and present.
- Determine the test status or the collection priority (see **Table 12–1**).
- Identify any special circumstances or dietary restrictions that must be addressed before collection.
- Verify which tests are needed and the date and time of their collection.

To *accession* a specimen means to record in the order received so that the specimen and accompanying paperwork for a specific patient can be matched. This involves assigning a unique number that identifies the specimen and all processes and paperwork related to the patient. It ensures prompt, accurate processing all the way through the testing and reporting process.

Patient Preparation

Every blood collection procedure begins with a requisition form from a patient's physician, requesting specific tests. Physicians or other health professionals who are licensed to practice are legally authorized to order laboratory testing. If a laboratory requisition indicates that the phlebotomist must collect a venous blood specimen for hematology testing, serum chemistry testing, or coagulation studies, the phlebotomist must select the proper tubes. For these tests, the proper order of collection would be tubes with stoppers that are colored light blue, red, and lavender. Requisition forms may be computer-generated or handwritten and should include the following:

- The patient's name and date of birth
- An identification number
- The name of the physician making the request
- The type of test requested and its status (timed, fasting, stat, etc.)

After the phlebotomist introduces herself or himself, she or he should greet and identify the patient according to Joint Commission standards. This includes obtaining the patient's full name, address, birth date, and any other identification numbers. The use of bar-coded identification wristbands is recommended. Then the patient's information should be compared with the information listed on the requisition form. It should also be compared with information on any identification bracelets the patient is wearing. If there is any language difficulty or situation that may inhibit the information's being discussed correctly, a family member or caregiver

LABORATORY ORDER FORM

Notification to Physicians and Other Persons Legally Authorized to Order Tests for Which Medicare Reimbursement Will Be Sought. *Medicare will pay only for tests that meet the Medicare coverage criteria and are reasonable and necessary to treat or diagnose an individual patient. Medicare does not pay for tests which documentation, including the patient record, does not support that the tests were reasonable and necessary. Medicare does not cover routine screening tests even if the physician or other authorized test orderer considers the tests appropriate for the patient.*

☐ STAT   ☐ ASAP   ☐ ROUTINE   ☐ CALL _____   ☐ FAX _____

BILLING: ☐ BILL FACILITY   ☐ BILL INSURANCE   ☐ BILL PATIENT   ☐ HMO   ☐ PPO   ☐ Health First HMO

PATIENT NAME: (LAST)   (FIRST)   NAME OF INSURANCE: GROUP #:   POLICY #:

SEX: SS#:   BIRTHDATE: PHONE NUMBER: AUTHORIZATION #:   GUARANTOR: GUARANTOR'S SS#:   GUARANTOR'S BIRTHDATE:

ADDRESS/ROOM #:   ZIP CODE: SPECIMEN COLLECTED BY: DATE/TIME OF COLLECTION: PHYSICAN'S/AUTHORIZED SIGNATURE:

	TESTS	*DX
10080CBC	CBC w/automated differential	
10200HEMGR	Hemogram	
10190HH	Hematocrit & Hemoglobin	
10490RETIC	Reticulocyte	
10500ESR	Sed Rate (ESR)	
10010ATIII	Anti Thrombin III	
10111DIMER	D DIMER Quant	
10258LUPUS	Lupus Panel	
10440PT	Protime/INR	
10450PTT	PTT (Activated)	
10460PTTTH	PTT Therapeutic	
20120NH3	Ammonia (On ICE)	
20140AMY	Amylase	
20270BILID	Bilirubin, Direct	
20280BILIT	Bilirubin, Total	
21910BUN	BUN	
20360CA	Calcium	
20540CPK	CK	
20500CKMB	CK & MB	
20550CREAT	Creatinine	
20300CRP	CRP	
20640FER	Ferritin	
20700GLU	Glucose	
20870HA1C	Hgb A1C	
20920HBSAB	Hep B Surf Ab (HBsAb)	
20930HBSAG	Heb B Surf Ag (HBsAg)	
20820HCGQ	Preg Test (HCG) Quant.	
20830PREG	Preg Test (HCG) Qual., Serum	
20963HMCYT	Homocysteine (On ICE)	
21060IRONP	Iron Package	
21460K	Potassium	
21090LACID	Lactic Acid (On ICE)	
21150LIPAS	Lipase	
21210MG	Magnesium	
20260PBNP	PBNP	
21410PHOS	Phosphorus	
21615PSASN	PSA Screen	
21614PSA3	Prostate Specific Ag 3rd	
21365PTH	PTH Intact	
21360PTHP	PTH Pkg (Phos, Ca, Mg, Ionized Ca)	
21720T3UP	T₃ Uptake	
21750T4	T₄ Total	
20670FTIP	FTI, T₄, T₃ Uptake	
21895TROP	Troponin	
21790TSH	TSH	
21990B12	Vitamin B12	
20650FOLAT	Folate	

	ELECTROPHORESIS	*DX
21540SPEPI	SPEP/Reflex SIFE	
21545SPEP	Serum Electro NO Interp	
21550UPEPI	UPEP/Reflex UIFE	
21555UPEP	Urine Electro NO Interp	
20990SIFEI	Serum IFE/Interp	

	ELECTROPHORESIS (CON'T)	*DX
20995SIFE	Serum IFE/NO Interp	
21000UIFI1	Urine IFE/Interp	
21605UIFE1	Urine IFE/NO Interp	
20880HGBEI	HGB Electro/Interp	
215600LIGI	CSF Olig/Interp	
	(SERUM Spec Also REQUIRED)	

	DRUG LEVELS	
LAST DOSE _____	NEXT DOSE _____	
20400CRBM	Carbamazepine (Tegretol)	
20600DIG	Digoxin	
20695GENTR	Gentamicin Trough	
20690GENPK	Gentamicin Peak	
21170LITH	Lithium	
21380PHNO	Phenobarbital	
21390PTN	Phenytoin (Dilantin)	
21985VANTR	Vancomycin Trough	
21980VANPK	Vancomycin Peak	
21780THEOP	Theophylline	
21970VALPR	Valproic Acid (Depakene)	

	PROFILES	*DX
20470BMP	Basic Metabolic (Na, K, CL, CO2, Glu, Bun, Creat, Ca)	
21230CMP	Metabolic Panel (Na, K, Cl, CO2, Glu, Bun, Crea, Ca, TP, Alb, ALT, AST, AiP, TBili)	
20885LIVER	Hepatic (Liver) Panel (Alb, AST, ALT, Alk Phos, TBili, DBili, Tot Protein)	
20980HYPOT	Hypothyroid Profile (T3 Uptake, T4 Total, TSH)	
21160LIPID	Lipid Profile (Chol, Trig, HDL, LDL calc, Chol/HDL Ratio)	
21630RENAL	Renal Function Panel (Na, K, Cl, CO2, Glu, Bun, Crea, Ca, Alb, Pho)	
20945HPACU	Acute Hepatitis Panel (Anti-HAV IgM, Anti-HBC IgM, HBS ag, Hepatitis C)	
20950HPPR	Hepatitis Profile (Anti-HBe & HBeAg will be performed if HBsAG Anti-HBc or Anti-HBc-Igm are positive)	

	URINE TESTS	*DX
Source: ☐ Foley Cath ☐ Midstream ☐ Straight Cath ☐ Suprapubic		
20560UCRCL	Creatinine Clearance 24 hr Blood & Urine Ht. ___ Ft. ___ In ___ Wt. ___ Total Volume ___	
21600UTP24	Protein, Urine 24 hr. Total Volume ___	
10571UA	Urinalysis	
10581UAMIC	Urinalysis w/Microscopic	
30400CXURN	Culture Urine	
10576UACXI	Urinalysis/Culture if (culture performed if > 5 wbc and/or 2+ Bacteria, Positive Leukocyte Esterase, Positive Nitrite)	
10420UHCG	Preg Test (HCG) Urine	

ADDITIONAL TESTS   DIAGNOSIS:

	MICROBIOLOGY CULTURE/VIROLOGY/MISC	*DX
30180CXAEN	Culture & Gram Stain Aerobic & Anaerobic Source	
30120CXBLD	Culture Blood	
30240CXCSF	Culture CSF & Gram Stain	
30220CXFLD	Culture Sterile Body Fluid Source	
30290CXFUN	Culture Fungus/Other Source	
30290CXFNS	Culture Fungus Skin, Hair, Nail Source	
30330CXGAS	Culture Group A Strep	
30820STRA	Strep Group A Antigen	
30340CXGBS	Culture Group B Strep Source	
30360CXLRT	Culture Gram Stain Lower Respiratory (Sputum, etc) Source	
30320CXGOT	Culture Other Source	
30380CXSTO	Culture Stool	
30710OVAP	Ova and Parasites	
30390CXURT	Culture Upper Respiratory (Throat/Nose) Source	
30420CXWND	Culture & Gram Stain Wound Source	
30410CXVIR	Culture Virus Comprehensive Source	
30350CXHSV	Culture Herpes Virus	
30740RSV	RSV Direct Antigen	
30930VRP	Viral Respiratory Direct Panel	
30570FLUAB	Influenzae A& B Antigen	
30760ROTA	Rotavirus Antigen	
030650CBLD	Occult Blood - Single Specimen	
306500CBLM	Occult Blood - Multiple Specimens	
30121CDIF	Clostridium difficile Toxin A & B	
30101CHLGC	Chlamydia & GC Amplification	
30500GIARD	Giardia lamblia Direct Antigen	
30940WETPR	Wet mount	

	IMMUNOLOGY	*DX
30060ANA	ANA	
30755RF	RA Factor	
30020DSDNA	Anti-dsDNA	
30030AMA	Anti-Mitochondrial Antibody	
30050ASMA	Anti-Smooth Muscle Antibody	
30072ENA	ENA Antibodies (Anti-Sm & Sm/RNF)	
30035ANCA	Neutrophil Cytoplasmic Antibodies (ANCA)	
30078SCL70	SCL-70 (Scleroderma) Antibody	
30070SSAB	SSA/RO and SSB/LA Antibodies (Sjogrens)	
30550HIVAB	HIV-1/2 Screening Antibody (Western Blot if positive)	
30630MONO	Mono Screen	
30770RPR	RPR	
20780RUBG	Rubella Antibody, IgG	
30790MEASG	Rubeola (Measles) Antibody, IgG	

	RANDOM URINE TESTS	*DX
21240MABR	Microalbumin Random	
21470UK1	Urine Potassium	
20580UCRE1	Urine Creatinine	
21820TOXIV	Toxi IV Screen	

*PLEASE provide narrative diagnostic information for each ordered test. However, if the test is marked as subject to the carrier's Local Medical Review Policy, please provide Medical Necessity.

Figure 12–1 Manual requisition form.

002390-11315
Doe, John
0004062352 09/19/1982 M
Col: 11/11/2011 3:22:00 PM
Sputum Cult
Provider, Test, MD

002360-11315
Doe, John
0004062352 09/19/1982 M
Col: 11/11/2011 3:22:00 PM
PT, Hemo, DIFF, Chem 14,
Venipuncture Fee
Provider, Test, MD

113151548
Doe, John
0004062352 09/19/1982 M
Col: 11/11/2011 3:22:00 PM
Sputum Cult
Provider, Test, MD

113151533
Doe, John
0004062352 09/19/1982 M
Col: 11/11/2011 3:22:00 PM
PT MIMA Blue
Provider, Test, MD

002378-11315
Doe, John
0004062352 09/19/1982 M
Col: 11/11/2011 3:15:00 PM
Chem 14, Hemo, Diff, PT,
Venipuncture Free
Provider, Test, MD

113151534
Doe, John
0004062352 09/19/1982 M
Col: 11/11/2011 3:15:00 PM
Hemo, DIFF, MIMA Lav
Provider, Test, MD

113151537
Doe, John
0004062352 09/19/1982 M
Col: 11/11/2011 3:15:00 PM
Chem 14 MIMA Green
Provider, Test, MD

113151535
Doe, John
0004062352 09/19/1982 M
Col: 11/11/2011 3:12:00 PM
Chem 14 MIMA Green
Provider, Test, MD

113151538
Doe, John
0004062352 09/19/1982 M
Col: 11/11/2011 3:15:00 PM
Hemo, DIFF, MIMA Lav
Provider, Test, MD

F113150702
Doe, John
0004062352 09/19/1982 M
Col: 11/11/2011 3:12:00 PM
Venipuncture Fee No Container
req'd
Provider, Test, MD

113151539
Doe, John
0004062352 09/19/1982 M
Col: 11/11/2011 3:15:00 PM
PT MIMA Blue
Provider, Test, MD

002390-11315
Doe, John
0004062352 09/19/1982 M
Col: 11/11/2011 3:22:00 PM
Sputum Cult
Provider, Test, MD

F113150704
Doe, John
0004062352 09/19/1982 M
Col: 11/11/2011 3:15:00 PM
Venipuncture Free No Container
req'd
Provider, Test, MD

113151548
Doe, John
0004062352 09/19/1982 M
Col: 11/11/2011 3:22:00 PM
Sputum Cult Sputum Cult
Provider, Test, MD

Figure 12–2 A computer requisition with a bar code.

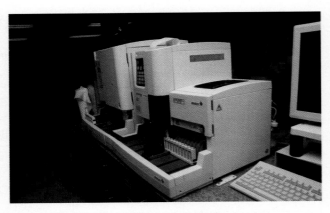

Figure 12–3 A special phlebotomist computer terminal.

should supply the information. The name of this other person must also be documented.

It is then time to explain the purpose for the procedure and what will occur. If the patient or his or her representative asks for any further information other than that which can be supplied briefly, ask if the representative would like to speak to the patient's physician prior to the procedure's being performed. Always obtain verbal permission to draw blood, from the patient or her or his representative, just prior to beginning the procedure. Remember to ask if the patient has experienced any problems involving venipuncture procedures in the past, and prepare for any possible problems. Examples of these problems include **syncope**, needle phobia, latex allergy, and patient trust. It is important that the phlebotomist show self-confidence and professionalism, which will help to calm and comfort the patient. *Needle phobia* is defined as an intense fear of needles. If a patient complains of needle phobia, the phlebotomist should not take this matter lightly. Symptoms of needle phobia include profuse sweating, paleness, light-headedness, nausea, and fainting. In severe conditions, patients may demonstrate dysrhythmia or even cardiac arrest.

The most critical errors that a phlebotomist can make are either to misidentify a patient or to mislabel a specimen. Both can lead to an additional, life-threatening error. An example might be specimens for typing and cross-matching before blood transfusion. Misidentifying a patient or specimen may

Table 12–1 Common Designations of Test Statuses

Test Status	Definition	Examples
STAT (stat)	Immediately	Cardiac enzymes, electrolytes, glucose, hemoglobin and hematocrit (H&H)
Med Emerg	Medical emergency (used instead of STAT)	Same as STAT
Timed	Collect at a specific time	Blood cultures, cardiac enzymes, cortisol, GTT, TDM, 2-h PP
ASAP	As soon as possible	Electrolytes, glucose, H&H
Fasting	No food or drink except water for 8–12 h prior to specimen collection	Cholesterol, glucose, triglycerides
NPO	Nothing by mouth	N/A
Preop	Before an operation	CBC, platelet function studies, PTT
Postop	After an operation	H&H
Routine	Relating to established procedure	CBC, chemistry profile

be punishable by dismissal of the responsible person. It may lead to a malpractice lawsuit against that individual. To prevent misidentification, the patient should be asked to state his or her name for proper identification. It is not appropriate to ask for identification in a way that requires a "yes" or "no" answer, such as "Are you Mr. Jones?" This must be avoided.

Preparing for the Venipuncture

The patient should be seated in a comfortable chair. Ask the patient to extend his or her arms downward in a straight line from shoulder to wrist with the palms up, and then inspect both arms. Ask if there is a preferred arm to use for the procedure. The veins of the forearm or elbow are usually used for venipuncture (see **Figure 12–4**). If the patient has no preference, after washing the hands, the phlebotomist selects the arm with the more prominent veins in the **antecubital** area. If this area is cyanotic, bruised, edematous, burned, or scarred on both arms, use the veins on the lower forearm, back of the hand, or side of the wrist instead (the inside portion of the wrist should not be used).

Apply a tourniquet (after making sure the site is clean and dry) and request that the patient make a fist. The tourniquet should be tied so that it can be easily released with one hand. Tie the tourniquet 3 to 4 in above the site of the draw immediately before beginning venipuncture. Tourniquets should never be left on for longer than 1 min, to avoid **hemoconcentration** and inaccurate test results.

If no tourniquet is available, a blood pressure cuff can be used for a multitube draw, being released and reinflated as needed. To make sure that the tourniquet is not too tight (causing stopping of arterial blood flow), check the pulse at the wrist. If a tourniquet is too tight, it may increase the effects of hemoconcentration, prevent arterial blood flow into the area, and result in failure to obtain blood. A tourniquet that is too tight will pinch and hurt the patient, and it may cause the arm to turn red or purple. A tight tourniquet will not allow for an increase in venous blood flow.

Tourniquets should be flat against the skin, and they may be tied over clothing if the patient is overweight or has hairy upper arms, in order to avoid discomfort. If a reusable tourniquet is used, make sure that it has been cleaned with soap and water or disposable antiseptic towelettes. Tourniquets can also be used when drawing blood from veins of the hand or foot (tying them on the wrist or ankle, respectively).

Before putting on gloves, the phlebotomist should use an index finger to palpate (feel) the patient's arm for an acceptable vein. Survey both arms thoroughly if the patient has no arm preference. Veins will "bounce" when palpated. The vein of first choice is the *median cubital vein*, which runs at slight angles to the antecubital fold. The main superficial vessels in the arms are the **basilic vein** and the **cephalic vein**. The basilic vein ascends from the forearm to the middle of the arm. It then penetrates deeply to join the brachial vein. The brachial and basilic veins merge to form the *axillary vein*. The cephalic vein runs upward from the hand to the shoulder, where it pierces the tissues to empty into the axillary vein. Past the axilla, the axillary vein becomes the *subclavian vein*. The median cephalic vein is the second choice of vein for drawing blood. The basilic vein, on the inside part of the antecubital area, should be used only if the medial, cephalic, or hand veins are not accessible. Among these, the median cubital vein is the preferred site for venipuncture in adults and is most commonly used.

Injury during phlebotomy usually occurs due to nerve injury. The phlebotomist should discontinue the procedure if the patient complains of tingling, numbness, or "shooting" pains. Never probe for a vein with the needle—this greatly increases the chance for nerve injury. Instead, choose another venipuncture site.

Use the veins of the foot only if the patient has good circulation in these areas and the physician (or a supervisor) has given approval for venipuncture there. If the patient is diabetic, blood may never be drawn from the feet or ankles. In general, most hospitals forbid ankle phlebotomy, and it is used only rarely, when other sites cannot be used. Usually only highly experienced phlebotomists perform this type of phlebotomy.

Performing the Venipuncture

There are three methods used to perform phlebotomy. Each depends on the patient's condition, the patient's age, and the amount of blood to be drawn. Phlebotomists may use the syringe, evacuated tube, or butterfly set method. The basic concepts of venipuncture are described in the following paragraphs.

The first step in performing the venipuncture is to identify the patient and to introduce yourself. Assemble the needed equipment within easy reach, and tear open sterile packets so that they can be used. Wash the hands. Apply the tourniquet in order to palpate the proper vein.

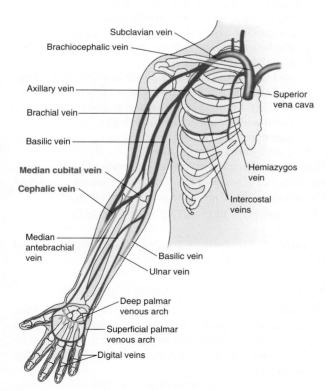

Figure 12–4 The veins of the arm that may be used for venipuncture.

Wash the hands and apply gloves. Phlebotomists must wear eye protection while performing venipuncture because the splashing of blood into the eyes could transfer biohazards to the phlebotomist. The phlebotomist must also be cautious about touching his or her eyes because the hands or gloves may be contaminated with blood or body fluids.

Cleanse the antecubital area with alcohol (or povidone-iodine in the case of blood alcohol testing), working outward and rubbing in a circular motion. Allow the alcohol to evaporate completely. If a blood culture is being performed, the area should be cleaned first by alcohol and then again by povidone-iodine. Never touch this area after it has been cleansed. Reapply the tourniquet after the area has dried. Ask the patient to again clench his or her hand into a fist. Do not have the patient "pump" the fist—he or she should simply hold it clenched. Stretch the skin downward below the collection site with the thumb of the nondominant hand—this will anchor the vein in place. Regardless of the method used for blood collection, the vein should be anchored *below the site of the draw.*

Quickly insert the needle into the vein at a 15° to 30° angle with the bevel facing up. Never exceed 30° because this will cause the needle to penetrate through the vein and potentially enter nerves or the brachial artery. Pull back on the syringe plunger or push an evacuated tube onto the double-pointed needle. As blood enters the tube or barrel, ask the patient to unclench the fist. According to the Clinical and Laboratory Standards Institute (CLSI), the tourniquet should be removed when the first tube begins to fill, but may be left on longer to assist the filling of additional tubes (never greater than 1 min).

As the specimen is drawn, the patient's condition must be continually checked. As each required tube is removed from the needle holder, it should be gently inverted. It can then be placed in the holding rack. Tubes with clot activator must be inverted 5 times. Those for coagulation studies (light-blue stoppers) should be inverted 3 to 4 times. All other anticoagulant tubes should be inverted 8 to 10 times. If the tubes are not inverted immediately after collection, small clots may form in the specimen. Nonadditive tubes should not be mixed because mixing may cause hemolysis if the sample has already begun to clot.

Throughout the procedure, make sure not to disturb the needle's position. After the final tube has been put in the rack, quickly remove the needle and apply gauze, with pressure, to the puncture site. Then ask the patient to apply direct pressure to the gauze but not to bend the arm. Activate the safety device to cover the needle immediately. Dispose of the entire assembly into a sharps container.

Conduct a two-point check to make sure that the vein is not leaking, and then apply the bandage. To do this, observe the site for 5 to 10 s after releasing pressure and removing the gauze. If visible bleeding occurs or if the tissue surrounding the puncture rises up, keep applying pressure until the bleeding is stopped. Apply the bandage and dispose of the gauze in a biohazard waste container. Instead of a bandage, clean gauze (never a cotton ball) may be taped over the site. Label all of the collection tubes, and never leave the room or release the patient until the tubes are labeled. Check the patient's status again, then leave the room or dismiss the patient. *Note:* In patients who have fragile veins, either the syringe method is used to draw blood from the antecubital space, or the blood is drawn from the veins in the hand instead.

The phlebotomist must sign all tubes collected for blood bank testing using first and last name—no initials. This is important for blood bank specimens so that the actual phlebotomist who performed the blood collection may be clearly and accurately identified. However, the emergence of computer systems, employee signature sheets, and other regulatory requirements may now allow the use of initials and/or computer identification numbering for these procedures.

The Order of the Draw

It is very important that, regardless of the method of blood collection used, tubes be collected in the correct order. If tubes are filled in the wrong order, the testing required may be interfered with due to specimen contamination by additive carryover, tissue thromboplastin, or microorganisms. The *order of the draw* is a specific sequence of tube collection that minimizes potential problems.

Carryover is also known as *cross-contamination*. It is the transfer of additive from one tube to the next. It may occur when blood in an additive tube touches the needle during evacuated tube system (ETS) blood collection, or when blood is transferred from a syringe into ETS tubes. If blood remains on or within the needle, it can be transferred to the next tube that is drawn or filled. This may contaminate that tube with additive from the previous tube, potentially affecting test results on the specimen. The most common tests affected by additive contamination are listed in **Table 12–2**.

To minimize the chance of specimen contamination, the CLSI recommends the following order of draw when ETS collection is done or when tubes are filled from a syringe:

1. Sterile tube (blood culture) (light-yellow SPS)
2. Light blue (coagulation tube)
3. Red (glass nonadditive or plastic clot activator tubes)
4. SST (gold plastic serum separator tubes)
5. PST (light-green plasma separator tubes)
6. Green (darker green heparin tubes)
7. Lavender (EDTA tubes)
8. Gray (oxalate/fluoride tubes)

One way to remember this order is to remember the following sequence of words, each of which corresponds to one of the specific eight tubes in the previously listed order:

STOP – LIGHT – RED – STAY – PUT – GREEN – LIGHT – GO

Table 12–3 shows more detailed information about blood collection tubes and order of draw.

Venipuncture with the Evacuated Tube Method

Required Equipment: Vacutainer® needle, needle holder, proper tubes for requested tests, 70% isopropyl alcohol, gauze pads, tourniquet, nonallergenic tape or bandage, transfer device, permanent marking pen, and biohazard bag or disposal container.

Check the requisition to determine the ordered tests. Gather the needed tubes and supplies. The expiration dates of all blood collection tubes and supplies must be checked. If

Table 12–2 Effects of Additive Contamination on Common Blood Tests

Contaminating Additive	Tests That May Be Affected
Citrate	Alkaline phosphatase Calcium Phosphorus
EDTA	Alkaline phosphatase Calcium Creatine kinase Partial thromboplastin Potassium Pro-time Serum iron Sodium
Heparin (all types)	Activated clotting time Acid phosphatase Calcium (certain tests) Partial thromboplastin Pro-time Sodium formulations Lithium formulations
Oxalates	Acid phosphatase Alkaline phosphatase Amylase Calcium Lactate dehydrogenase Partial thromboplastin Potassium Pro-time Red cell morphology
Silica (clot activator)	Partial thromboplastin time Pro-time
Sodium fluoride	Sodium Urea nitrogen

they are out of date, they cannot be used. This is in compliance with quality control and quality assurance regulations. Wash and dry the hands. Identify the patient, explain the procedure, and obtain permission for the procedure (see **Figure 12–5**). Help the patient to sit comfortably with the selected arm supported, in a slightly downward position. Assemble the equipment. Choose the needle based on inspection of the veins. Attach the needle firmly to the Vacutainer holder while keeping the cover on the needle.

Apply the tourniquet around the patient's arm, 3 to 4 in above the elbow (see **Figures 12–6A** and **12–6B**). Do not tie the tourniquet so tightly that blood flow in the artery is restricted. The tourniquet should not remain in place for more than 1 min. Ask the patient to make a fist. Select the site for venipuncture by palpating the antecubital space with an index finger (see **Figure 12–7**).

Wash the hands, and apply gloves. Cleanse the site with an alcohol pad, starting in the center and working outward in a circular pattern (see **Figure 12–8**). The site should be allowed to air-dry. Hold the Vacutainer assembly in the dominant hand, with the thumb on top and fingers underneath. The first tube to be drawn may be positioned in the needle holder. It should not, however, be pushed onto the double-pointed needle past the marking on the holder. The needle sheath should be removed.

Grasp the patient's arm with the nondominant hand, using the thumb and forefinger to draw the skin tight over the site (see **Figure 12–9**). Insert the needle through the skin, into the vein, with the bevel facing up. Use a 15° to 30° angle (see **Figure 12–10**).

Place two fingers on the flanges of the needle holder. Use the thumb to push the tube onto the double-pointed needle,

Table 12–3 Draw Order, Stopper Color, and Rationales for Collection

Draw Order	Stopper Color	Rationale for Collection Order
Sterile collections (blood cultures)	Yellow SPS, sterile media bottles	It minimizes chance of microbial contamination.
Coagulation tubes	Light blue	It is the first additive tube in the order because all other additive tubes affect coagulation tests.
Glass nonadditive tubes	Red	They prevent contamination by additives in other tubes.
Plastic clot activator tubes Serum separator tubes (SSTs)	Red Red and gray rubber, or gold plastic	They are filled after coagulation tests because silica particles activate clotting and affect coagulation tests (the carryover of silica into subsequent tubes can be overridden by the anticoagulant in them).
Plasma separator tubes (PSTs)	Green and gray rubber, or light-green plastic	Heparin affects coagulation tests and interferes in collection of serum specimens; it causes the least interference in tests other than coagulation tests.
Heparin tubes	Green	It is the same as for plasma separator tubes.
EDTA tubes	Lavender, or pink	These are responsible for more carryover problems than any other additive: EDTA elevates sodium and potassium levels, chelates and decreases calcium and iron levels, and elevates prothrombin time and partial thromboplastin time results.
Plasma preparation tubes (PPTs)	Pearl top	It is the same as for EDTA tubes.
Oxalate/ fluoride tubes	Gray	Sodium fluoride and potassium oxalate affect sodium and potassium levels, respectively. They must be filled after hematology tubes because oxalate damages cell membranes and causes abnormal red blood cell morphology; oxalate interferes in enzyme reactions.
Citrate ACD	Light yellow (ACD)	Blood banking and histocompatibility testing.

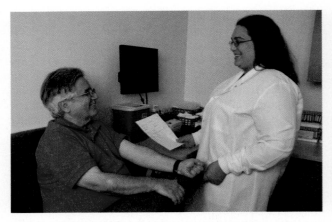

Figure 12–5 Identify the patient, explain the procedure, and obtain permission for the procedure.

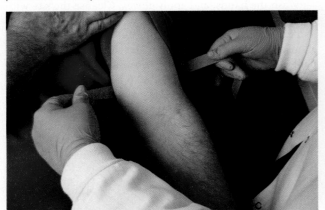

Figure 12–6A Tourniquet around the patient's arm.

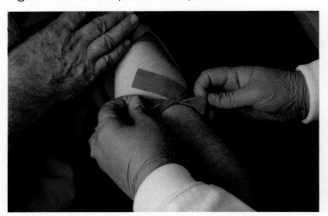

Figure 12–6B Tourniquet around the patient's arm.

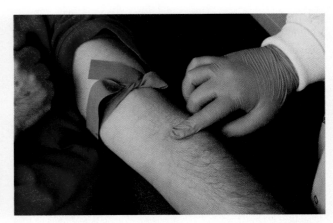

Figure 12–7 The venipuncture site being selected by palpating the vein.

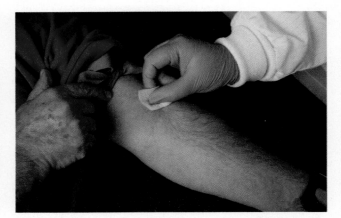

Figure 12–8 The cleansing of the venipuncture site.

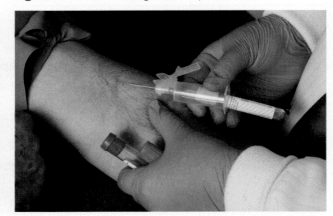

Figure 12–9 Grasp the patient's arm with the nondominant hand, using the thumb and forefinger to draw the skin tight over the site.

making sure not to alter the needle's position in the patient's vein. As blood begins to flow into the tube, ask the patient to release his or her fist. Allow the tube to fill to its maximum capacity. Curl the fingers underneath and push on the needle holder with the thumb to remove the first collection tube. Make sure not to move the needle in the patient's vein while you are removing the tube (see **Figure 12–11**).

Insert the second tube into the needle holder, following the previously mentioned steps (see **Figure 12–12**).

Continue filling, removing, and replacing tubes as needed. After each tube is removed, remember to gently invert it to mix blood with anticoagulants. For collecting blood in multiple tubes, the tourniquet should remain tied on the patient's arm no longer than 1 min. Remove the last tube from the holder. Place gauze over the puncture site (see **Figure 12–13**), and quickly remove the needle while engaging the safety device. Dispose of the entire unit in a sharps container.

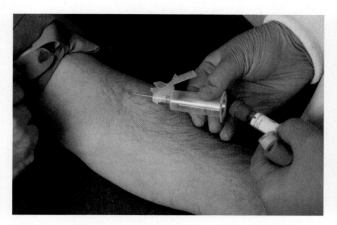

Figure 12–10 Inserting the needle at a 15 to 30 degree angle.

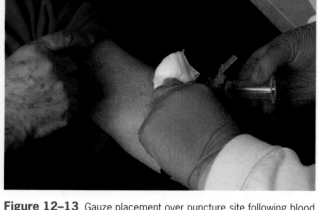

Figure 12–13 Gauze placement over puncture site following blood collection.

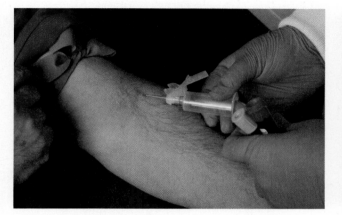

Figure 12–11 Make sure not to move the needle in the patient's vein while you are removing the tube.

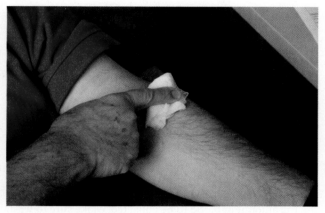

Figure 12–14 Apply pressure to the gauze, and then ask the patient to do so, while not bending his or her arm.

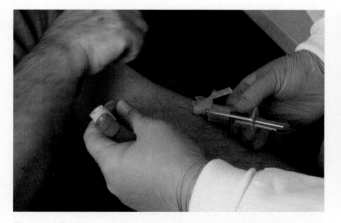

Figure 12–12 Insert the second tube into the needle holder, following the previously mentioned steps.

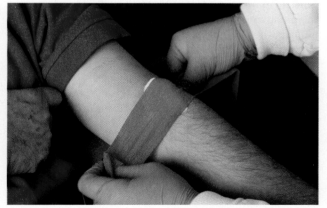

Figure 12–15 Apply a hypoallergenic bandage. Check the patient's status, and if it is normal, release the patient.

Apply pressure to the gauze, and then ask the patient to do so, while not bending his or her arm (see **Figure 12–14**). This should last for between 3 and 5 min to avoid disruption of the clotting process. Apply a hypoallergenic bandage. Check the patient's status, and if it is normal, release the patient (see **Figure 12–15**). Label the tubes with the patient's name, phlebotomist's initials, date, and time of collection (see **Figure 12–16**). Inpatient blood specimens should be labeled at the bedside immediately following collection. Check the puncture site for active bleeding prior to bandaging (the gauze remaining in place under the bandaged site).

Clean the work area, remove gloves, and wash the hands. Clean the tourniquet if it is reusable. Dispose of all blood-contaminated materials in a biohazard container. Complete the requisition for the laboratory, and route it to the proper location. Record the procedure in the patient's chart.

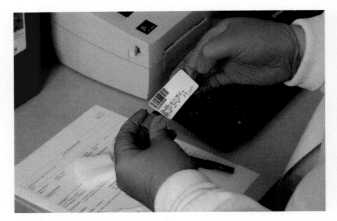

Figure 12–16 A fully labeled blood collection tube.

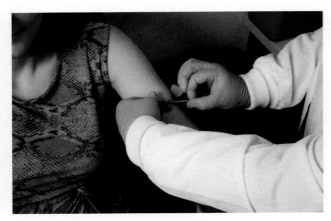

Figure 12–17 The tourniquet in place on the arm.

Venipuncture with the Syringe Method

Required equipment: Syringe with 21- or 22-gauge safety needle, required Vacutainer tubes, 70% isopropyl alcohol, sterile gauze pads, tourniquet, syringe adapter, nonallergenic tape or bandage, permanent marking pen, and biohazard bag or disposal container.

First, check the requisition form to verify the ordered tests. Gather the correct tubes and supplies. Identify the patient, explain the procedure, and obtain permission for the procedure. Have the patient sit comfortably with the arm well supported, pointing slightly downward. Assemble the needed equipment, with the correct syringe and needle chosen after inspecting the patient's veins and ascertaining the amount of blood to be collected. Make sure to wash your hands before inspecting the patient's veins. Attach the needle to the syringe. Pull and depress the plunger several times to make sure it is loose in the barrel. This is known as "breaking the seal." This helps to avoid any "jerking" of the plunger when the phlebotomy procedure is being performed, ensuring greater comfort to the patient and accuracy in the amount of blood drawn. When the plunger of the syringe is pulled back, a vacuum is created.

During this entire time, make sure that the needle cover is in place. Apply the tourniquet around the arm 3 to 4 in above the elbow, never tying it so tightly that it restricts blood flow to the artery (see **Figure 12–17**). The tourniquet should never remain in place longer than 1 min.

Ask the patient to make a fist. Palpate the antecubital space (usually utilizing the median cubital vein) with the index finger to trace the vein's path and judge its depth (see **Figure 12–18**).

Wash the hands again and put on the gloves. Cleanse the site with the alcohol pad, starting at the center and moving outward in a circular motion (see **Figure 12–19**). Allow the area to air-dry before continuing.

Remove the needle sheath. Hold the syringe in the dominant hand with the thumb on top and fingers underneath. Grasp the patient's arm with the nondominant hand while using the thumb and forefinger to draw the skin tight over the site (to anchor the vein). Insert the needle through the skin into the vein, with the bevel of the needle pointed up. The needle should be aligned parallel to the vein, at a 15° angle (see **Figure 12–20**). Watch for a quick "flash" of blood

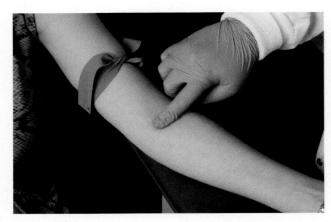

Figure 12–18 Palpate the antecubital space (usually utilizing the median cubital vein) with the index finger to trace the vein's path and judge its depth.

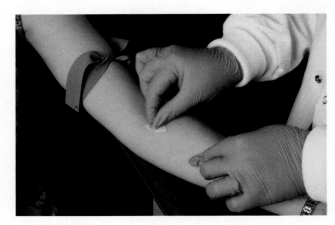

Figure 12–19 Cleanse the site with the alcohol pad, starting at the center and moving outward in a circular motion.

in the hub of the syringe, and then ask the patient to release her or his fist.

Pull back the plunger slowly with the nondominant hand. Do not allow more than 1 mL of space between the blood and the top of the plunger. Do not move the needle after entering the vein, and fill the barrel to the required volume (see **Figure 12–21**).

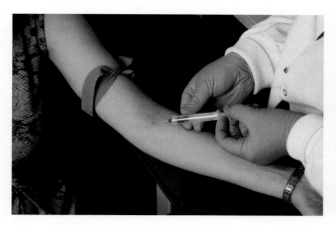

Figure 12–20 The needle should be aligned parallel to the vein at a 15 degree angle.

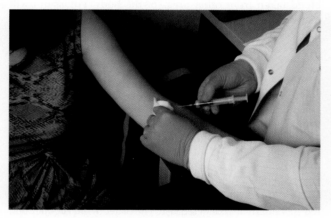

Figure 12–21 Do not move the needle after entering the vein, and fill the barrel to the required volume.

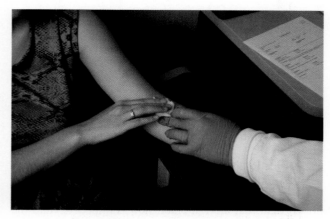

Figure 12–22 Place a gauze pad over the venipuncture site at the moment of needle withdrawal.

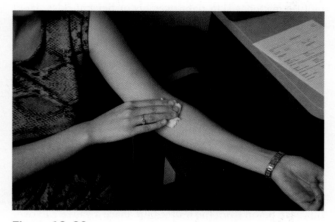

Figure 12–23 Ask the patient to apply direct pressure to the puncture site with the gauze pad, and not to bend the arm.

When approximately 1 min has elapsed, release the tourniquet. This must occur before the needle is removed from the vein in order to avoid blood leaking into adjacent tissues.

Place a gauze pad over the venipuncture site at the moment of needle withdrawal (see **Figure 12–22**), and immediately activate the needle safety device.

Ask the patient to apply direct pressure to the puncture site with the gauze pad, and not to bend the arm (see **Figure 12–23**). Transfer the blood to the required tube or tubes, using a safety transfer device, immediately after the procedure (see **Figure 12–24**). Do not press on the plunger during the transfer. Discard the entire assembly once transfer is complete. Invert tubes after blood has been added, and label them with the patient information. Inspect the puncture site for bleeding. Apply a hypoallergenic bandage.

Be sure that the patient's condition is normal before he or she is released. Clean the work area, remove the gloves, and wash the hands. Clean the tourniquet if it is reusable. Dispose of any blood-contaminated materials in a biohazard container. Complete the requisition form for the laboratory. Route the specimen(s) to the proper location. Record the procedure in the patient's record.

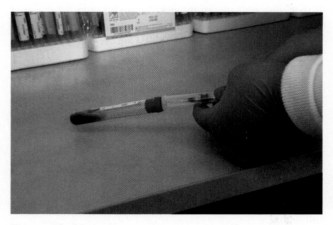

Figure 12–24 Transfer the blood to the required tube or tubes, using a safety transfer device, immediately after the procedure.

Venipuncture with the Butterfly Set (Winged Infusion Set)

Required equipment: Winged infusion ("butterfly") needle set, appropriate tubes with needle and needle adapter, syringe with needle, tourniquet, alcohol pads or other antiseptic preps, gauze pads, sharps disposal container, nonallergenic bandage, permanent marking pen, and biohazard bag or disposal container.

Check the requisition form and gather the required tubes. Assemble the rest of the supplies. Wash the hands and put on gloves. Identify the patient and explain the procedure. Remove the butterfly device from its packaging. Stretch the tubing slightly, making sure not to accidentally activate the needle retractor device. Attach the butterfly device to the syringe. Draw blood into the syringe or push the blood collecting tube onto the end of the holder.

Seat the first tube into the tube holder, placing the unit in a location where it cannot roll. Apply a tourniquet to the patient's wrist, proximal to the wrist bone. Make sure it is not so tight that arterial blood flow is impeded. Hold the patient's hand in the nondominant hand, keeping his or her fingers lower than the wrist. Select a vein. Cleanse the site at the forking (**bifurcation**) of the veins. Use the thumb to pull the patient's skin tight over his or her knuckles. Hold the needle at a 10° to 15° angle with the bevel facing up, and align it with the vein.

Insert the needle while holding the wings or the rear portion of the assembly. After insertion, do not touch the wings again, and ensure that the safety device is not activated. Draw blood into the syringe, or push the blood-collecting tube onto the end of the holder. When you draw blood into the syringe, make sure that the vacuum that is created is slow and steady. There should be no more than 1 mL of space between the blood and the plunger.

When the blood appears in the tube or a "flash" of blood is seen in the hub of the syringe, release the tourniquet. Keep the tube and holder in a downward position so that the tube fills with blood from the bottom up. Place a gauze pad over the puncture site. Gently remove the needle.

The final steps in this procedure are identical to the procedures listed previously. The advantage of a butterfly set is that the small size of the needle can be used for drawing blood from small, difficult, or hand veins.

Performing Capillary Puncture

Capillaries connect small arterioles to small venules. These tiny vessels may be punctured to efficiently collect blood specimens when only a small amount of blood is required. **Capillary puncture** (also known as *dermal puncture*) is also done when venipuncture would be difficult because of certain conditions. The requisition will not indicate that capillary puncture is to be used, so it is up to the phlebotomist to make an accurate decision.

Most commonly, capillary puncture is used for the following:

- Neonates, infants, and young children
- Obese patients
- Older patients
- Patients who need frequent glucose monitoring
- Patients with burns or scars in venipuncture sites
- Patients on intravenous therapy
- Patients who have had a mastectomy
- Patients at risk for venous thrombosis
- Patients who are severely dehydrated
- Tests that only require a small volume of blood

- When venous blood and capillary blood are not identical

Capillary puncture blood is a mixture of arterial blood and venous blood, along with interstitial fluids from the surrounding tissues. In the first drop of capillary blood, small amounts of tissue fluid are concentrated. The composition of blood obtained by capillary puncture more closely resembles arterial blood than venous blood. Capillary blood usually contains higher levels of hemoglobin and glucose, but venous blood has higher levels of potassium, calcium, and total protein. However, analyte levels (the samples being analyzed) are usually the same in capillary and venous blood. Capillary puncture is generally not appropriate for patients who are dehydrated because specimens may be hard to obtain. Also the results may not be representative of blood elsewhere in the body.

Capillary blood will contain higher levels of glucose, but lower levels of total protein, calcium, and potassium than blood taken from other areas of the body. Potassium will increase in capillary blood with the presence of hemolysis or excess tissue fluid. When sequential samples of these substances are collected, the same collection method should be used. This is primarily significant when a series of timed glucose tests are conducted, such as in a glucose tolerance test.

Specimens that are free from clots are required. If blood collection from an infant is too slow, platelets clump and cause incorrect platelet counts in the complete blood cell count. Additional clotting causes erroneous white and red blood cell counts. If an **ethylenediaminetetraacetic acid (EDTA)** specimen is needed, the EDTA specimen is drawn first so that enough volume can be obtained before clotting starts. Other additive specimens are collected next, and clotted specimens are collected last. The order of **microcollection** is as follows: blood gases, lavender-stoppered (EDTA) microcontainers, green-stoppered (sodium heparin) microcontainers, other additive microcontainers, and red-stoppered (nonadditive) microcontainers.

Routine Capillary Puncture

Routine capillary puncture involves proper site selection, patient preparation, specimen collection, and specimen handling. Generally, for routine capillary puncture, the fingers are used for this purpose in adults and children over the age of 1 year. For children younger than 1 year, dermal puncture is performed on the heel.

If the intent is to puncture the finger and the patient's hands are cold, the patient should warm them in warm water and then dry them thoroughly. To prepare the patient for capillary puncture, cleanse the puncture site well with an alcohol prep pad. The phlebotomist must be efficient when doing a capillary puncture because blood flow usually stops very quickly. Make sure the supplies are organized nearby before beginning. Grasp the finger firmly and apply gentle intermittent pressure, without squeezing the finger. Press the puncture device firmly against the skin, and quickly depress its plunger.

Heel Puncture in Infants

Capillary punctures are often performed on the bottom of the heel of the foot, on the medial and **lateral** surfaces (see **Figure 12–25**). According to the CLSI, the safest areas for

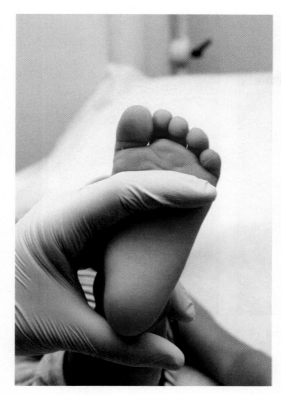

Figure 12–25 The area of the foot used for heel puncture.

performing heel puncture are on the **plantar** surface of the heel (the medial or lateral plantar edges of the heel). This area prevents bone or nerve damage from occurring. The depth of the lancet insertion must be controlled to avoid injuring the heel (calcaneus) bone, because it may cause osteomyelitis. Studies have shown that heel punctures deeper than 2 mm risk injuring the calcaneus bone. Deep heel puncture may also damage an artery or nerve. The center of the plantar surface should never be used for heel puncture.

A deep puncture does not necessarily produce more bleeding. Blood flow can be increased by applying a heel warmer. After the procedure, the area should not be bandaged because of the potential of its peeling off. A loose bandage may become a choking hazard.

The actual puncture will be on the plantar surface of the heel. This should be medial to a line drawn posteriorly from the middle of the great toe to the heel, or lateral to a line drawn posteriorly between the fourth and fifth toes. This site is chosen because most infants have no arteries, bones, or nerves in this area. The inside of the heel contains the posterior tibial artery. Therefore, the outside of the heel is often suggested for puncture. Proper incision devices guarantee a controlled depth of puncture. Previous puncture sites should be avoided to keep infections from occurring. Do not perform any puncture in the central arch area of the foot, which can result in cartilage, nerve, or tendon damage.

Optimal depth of puncture is 2 mm because the capillary bed of the infant is 0.35 to 1.6 mm beneath the skin surface. This will puncture the major capillary beds but not injure the bone or nerves of the heel. The infant's fingers should not be punctured because many lancets are longer than the short

distance to the finger bones and nerves. The fingers of infants also do not produce adequate blood specimens.

Excessive crying by an infant elevates leukocyte counts, which do not return to normal for nearly 60 min. Blood samples should not be taken until at least 60 min has passed because the infant has cried. **Figures 12–26 A through H** show the procedure for performing blood collection from an infant's heel.

The greatest concern of infant heel puncture is **hemolysis** of microcollection samples. Hemolysis may be caused by alcohol not being allowed to dry after the skin is cleaned prior to puncture, squeezing of the area to a greater degree than necessary to ensure blood flow, increased red cell fragility or high red blood cell volume in newborns, and blood

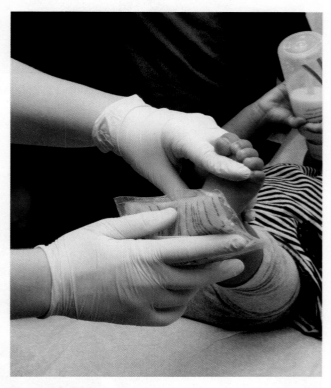

Figure 12–26A Warming the heel with a heel warmer.

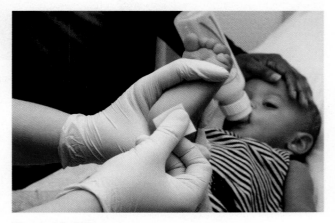

Figure 12–26B Cleaning the puncture site with alcohol.

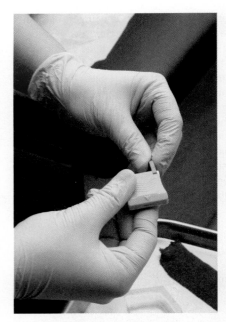

Figure 12–26C Prepping the lancet.

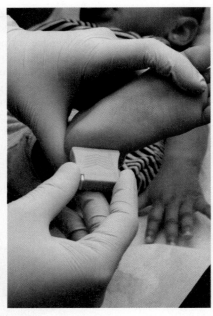

Figure 12–26D Puncturing the heel with a lancet.

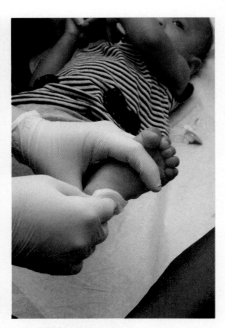

Figure 12–26E Wiping away the first drop of blood.

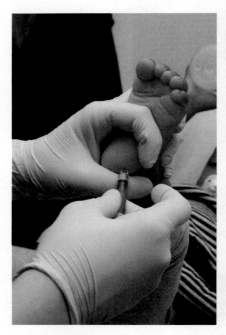

Figure 12–26F Applying the blood to the microtainer while squeezing the heel.

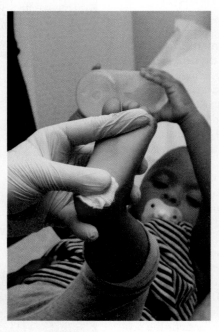

Figure 12–26G Applying gauze to stop the bleeding.

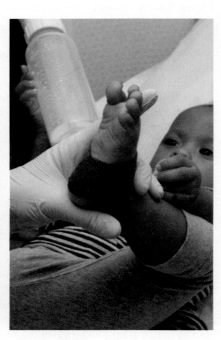

Figure 12–26H Bandaging the wound.

Table 12–4 Heel Stick Skin Puncture

Procedures	Materials
Apply gloves before touching the patient.	Gloves
Identify the patient. If an inpatient, verify the identification bracelet name, hospital number, computer label, and requisition information. If an outpatient, ask the name of the patient bringing the infant in for testing. Verify this with the computer label or requisition.	ID bracelet, computer label, requisition form
Verify collection orders.	Requisition form
Choose the heel for puncture—it should not be cold or swollen.	
Warm the heel for 3 min.	Heel warmer
Select appropriate containers for blood collection.	Microcontainers
Clean the puncture site and allow to dry.	Alcohol, alcohol wipes, sterile gauze pad
Puncture the heel and dispose of puncture device.	Lancet, sharps container
Wipe away the first drop of blood.	Sterile gauze pad
Collect specimen, touching only the tip of the collection tube to the drop of blood—the puncture site should be held in a downward angle and gentle pressure should be applied to the foot.	Collection tube, specimen container
Seal the container.	Specimen container
Mix anticoagulant specimens 8 to 10 times.	Specimen container
Hold gauze or cotton ball to puncture site until bleeding stops.	Gauze or cotton ball
Label containers.	Specimen container
If sample is insufficient, repeat puncture at a different site.	New sterile lancet required

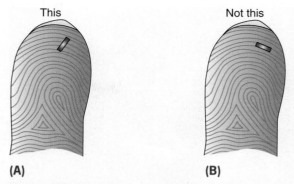

This **Not this**

(A) **(B)**

Figure 12–27 (A) The correct area for capillary puncture and (B) the incorrect area for capillary puncture.

the ring finger, aiming at the fleshy area closer to the center of the finger to protect the underlying bone. The puncture should be made perpendicular to the grooves of the *whorls* (spiral patterns) that make up the fingerprint (see **Figure 12–27**). As always, areas that are callused, burned, infected, cyanotic, edematous, or scarred must be avoided.

Wipe away the first drop of blood because it will contain tissue fluid that can interfere with the accuracy of test results. Fill the containers according to the manufacturer's directions by touching the first container to the next drops of blood, while not touching the skin with the container. Should blood flow stop before the procedure is finished, wipe the site with clean gauze. This should initiate additional blood flow. If blood contaminates gloves or surfaces, keep spare gloves, extra gauze pads, and disinfectant close at hand. Once the containers are filled, ask the patient to apply pressure to the gauze over the puncture site if she or he is able to do so. If required, seal containers in the proper manner.

Many capillary collection containers are too small to have labels applied. The best way to transport them when they are full is to place them inside red-stoppered tubes with the sealed ends down, replace the stopper, and label the tube. Plastic plugs are used to fit over the tops of **Microtainer** tubes that can be placed in either labeled tubes or labeled zipper-lock bags. Make sure to decontaminate collection containers before they are delivered to the laboratory if blood was deposited on their surfaces during collection. **Figures 12–28 (A through G)** show the procedures for performing blood collection from a finger puncture.

Postcollection Specimen Handling

It is vital to handle specimens properly after collection to maintain their quality for accurate test results. It may be necessary to process the blood before the sample is sent to the laboratory. This often involves separating the plasma or serum from the red blood cells. If there is no anticoagulant in the collection devices, the blood will immediately begin to clot. Tubes with speckled tops have silica additives to accelerate clotting, and they should be allowed to sit upright in a

being scraped off rather than allowing it to flow into micro-collection containers. **Table 12–4** lists the requirements for a **heel stick** skin puncture.

Finger Punctures

The medical term used to describe a finger or toe is *phalanx*, with the plural being *phalanges*. The thumb is avoided because of common calluses, the index finger has more nerve endings (making puncture more painful), and the fifth finger does not have sufficient tissue for a successful puncture. Usually, the puncture is made at the tip and slightly to the side of

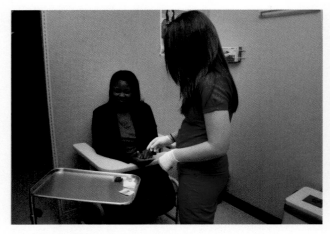

Figure 12–28A Greeting and identifying the patient.

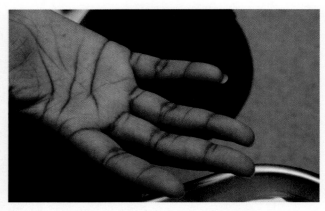

Figure 12–28B Examining the patient's fingers for wounds or lesions.

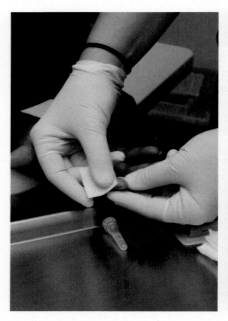

Figure 12–28C Cleaning the puncture site.

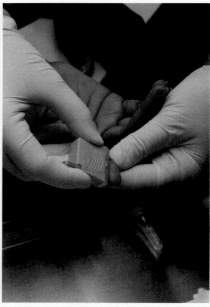

Figure 12–28D Puncturing the finger.

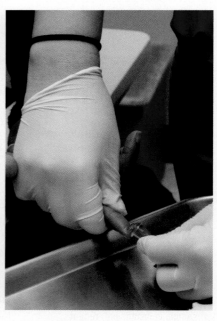

Figure 12–28E Blood collection into the microcontainer.

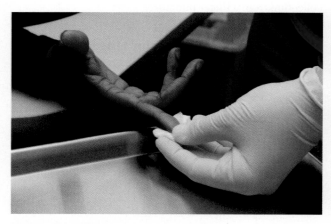

Figure 12–28F Using gauze to stop bleeding.

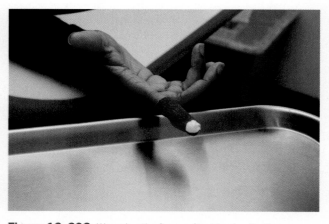

Figure 12–28G Wrapping the finger after blood collection.

rack for 30 to 60 min in order for a solid clot to form. Clot accelerators cause dense clots to form within 30 min. Clotting may be delayed by anticoagulants such as warfarin or heparin in the tubes. When a clot has formed, the clot should be removed from the serum within 2 h.

To remove clots from serum, a centrifuge is required. It must be set at a certain **g force** (minimum of 1,000g), time (10 to 15 min), and temperature (25°C). After centrifugation, there is no need to remove the serum from the tube because the **thixotropic gel** inside will form a barrier over red blood cells. These tubes cannot be centrifuged again, although the serum can be decanted and recentrifuged in another tube.

Plasma tests require that the plasma be removed from the cells as soon as possible. Centrifugation is used, followed by aspiration of the plasma and transfer to another tube by using a disposable pipette. Green-gray marble-topped tubes contain a lithium heparin anticoagulant and thixotropic gel that will form the needed barrier after centrifugation. If testing cannot be immediately performed, serum is usually refrigerated or even frozen.

Complete blood counts require whole blood. The laboratory will conduct the transportation and storage of these specimens. The College of American Pathologists (CAP) recommends that whole blood needed for automated blood counts be refrigerated and tested within 72 h. Couriers are often used to transport specimens, regulated by the Department of Transportation (DOT) Hazardous Materials Shipping Regulations. Those who ship such materials must be fully trained in the handling, packing, and shipping of biohazardous materials.

Routine Blood Film (Smear)

A *blood film* or *smear* is a drop of blood that is spread thinly on a microscope slide. These are required to perform manual *differential* (diff) tests, in which the number, type, and characteristics of the blood are determined by microscopic examination. This may be done as part of a complete blood count or to verify the accuracy of machine-generated differential or platelet counts. Usually, two blood smears are prepared to be tested. Today, blood smears are not usually made at the patient's bedside, but rather in the hematology department from blood that was collected in a tube containing EDTA. Blood smears and EDTA specimens are obtained before other specimens to minimize the effects of platelet aggregation. This may be done by hand or via an automated machine that makes a uniform blood smear from just a single drop of blood.

Specimen Recollection

Occasionally, after laboratory analysis, problems with the sample are discovered. Recollection may then be required. Reasons for rejection of a specimen include the following:

- Clotted blood in an anticoagulated specimen
- Defective tube
- Hemolysis
- Improper handling
- Incorrect tube used for the ordered test
- Insufficient quantity
- Mislabeled (or unlabeled) specimen

The major cause of specimen rejection is hemolysis, which cannot be detected until blood cells separate from the plasma or serum. Therefore, the phlebotomist must take the proper steps to make sure that red blood cells are not damaged during collection. If serum or plasma is hemolyzed, it will appear "rosy" to bright red as hemoglobin is released from the cells. Tests that are more greatly affected by hemolysis include tests for electrolytes, bilirubin, many liver enzymes, and total protein.

Summary

Venipuncture requires the use of a tourniquet to prevent venous blood flow, which makes the veins easier to locate and puncture. Syringes are commonly used for blood collection for elderly patients (because their veins tend to be more fragile), for children (because their veins are smaller), and for obese patients (because their veins tend to be deeper). The blood collection process begins with a test requisition that is usually made by a physician or other qualified healthcare professional. A requisition is a form on which test orders are entered—it can be done manually or it can be computerized. In general, for blood collection, needles should be inserted into veins at angles between 15° and 30°. The patient should always be greeted and identified before any blood collection procedure is begun. The median cubital vein is the vein of first choice for phlebotomy. Capillary puncture is also known as dermal puncture. It is often done when venipuncture will be difficult, because of certain conditions. Capillary puncture blood is a mixture of arterial blood and venous blood. Routine capillary puncture involves proper site selection, patient preparation, specimen collection, and specimen handling.

CRITICAL THINKING

Marshall went to the fifth floor of the hospital to draw the blood of a 75-year-old man, using a Vacutainer system. He had difficulty in getting enough blood for the required test. After two attempts, he called his supervisor for help. When the supervisor arrived in a half hour, she noticed a complication in the patient.

1. What would be the most common complication related to his venipuncture?
2. What would be the best method for collecting blood from this patient?

WEBSITES

http://findarticles.com/p/articles/mi_qa3689/is_199809/ai_n8811248/pg_3/

http://home.caregroup.org/departments/pathology/lab_manual/PLM_specimen_venipuncture.pdf

http://www.aacc.org/publications/cln/2010/January/Pages/safety3.aspx

http://www.austincc.edu/health/phb/documents/phbFingerstick.pdf

http://www.austincc.edu/mlt/phb_tubes

http://www.bd.com

http://www.bd.com/vacutainer/labnotes/Volume20Number1/

http://www.cap.org/apps/docs/pt_checkup/pol_library/patient_identification_specimen_collection.pdf

http://www.doh.state.fl.us/disease_ctrl/std/prevent/MODULE_2_V2.1.pdf

http://www.duiattorney.com/dui-basics/chain-of-custody

http://www.enotes.com/nursing-encyclopedia/blood-specimen-collection

http://www.medialabinc.net/venipuncture-keyword.aspx

http://www.nytimes.com/2006/05/30/health/30case.html

http://www.phlebotomycert.com/cap_puncture.htm

http://www.phlebotomycert.com/veni_technique6.htm

http://www.questdiagnostics.com/hcp/testmenu/Order_of_Draw.pdf

http://www.scribd.com/doc/3772478/Collection-of-Blood-Samples

http://www.uams.edu/clinlab/venipuncture.htm

REVIEW QUESTIONS

Multiple Choice

1. When performing a venipuncture, it is necessary to
   A. use an assistant
   B. place the patient in the Trendelenburg position
   C. perform a surgical scrub at the venipuncture site
   D. use a tourniquet

2. The venipuncture site most commonly used on adults is the
   A. brachial vein
   B. cephalic vein
   C. median cubital vein
   D. basilic vein

3. How should the patient's arm be positioned when blood is drawn in phlebotomy?
   A. bent at the elbow
   B. slightly downward
   C. slightly upward
   D. hanging down

4. A phlebotomist should not attempt to obtain blood from any patient more than
   A. one time
   B. two times
   C. three times
   D. four times

5. In phlebotomy, approximately what is the smallest desirable angle for insertion of the needle into the vein?
   A. 10°
   B. 15°
   C. 30°
   D. 45°

6. The common range of needle gauge for performing a venipuncture is
   A. 13 to 20
   B. 15 to 23
   C. 19 to 20
   D. 20 to 30

7. Which of the following is the last step for a phlebotomist after a venipuncture is done?
   A. Release the tourniquet.
   B. Draw the last tube.
   C. Apply pressure to the gauze at the site of needle insertion.
   D. Apply a hypoallergenic bandage.

8. What is the longest time that a tourniquet should remain on a patient's arm?
   A. 1 min
   B. 2 min
   C. 3 min
   D. 4 min

9. Which of the following statements is true about the advantage of using a butterfly set?
   A. They are the most common method to draw blood.
   B. They have less risk of needlesticks.
   C. They are less expensive than other needles.
   D. They make it easier to draw blood from difficult veins.

10. The temperature of heel warming devices should NOT exceed
    A. 98°F
    B. 101°F
    C. 108°F
    D. 115°F

11. The greatest concern of infant puncture for microcollection samples is
    A. contamination
    B. hemolysis
    C. accuracy
    D. clotting

12. Which of the following tests should NOT be collected via capillary puncture?
    A. hemoglobin
    B. electrolytes
    C. blood glucose
    D. blood culture

13. Which of the following steps is NOT recommended in capillary puncture on the heel of an infant?
    A. cleaning the site
    B. applying a bandage
    C. warming the site
    D. using isopropyl alcohol

14. How long should a blood collection specimen be centrifuged?
    A. 3 to 5 min
    B. 7 to 10 min
    C. 10 to 15 min
    D. 20 to 30 min

15. Reasons for rejection of a specimen include all of the following, EXCEPT
    A. hemolysis
    B. insufficient quantity
    C. nonclotted blood
    D. improper handling

CHAPTER 13

Specimen Collections and Special Procedures

OUTLINE

Introduction
Glucose Testing
    Glucose Tolerance Testing
    Fasting Blood Glucose Test
    A 2-h Postprandial Blood Glucose Level Test
    Hemoglobin (HbA1c) Testing
Timed Specimens
    Fasting
Platelet Function Assay
Blood Donation
Therapeutic Collection
Chain of Custody
Specimen Tampering
Blood Alcohol Testing
Employee Testing
Athletic Testing
Forensic Specimens
Toxicology
Therapeutic Drug Monitoring
Alternative Collection Sites
    Arterial Punctures
    Venous Access Devices
Summary
Critical Thinking
Websites
Review Questions

OBJECTIVES

After studying this chapter, readers should be able to:
1. Define *timed specimens* and list when these tests are used.
2. Define *fasting* and how it relates to blood testing.
3. Explain fasting blood glucose.
4. Discuss the purpose of bleeding time.
5. Explain therapeutic collections and list two most commonly used as methods of treatment.
6. Describe blood donation and factors that affect a person donating blood.
7. Explain the purpose of drug monitoring.
8. Describe the glucose tolerance test.
9. Discuss blood alcohol testing.
10. Explain forensic specimens.

KEY TERMS

Analytes: Substances being chemically analyzed.
Assays: Tests to determine the purity or concentration of substances.
Cannula: A flexible tube that is inserted into a duct or cavity to deliver medication or to drain fluid.
Central venous therapy lines: Venous access devices involving the introduction of a cannula into a vein other than a peripheral vein.
Chain of custody: Chronological documentation, or paper trail, describing both the movement of evidence or other information and who has come into contact with it.
Cushing's syndrome: A metabolic disorder resulting from either the chronic and excessive production of cortisol by the adrenal cortex or the administration of glucocorticoids in large doses for several weeks or longer.
Diabetes mellitus: A condition caused by the inability to properly metabolize sugars; type 1 is characterized by the inability to form insulin, and type 2 is characterized by the inability to make enough insulin.
Diurnal variation: The time at which an organism's functions are active, change, or reach certain levels.
Gestational diabetes: A disorder characterized by an impaired ability to metabolize carbohydrates, usually caused by a deficiency of insulin or insulin resistance, occurring in pregnancy. It usually disappears after delivery of the infant, but may recur years later as type 2 diabetes mellitus.
Glycolysis: The metabolic process in which glucose is converted, by a series of steps, to pyruvic acid.

KEY TERMS CONTINUED

Hemochromatosis: A disorder that causes deposition of hemosiderin in the body tissues, leading to cirrhosis of the liver, heart failure, and destruction of the pancreas.

Hemostasis: The body's mechanism for controlling bleeding; normal hemostasis involves the proper functioning of the platelets and clotting factors.

Heparin lock: The most commonly used type of venous access device for administering medications over a longer period of time (also used for obtaining blood samples); it is a special winged needle set left in a patient's vein for between 48 and 72 h.

Insulinoma: A tumor of the pancreas that produces too much insulin, resulting in hypoglycemia.

Lipemic: Related to lipemia, the presence of larger than normal amounts of fat in the blood.

Peak: The expected highest level of serum concentration of medications.

Platelet function assay: A test that measures both platelet adhesion and aggregation (primary hemostasis).

Polycythemia: An abnormal increase in production of red blood cells.

Reclined position: Lying back or down.

Reference values: Ranges used for various tests in determining how results relate to normal, healthy ranges.

Salicylates: Widely prescribed drugs derived from salicylic acid; they exert analgesic, antipyretic, and anti-inflammatory actions.

Shunts: Devices inserted into the forearm to allow hemodialysis to occur; shunts are connected to machines that filter the blood.

Therapeutic medication: A medicine needed to properly treat a condition.

Trough: The expected lowest level of serum concentration of medications.

Introduction

There are special types of specimen collection procedures that physicians order, and phlebotomists should be familiar with them. Glucose testing is used to diagnose various types of diabetes. Timed specimens can detect changes in patient conditions, therapeutic medication blood levels, and metabolic rates of substances and can measure analytes exhibiting diurnal variation. Patients must fast for certain tests in order to achieve accurate results. Preoperative states and certain bleeding disorders require bleeding time tests or platelet function assays. For the purpose of blood transfusion, blood donors must pass specific criteria to be qualified to donate. Phlebotomists must be specially trained for blood donation. For blood alcohol testing and toxicology studies, there are legal and ethical aspects that must be understood and followed. The procedures discussed in this chapter correspond to those set forth by the Clinical and Laboratory Standards Institute (CLSI).

Glucose Testing

The testing of glucose levels helps to diagnose **diabetes mellitus**, gestational diabetes, hyperinsulinism, and other related conditions. Glucose testing is probably the most frequently ordered type of blood test. An increase in blood glucose may indicate the development of diabetes, which can cause kidney failure, blindness, and circulatory problems that have the potential to result in amputations. Glucose meters (*glucometers*) are available in many different varieties, as shown in **Figure 13–1**. Many patients utilize these devices at home for simple and accurate glucose testing. **Table 13–1** summarizes various types of glucose tests.

Glucose Tolerance Testing

A glucose tolerance test determines the body's ability to metabolize carbohydrates by administering a standard dose of glucose. The blood and urine are then measured for glucose levels at regular intervals. The patient usually must eat a high-carbohydrate diet for 3 days prior to the test and then fast the night before the test.

On the morning of the test, a fasting blood glucose level is obtained. If the patient's fasting blood sugar is 150 milligrams

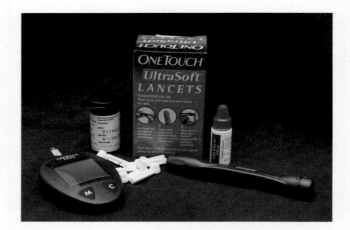

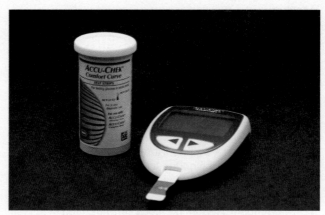

Figure 13–1 Several different glucometers.

Table 13–1 Glucose Tests

Type	Purpose	Timing	Comments
Fasting blood sugar (FBS)	To identify diabetes risk	No intake of food or drink for 8–12 h prior	Single blood sample
Glucose challenge screening test	To identify gestational diabetes risk (1 h) or polycystic ovary syndrome risk (2 h)	1 or 2 h after oral glucose intake	Blood sample; if the test is positive, a complete GTT is done
Intravenous glucose tolerance test (IVGTT)	To evaluate insulin secretion in prediabetes	N/A	Blood samples taken after administration of glucose through an IV or directly into bloodstream
Random blood sugar (RBS)	To identify diabetes or hypoglycemia risk	Throughout the day	Random samples taken; a wide variety of results indicate a possible problem
2-hour postprandial blood sugar (2-h PP)	To identify diabetes risk	Exactly 2 h after a meal	Now used less frequently because of inconsistent results
2- or 3-hour oral glucose tolerance test (2- or 3-h OGTT)	To diagnose diabetes mellitus, gestational diabetes, hypothalamic obesity, and reactive hypoglycemia	30 min, 1 h, 2 h, and 3 h after ingesting oral glucose	Fasting blood sugar

per deciliter (mg/dL) or above, the glucose load should not be administered, because this could be very dangerous. The phlebotomist should inform the patient's physician of this situation.

When the patient's fasting blood glucose is within normal limits, the glucose tolerance test may proceed. The test requires that the patient drink a 100-g dose of glucose (this is adjusted according to the weight of the patient). Blood and urine are collected periodically for up to 6 h. The glucose tolerance test is most often used to assist in the diagnosis of diabetes, hypoglycemia, or other disorders affecting carbohydrate metabolism. A normal fasting blood glucose range is between 70 and 126 mg/dL. This test is administered when a patient has a consistently high fasting blood sugar.

All of the glucose solution must be swallowed within 5 min, and no vomiting can have occurred. When blood specimens are taken, they are usually collected into gray-topped tubes containing a substance (sodium fluoride) that prevents the breakdown of glucose, ensuring accuracy. The tubes also contain potassium oxalate, which binds with calcium to prevent clotting.

If the glucose level does not exceed 100 grams per deciliter (g/dL) at the onset of the test period, or 180 g/dL at 1 h after the glucose is ingested, the patient is believed to have a normal glucose level. Should the blood glucose level exceed 200 g/dL, glucose will escape into the urine because damaged renal tubules are not able to absorb the excessive amounts.

Urine samples are also collected concurrently with the blood samples, at 30 min, 1 h, 2 h, and 3 h after drinking the glucose solution. Care must be taken to ensure accurate labeling of all samples. The patient must remain at the testing location throughout, and no food, smoking, alcohol intake, or chewing gum is allowed. Water may be consumed, however. Each specimen should be centrifuged after clotting has occurred to prevent **glycolysis**. Both urine and serum glucose levels should be run soon after collection, and not as part of the routine laboratory specimens.

An alternative test called the oral glucose tolerance test (OGTT) is used if the patient is diabetic. The patient fasts only overnight, and his or her fasting blood glucose is collected in the morning, followed by the patient drinking 75 g of glucose within 5 min. The patient's glucose is again checked 2 h after the drink, with normal blood glucose being below 140 mg/dL. Prediabetes is indicated if the 2-h blood glucose is 140 to 200 mg/dL. Diabetes is indicated if the 2-h blood glucose is greater than or equal to 200 mg/dL.

Fasting Blood Glucose Test

A fasting blood glucose level is determined via a blood glucose tolerance test. Glucose testing measures the blood glucose levels after a 12-h period of fasting. Blood glucose may be measured with venous whole blood or finger puncture blood as a quick way to diagnose hypoglycemia and hyperglycemia. It may also be used for self-adjustment of insulin dosage at home. Glucose is the most important carbohydrate in the body metabolism. Glucose is the primary source of energy within most cells. Elevated levels are found with diabetes mellitus, hyperthyroidism, **Cushing's syndrome**, pancreatitis, pregnancy (**gestational diabetes**), severe liver disease, shock, and trauma. Also drugs such as glucagon, corticosteroids, oral contraceptives, and certain diuretics may cause higher levels of blood glucose.

Hypoglycemia is found with Addison's disease, **insulinoma**, hypopituitarism, insulin-producing tumors, **salicylates**, and sulfonamide. The patient must fast for 8 to 12 h before blood is collected. Patients who are taking injectable insulin or oral hypoglycemics will need to have the test performed prior to administration of these medications.

A fasting blood glucose level is determined via a blood glucose tolerance test. The patient must fast for a 12-h period and then drink a mixture of 100 g of glucose, adjusted slightly according to the patient's weight. If the glucose level does not exceed 100 g/dL at the onset of the test period, or 180 g/dL at 1 h after the glucose is ingested, then the patient is believed to have a normal glucose level. Should the blood glucose level exceed 200 g/dL, glucose will escape into the urine because damaged renal tubules are not able to absorb the excessive amounts. A gray-stoppered collection tube must be selected for this test. It contains two additives: sodium fluoride, which prevents red blood cells from metabolizing glucose as a food source after collection, and potassium oxalate, which binds with calcium to prevent clotting.

A 2-h Postprandial Blood Glucose Level Test

A physician may order a 2-h postprandial blood glucose level test instead of a standard glucose tolerance test. The postprandial test involves blood sugar being drawn 2 h after eating a meal. If the patient is healthy, the blood glucose level should not be elevated 2 h after a meal. If it is elevated, diabetes is indicated. This test is used for screening after a patient has exhibited elevated levels in a fasting blood glucose test. It is important for patients with diabetes mellitus to monitor glucose testing. The most common method for performing glucose testing is point-of-care testing (POCT).

Hemoglobin (HbA1c) Testing

Glycosylated hemoglobin (also known as G-hemoglobin or G-Hgb) is hemoglobin that has an attached glucose residue. The hemoglobin *HbA1c* test is relatively new, and it is based on the amount of this substance in the blood. It detects hyperglycemia that may not been seen in type 1 diabetes patients who experience large swings in their blood glucose levels. The amount of hemoglobin A1c is directly related to the average glucose levels in the blood over a 3-month period before the test.

A glucose tolerance test determines the body's ability to metabolize carbohydrates by administering a standard dose of glucose. The blood and urine are then measured for glucose levels at regular intervals. The patient usually must eat a high-carbohydrate diet for 3 days prior to the test and then fast the night before the test. On the morning of the test, a fasting blood glucose level is obtained. The patient then drinks a 75-g dose of glucose (this is adjusted according to the weight of the patient). Blood glucose levels in normal individuals typically peak 30 min to 1 h after glucose ingestion, and they return to normal fasting levels within 2 h. Glucose tolerance test (GTT) specimen results are plotted on a graph, creating GTT curves (see **Figure 13–2**). Blood and urine are collected periodically for up to 6 h. The glucose tolerance test is most often used to assist in the diagnosis of diabetes, hypoglycemia, or other disorders affecting carbohydrate metabolism.

All of the glucose solution must be swallowed within 5 min, and no vomiting can have occurred. If a patient undergoing a glucose tolerance test vomits within 30 min of drinking the glucose beverage, the phlebotomist must notify a nurse or the physician immediately to see if the test should be rescheduled. When blood specimens are taken, they are usually collected into gray-topped tubes containing a substance (sodium fluoride) that prevents the breakdown of glucose, ensuring accuracy. The tubes also contain potassium oxalate, which binds with calcium to prevent clotting.

Two hours after drinking the glucose solution, a normal blood glucose level is lower than 140 mg/dL. A blood glucose level between 140 and 199 mg/dL indicates prediabetes. A

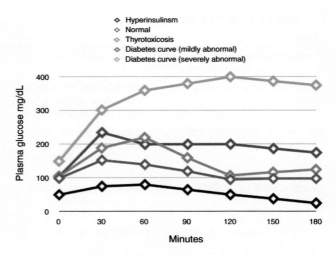

Figure 13–2 Glucose tolerance test specimen results.

blood glucose level of 200 mg/dL or higher indicates diabetes. Urine samples are also collected concurrently with the blood samples, at 30 min, 1 h, 2 h, and 3 h after drinking the glucose solution. Care must be taken to ensure accurate labeling of all samples.

The patient must remain at the testing location throughout, and no food, smoking, alcohol intake, or chewing gum is allowed. Water may be consumed, however. Each specimen should be centrifuged after clotting has occurred to prevent glycolysis. Both urine and serum glucose levels should be run soon after collection, and not as part of the routine laboratory specimens.

An alternative test called the oral glucose tolerance test (GTT) is used if the patient is diabetic. The patient fasts only overnight, and his or her fasting blood glucose is collected in the morning, followed by the patient drinking 75 g of glucose within 5 min. The patient's glucose is again checked 2 h after the drink, with normal blood glucose being below 140 mg/dL. Prediabetes is indicated if the 2-h blood glucose is 140 to 200 mg/dL. Diabetes is indicated if the 2-h blood glucose is greater than or equal to 200 mg/dL.

Timed Specimens

Timed specimens are defined as specimens that are collected at a specific time because timing of collection is critical for any of various reasons. The results of these tests will be most accurate at that specific moment. The reasons for certain blood samples to be taken at specific times include the following:

- blood cultures
- cardiac enzymes
- **therapeutic medication** blood levels, such as lithium levels
- measurement of metabolism rates of various substances
- measurement of **analytes** that exhibit **diurnal variation**

Special patient preparation and timing may be required for certain laboratory tests, including those that test for the highest and lowest medication level times during the day. Other timed specimens include glucose tolerance tests, iron levels, cortisol levels, hormone **assays**, and cardiac enzymes. Phlebotomists must understand how critical the preparation of the patient is prior to collection as well as the timing requirements for collection.

Specifics for therapeutic drug monitoring include correlation of timing for the last dose and time of collection. Drugs that are monitored tend to have a narrow therapeutic index—the blood level required is close to the level that causes significant side effects and/or toxicity. Some drugs have short half-lives, such as amikacin, tobramycin, and gentamicin. Others have longer half-lives, such as digoxin, methotrexate, and phenobarbital. Rates of drug metabolism differ among individuals as well as over time. Indications for therapeutic drug monitoring include the following:

- Knowledge of the drug level influences management.
- The drug dose cannot be optimized by clinical observation alone.
- There are potential patient compliance problems.
- There is an experimentally determined relationship between plasma drug concentration and the pharmacological effect.
- There is a narrow therapeutic window.

Fasting

The **reference values** or expected values published for many laboratory tests are determined from normal volunteers who are in good health. These volunteers are tested after abstaining from food and exercise for a short time. These states are referred to as *fasting* and *basal state specimens*, and they are usually drawn first thing in the morning, after sleeping and very little physical activity. Fasting is the most common timed specimen request, and it means abstaining from food and beverages, except water, for 8–12 h before the test. All strenuous activity should be avoided as well. It is important to avoid eating (patients must fast) because glucose and triglyceride levels are affected by eating.

Blood drawn shortly after a meal may appear cloudy (**lipemic**). Lipemia is caused by a large amount of fatty compounds in the blood after a meal, and it interferes with many laboratory tests. When lipemia is severe, blood serum appears similar to milk instead of its normal clear yellow appearance.

Platelet Function Assay

The **platelet function assay** (PFA) test is used to determine platelet adhesion and aggregation (also called *primary hemostasis*). When platelet function is not normal, it is most commonly caused by uremia, von Willebrand disease (the most common hereditary bleeding disorder), and exposure to various agents, including aspirin. The PFA test is replacing the *bleeding time test* because that test is not useful in patients who use aspirin or nonsteroidal anti-inflammatory agents (NSAIDs), which alter the results. The PFA test requires only a simple venipuncture and is less invasive. Collection is made into two light-blue-topped citrate tubes, which should not be refrigerated and must be delivered to the laboratory within 1 h after collection. A common type of platelet function assay is the *PFA-100*, which analyzes whole blood. PFA tests require the following procedures:

- Standard venipuncture is performed using a 21-gauge or larger needle, with blood being drawn directly into an evacuated plastic or siliconized glass tube or syringe that contains 3.8% buffered sodium citrate.
- If venous collapse or stoppage of blood flow during collection occurs, the sample must be discarded; hemolyzed blood samples cannot be used.
- Samples may be stored at room temperature for up to 4 h, but the PFA test should occur as soon as possible after collection.

In the laboratory, the testing procedures for the collected blood samples are as follows:

- The test cartridges should be allowed to reach room temperature before opening (this usually takes 15 m).
- The top foil from each cartridge is removed (see **Figure 13–3**), and each test cartridge required for use is placed in the cassette of the PFA-100 instrument and pushed until it snaps securely in place (see **Figure 13–4**).
- The tube is inverted by hand 3–4 times.
- Pipette 800 microliters of blood from the collection tube into the smaller opening (sample reservoir opening) of the cartridge, dispensing it slowly along one of the inside corners to reduce air entrapment (see **Figure 13–5**).

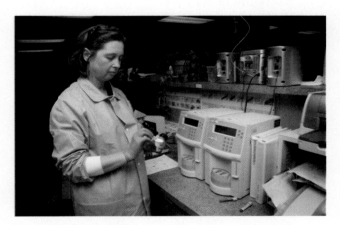

Figure 13–3 The top foil from each cartridge is removed.

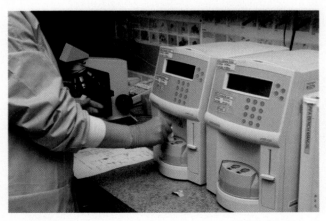

Figure 13–4 Each test cartridge required for use is placed in the cassette of the PFA-100 instrument and pushed until it snaps securely in place.

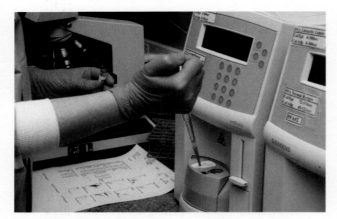

Figure 13–5 Pipette 800 microliters of blood from the collection tube into the smaller opening (sample reservoir opening) of the cartridge, dispensing it slowly along one of the inside corners to reduce air entrapment.

- Place the cassette with the test cartridge or cartridges into the incubation well(s) of the instrument, making sure the cassette is flush to the carousel surface—do not apply any pressure to the sample reservoir opening.
- The test is started within the PFA-100 machine, following the policies and procedures of the testing facility (see **Figure 13–6**).

The PFA-100 system analyzes small samples of anticoagulated whole blood, allowing for rapid evaluation of platelet function. Each test cartridge is designed for single use. Several chambers within each cartridge expose platelets to high shear flow conditions. A collagen coating, combined with either epinephrine or adenosine diphosphate (ADP), triggers the platelet activation process. The platelets form a thrombus at the aperture of the device, and the computer determines the time from the start of the test until this occurs. The time interval is reported as *closure time.*

Some healthcare organizations still utilize the bleeding time test, but it is becoming less common every year. The bleeding time test measures platelet plug formation in the capillaries, and was primarily used to test for **hemostasis.**

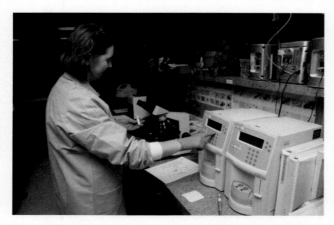

Figure 13–6 The test is started within the PFA-100 machine, following the policies and procedures of the testing facility.

This test involved making a minor standardized incision on the forearm and recording the length of time needed for bleeding to cease. This length of time depends on the quantity and quality of platelets, and the ability of the blood vessel wall to constrict.

Blood Donation

Phlebotomists perform blood donations, and the blood contains many products that may help save a life during blood transfusion. These products include plasma, platelets, red blood cells, blood clotting factors, blood typing reagents, proteins, and immunoglobulins. Blood products are separated into components at the donation facility, such as the American Red Cross. Labeling must be completely accurate so that each unit is traceable to its donor.

Not everyone is allowed to donate blood. Individuals must be of the appropriate age (between 17 and 66 years), weight (at least 110 lb), and health status. For minors, written parental consent is required. Hematocrit and hemoglobin levels should be high enough that the donor is not harmed by the donation. Before donation, a complete health history and physical examination is required. Recent foreign travel, IV drug use, recent tattoos, and certain sexual activities may cancel a person's ability to donate blood. The questions about sexual activity are in place to screen for human immunodeficiency virus (HIV) and sexually transmitted infections (STIs).

The blood supply available for transfusion must be kept safe. Sometimes people who are pressured into donating may lie during the questioning simply because they want to contribute to the blood supply. Admitting risky behaviors can be difficult. Staff members should inform donors that they will have a second chance to admit risky behaviors without any others hearing the information.

After the initial screening is accepted, the donor is placed in a sitting or **reclined position**. Donation collects between 450 and 500 mL of blood, which takes approximately 7 min. The skin is twice cleaned, in the antecubital area, and blood is collected in a sterile, closed collection system. This consists of a blood collection bag, tubing, and a 16-gauge needle. The blood flows via gravity from the vein into the bag, which is placed lower than the arm of the donor. The bag contains citrate phosphate dextrose, an anticoagulant. Sometimes the bag is placed on a mixing unit beside the patient so that its contents can be agitated, ensuring complete mixing of blood with the anticoagulant. It may also be mixed manually by manipulating the bag. These sterile closed collection systems are only for single use. If the bag does not fill properly, for any reason, all of the components of the system must be discarded. Another complete system must be used for a second attempt.

Blood donations for one's own future use can also be made, and they are known as *autologous blood donations.* These can be kept on reserve for use within a specified time period. If one is donating before an upcoming surgery, certain conditions must be met, including a written physician's order and the ability to normally regenerate red blood cells. Health status must be stable, and hemoglobin must be at least

11 g. The upcoming surgery must be more than 72 h from the time of blood donation. This type of donation is becoming more popular as people become more aware of the risks of blood-borne pathogens.

Patients must be monitored for dizziness, nausea, and other side effects. The donor should be kept in a reclining position, with the head lower than the heart. He or she should not walk or stand due to the likelihood of fainting and falling. After donation, the patient is given fruit juice or a small snack to keep blood glucose levels adequate.

Therapeutic Collection

Usually, therapeutic phlebotomy is used to treat **polycythemia**, a disease causing the overproduction or an abnormal increase in red blood cells. This condition can harm the overall health of the patient. It causes the heart and other organs to become very strained by attempting to circulate abnormally high amounts of cells. Another condition using therapeutic collection is **hemochromatosis**, wherein the body stores abnormal amounts of iron. This condition can lead to serious health problems, and therapeutic collection of blood is undertaken to reduce the levels of iron throughout the body.

Chain of Custody

Forensic laboratories are legally accountable for the documentation of evidence handling within the organization, while clinical laboratories are not. This documentation starts when specimens are received from a medical examiner or coroner's office. The **chain of custody** is a process that maintains control of, and accountability for, each specimen from the time of collection to the time of disposal. It documents both the identity of every individual who has handled a specimen and each time that the specimen is transferred. A chain of custody form is required, which also identifies the patient or subject from whom the specimen was collected; the person who obtained and processed it; and the date, location, and signature of the person who attests that the specimen is the correct one and matches its documentation.

Specimens are placed into specimen transfer bags and permanently sealed until the time of analysis. The seal ensures "tamper-evident" transfer. Many clinical laboratories, in actuality, also use the chain of custody. An example is for in-house drug-testing programs. Forensic specimens differ from clinical specimens because they are accepted in any condition. Employees of forensic laboratories must verify that requisitions match the labeled evidence collected, including names, ages, gender, case numbers, and types of specimens.

Specimen Tampering

Subjects being tested often tamper with their specimens in order to avoid being caught using various types of drugs. Most commonly, urine specimens are tampered with to make them test "negative" for drugs. The subject may ingest various substances that alter the urine or may add substances into the urine during the time of collection. Water is the most common substance used; subjects use it to dilute the urine so that drug concentrations are lower than the detection limit. Other added substances include bleach, liquid soap, ammonia, salt,

baking soda, vinegar, lemon juice, cologne, and products sold for this purpose (including UrinAid and Klear).

Drug testing of urine typically involves the collection of "split urine" in 45-mL increments into acceptable containers. Collectors must inspect the containers immediately to check for signs of tampering within 4 min of collection. The collector then pours at least 30 mL of urine from the collection container into a specimen bottle and seals it. This is labeled as the *primary* ("A") specimen bottle. Then at least 15 mL of the urine is poured into a second bottle and sealed. This is labeled as the *split* ("B") specimen bottle.

Detection of substances added into collected urine involves inspecting the specimen's color, odor, and temperature. Simple tests can also be used to determine the urine's specific gravity, creatinine level, and electrolyte level. Other precautions include the addition of a bluing agent to the toilet water, preventing the patient from taking unneeded items into the collection room, and direct observation of any devices concealed in the subject's clothing. If tampering is either suspected or observed, the collector may request another specimen and sometimes conduct another collection procedure under direct observation (according to strict federal guidelines).

Blood Alcohol Testing

Police may request blood alcohol level testing, such as in the case of a driving under the influence (DUI) charge. The patient must consent to having the blood test performed, and he or she may refuse it. If a phlebotomist attempts to collect a specimen without written consent, he or she may be guilty of assault and battery. The test will not be admissible in court. Great care must be taken by the phlebotomist during collection because these specimens are often used for legal cases. The chain of custody of these samples must be closely monitored. When blood alcohol testing is performed, the site from which blood will be taken must be cleaned by an appropriate antiseptic (for example, chlorhexidine) instead of alcohol, because alcohol used for cleaning the skin could give a false positive to the test. Iodine swabs also cannot be used because they contain alcohol.

Employee Testing

Employee testing began when the Department of Health and Human Services (HHS) established the first federal drug-testing programs. The *Custody and Control Form* (CCF) is used in these programs (see **Figure 13–7**). Compliance provides quality assurance and quality control, personnel, standards of testing of specimens, and results reporting. Other guidelines and forms are provided by the Department of Transportation (DOT). Individuals who collect samples for employee testing have direct contact with those being tested. They must ensure that specimen integrity and the collection process are adequately maintained and utilized.

Employee testing is used for many reasons, including the following:

- To comply with customer, contract, or insurance carrier requirements
- To comply with federal regulations

- To establish reasons for disciplinary actions
- To identify users and refer them for assistance
- To improve the safety and health of employees as well as to reduce addiction
- To minimize the chances of hiring drug users or abusers
- To reinforce "no drug use" policies

Common industries that DOT requires to participate in antidrug programs include aviation, highway, mass transit, railroad, hazardous materials transport, pipeline, maritime, and other safety-sensitive industries.

Drug testing may be utilized prior to employment, before a job promotion, as part of an annual physical test, for employees who are reasonably suspected of using drugs, as part of a

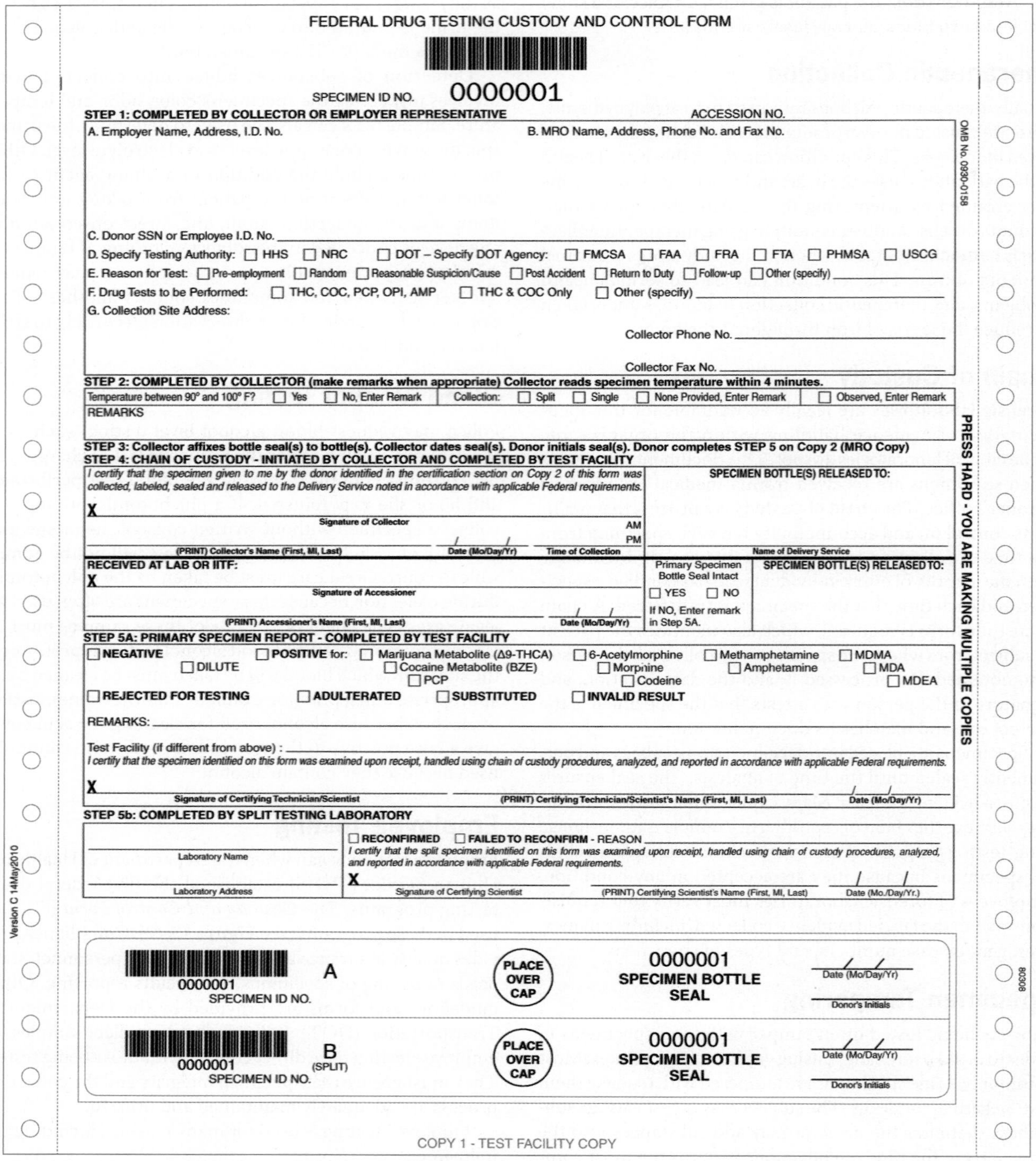

FEDERAL DRUG TESTING CUSTODY AND CONTROL FORM

SPECIMEN ID NO. 0000001

OMB No. 0930-0158

STEP 1: COMPLETED BY COLLECTOR OR EMPLOYER REPRESENTATIVE ACCESSION NO.

A. Employer Name, Address, I.D. No. B. MRO Name, Address, Phone No. and Fax No.

C. Donor SSN or Employee I.D. No. ______

D. Specify Testing Authority: ☐ HHS ☐ NRC ☐ DOT – Specify DOT Agency: ☐ FMCSA ☐ FAA ☐ FRA ☐ FTA ☐ PHMSA ☐ USCG

E. Reason for Test: ☐ Pre-employment ☐ Random ☐ Reasonable Suspicion/Cause ☐ Post Accident ☐ Return to Duty ☐ Follow-up ☐ Other (specify) ______

F. Drug Tests to be Performed: ☐ THC, COC, PCP, OPI, AMP ☐ THC & COC Only ☐ Other (specify) ______

G. Collection Site Address:

Collector Phone No. ______

Collector Fax No. ______

STEP 2: COMPLETED BY COLLECTOR (make remarks when appropriate) Collector reads specimen temperature within 4 minutes.

Temperature between 90° and 100° F? ☐ Yes ☐ No, Enter Remark | Collection: ☐ Split ☐ Single ☐ None Provided, Enter Remark | ☐ Observed, Enter Remark

REMARKS

STEP 3: Collector affixes bottle seal(s) to bottle(s). Collector dates seal(s). Donor initials seal(s). Donor completes STEP 5 on Copy 2 (MRO Copy)

STEP 4: CHAIN OF CUSTODY - INITIATED BY COLLECTOR AND COMPLETED BY TEST FACILITY

I certify that the specimen given to me by the donor identified in the certification section on Copy 2 of this form was collected, labeled, sealed and released to the Delivery Service noted in accordance with applicable Federal requirements.

X ______ Signature of Collector

______ (PRINT) Collector's Name (First, MI, Last) __/__/__ Date (Mo/Day/Yr) ______ AM PM Time of Collection

SPECIMEN BOTTLE(S) RELEASED TO: ______ Name of Delivery Service

RECEIVED AT LAB OR IITF:

X ______ Signature of Accessioner

______ (PRINT) Accessioner's Name (First, MI, Last) __/__/__ Date (Mo/Day/Yr)

Primary Specimen Bottle Seal Intact ☐ YES ☐ NO If NO, Enter remark in Step 5A.

SPECIMEN BOTTLE(S) RELEASED TO:

STEP 5A: PRIMARY SPECIMEN REPORT - COMPLETED BY TEST FACILITY

☐ NEGATIVE ☐ DILUTE ☐ POSITIVE for: ☐ Marijuana Metabolite (Δ9-THCA) ☐ Cocaine Metabolite (BZE) ☐ PCP ☐ 6-Acetylmorphine ☐ Morphine ☐ Codeine ☐ Methamphetamine ☐ Amphetamine ☐ MDMA ☐ MDA ☐ MDEA

☐ REJECTED FOR TESTING ☐ ADULTERATED ☐ SUBSTITUTED ☐ INVALID RESULT

REMARKS: ______

Test Facility (if different from above) : ______

I certify that the specimen identified on this form was examined upon receipt, handled using chain of custody procedures, analyzed, and reported in accordance with applicable Federal requirements.

X ______ Signature of Certifying Technician/Scientist ______ (PRINT) Certifying Technician/Scientist's Name (First, MI, Last) __/__/__ Date (Mo/Day/Yr)

STEP 5b: COMPLETED BY SPLIT TESTING LABORATORY

______ Laboratory Name

______ Laboratory Address

☐ RECONFIRMED ☐ FAILED TO RECONFIRM - REASON ______

I certify that the split specimen identified on this form was examined upon receipt, handled using chain of custody procedures, analyzed, and reported in accordance with applicable Federal requirements.

X ______ Signature of Certifying Scientist ______ (PRINT) Certifying Scientist's Name (First, MI, Last) __/__/__ Date (Mo./Day/Yr.)

PRESS HARD - YOU ARE MAKING MULTIPLE COPIES

Version C 14May2010

0000001 SPECIMEN ID NO. A PLACE OVER CAP 0000001 SPECIMEN BOTTLE SEAL __/__/__ Date (Mo/Day/Yr) ______ Donor's Initials

0000001 SPECIMEN ID NO. B (SPLIT) PLACE OVER CAP 0000001 SPECIMEN BOTTLE SEAL __/__/__ Date (Mo/Day/Yr) ______ Donor's Initials

80308

COPY 1 - TEST FACILITY COPY

Figure 13–7 The Federal Drug Testing Custody and Control Form (CCF).

Source: Courtesy of the Substance Abuse and Mental Health Services Administration. Full form available at: http://www.reginfo.gov/public/do/PRAViewIC?ref_nbr=201007-0930-002&icID=193835

random testing program, after accidents or injuries, to clear an employee to return to work, in relation to investigations of child or elder abuse, and when operation of company vehicles is required.

Employers must explain what actions will be taken following a positive drug test. Institutional procedures for drug testing are usually a part of a workplace drug-testing program. Testing must be timely in order to produce accurate results. However, many drugs are detectable for several days after use. Employees must be aware and thoroughly trained in all of the procedures related to drug testing.

When an employee is tested, he or she must be correctly identified via driver's license, employee badge, or other issued picture identification. Alternatively, the employee may be identified by an employer or employer representative, or via any other identification that the employer allows.

Athletic Testing

Athletes have been in the news more frequently in recent years because of their use of various drugs to enhance physical performance. Agencies such as the National Collegiate Athletic Association (NCAA) are regularly involved in drug testing—in this case, of college athletes. Primarily, urinalysis is used to check for the presence of anabolic steroids and other performance-enhancing drugs. Also, the use of certain nutritional or dietary supplements may cause a positive drug test result. The NCAA and other organizations commonly ban the following substances: anabolic steroids, stimulants, diuretics, illegal drugs, peptide hormones and their analogs, and antiestrogens.

Another area of focus is "blood doping," wherein whole blood or other blood products are injected intravenously into athletes in order to increase blood oxygen-carrying capacity to increase endurance. Also, genetically engineered proteins such as recombinant human erythropoietin (rHuEPO) are used for the same effect. This form of erythropoietin is hard to detect, although newer detection methods are more effective.

Forensic Specimens

Forensic specimens, like legal specimens, must follow a special chain of custody procedure. Documentation must account for the specimen at every moment from collection until delivery. Each person who handles the specimen must sign and date a legal document that indicates both the person from whom the specimen was collected and the length of time each person in the chain had custody of the specimen. Forensic specimens must be kept in locked containers or sealed tubes so that unauthorized people cannot tamper with them.

The various types of samples collected for forensic purposes include blood, bones, hair, nails, saliva, skin, soil or mud, sperm, sweat, teeth, and vegetation. Usually, forensic specimens are collected to prove or disprove links between individuals, objects, or places. General guidelines for collecting forensic specimens are listed in **Table 13–2**. It is important to follow the guidelines for handling forensic specimens that are set forth by the employer. The employer should provide proper training concerning this work. Forensic evidence kits may be required.

Toxicology

Toxicology is the science that deals with poisoning, particularly with the effects of drugs or other chemicals upon the intracellular function of tissues and organs. Toxicologists study how poisons act and how they can be detected. They also focus on the treatment of medical conditions that poisons can cause. It is vital to follow laboratory protocols when handling toxicology specimens. Contamination can come from bacteria and oil on the hands, glass, and plastic materials, so great care must be taken in handling these specimens.

Therapeutic Drug Monitoring

A physician may use *therapeutic drug monitoring* to supervise a patient's drug or medication treatment. Each patient requires different dosages to produce desired effects. Monitoring medication levels helps to establish beneficial levels for the patient and helps to avoid toxicity. Common medications requiring therapeutic monitoring are listed in **Table 13–3**.

For therapeutic drug monitoring, specimens are obtained by routine venipuncture, but must be collected when medicines are at their highest serum concentration—usually 15 to 30 min after being administered. This is known as the **peak** level. **Trough** levels are also collected, when the serum concentrations of medications are expected to be at their lowest levels, usually immediately before administration of a scheduled dose. If a patient is hospitalized, the phlebotomist should double-check with the patient's nurse to verify that the dosage schedule is accurate.

Usually peaks and troughs are measured for antibiotics that are toxic at high levels, but not effective at lower levels. Drugs (such as antibiotics) with a short half-life make the time of collection more critical. Timing is less critical for drugs that have longer half-lives. The actual times that specimens are drawn must be documented. All drug-monitoring specimens must be labeled as either peak or trough to signify the levels that were established correctly.

Table 13–2 Collection of Forensic Specimens

Factor	Comments
Documentation	All specimen handling must be documented, usually on a chain of custody form.
Gloves	They should always be worn when handling specimens, to avoid contamination.
Handling	Specimens should be packed, stored, and transported correctly, such as by refrigeration, humidity control, or controlling room temperature.
Labeling	Specimens should be labeled with patient name, birth date, name of person performing the collection, type of specimen, date of collection, and time of collection.
Packaging	Packing of specimens should be secure and tamper-proof—only authorized people should touch specimens.
Timing	Collect specimens as soon as possible.

Alternative Collection Sites

Blood may also be collected from alternative sites other than the commonly used veins and capillaries. Arterial punctures and venous access devices are commonly used.

Arterial Punctures

Usually, arterial punctures are used to test arterial blood gases (ABGs), which measure the lungs' ability to exchange carbon dioxide and oxygen. Results may show the partial pressure of these substances in the arterial blood as well as the pH level of the blood. Because arterial blood is oxygenated, it has a bright red appearance (while venous blood has a dark red appearance because it carries carbon dioxide). Arterial puncture is usually not performed by a phlebotomist because it requires special training. Usually, arterial punctures are performed by members of the respiratory therapy department of a facility. Licensed personnel who are usually responsible for conducting arterial punctures include nurses, physicians, medical technologists, and respiratory therapists. Because blood pressure is much higher in the arteries, arterial blood will pulsate into the tube during the draw.

Actual steps for performing arterial puncture are as follows:

1. Cleanse the skin at the puncture site with the alcohol swab. The patient's hand should be bent back slightly, or a small rolled towel should be placed under the wrist. This brings the radial artery closer to the surface. Over-extending the wrist should be avoided, as this might occlude the pulse.

2. Palpate for the pulse with the index or middle finger. After locating the strongest pulse sensation, slightly anchor the artery with the index and middle fingers. This will prevent the artery from rolling when it is punctured.

3. The syringe should be held at a 45° angle or less in the opposite hand, similar to a person holding a pencil or a dart. This near-parallel insertion of the needle will minimize trauma to the artery and allow the smooth muscle fibers to seal the puncture hole after the needle is withdrawn.

4. While anchoring the artery and with the bevel of the needle turned upward, insert the needle to just under the skin surface. Now advance the needle slowly until a flashing pulsation of blood is seen in the hub of the needle. Stop and maintain this position until 2 to 4 cc of blood has been collected in the syringe. If the needle is advanced too far, withdraw it slowly until blood flows into the syringe. There should be no need to aspirate the blood into the syringe as arterial pressure will allow autofilling of the syringe. Only in the event that a small-gauge needle (e.g., 25 gauge) is used, or the patient is hypotensive, should the syringe be aspirated.

5. After obtaining the desired amount of blood, withdraw the needle and apply pressure to the puncture site with the 4×4 gauze. After pressure has been applied for 2 min, check the site for bleeding, oozing, or seepage of blood. If there are any signs present, apply pressure until all bleeding has stopped. A long compression time will be necessary for patients who are on anticoagulant therapy or who have bleeding disorders.

6. Remove the needle from the syringe. The needle should never be recapped, bent, or purposely broken because of the danger of self-puncture. All needles should be placed in designated, puncture-resistant containers (commonly known as sharps containers).

7. It is vitally important that air bubbles be removed from the blood gas syringe, as they may alter the blood gas results. Hold the syringe upright, and gently tap the syringe so that the air bubbles are forced to the top of the syringe where they can be expelled.

Cap the syringe and place it in a bag of ice (icing the sample will prevent any further metabolism of blood). Attach the lab slip to the bag, and have the sample transported to the laboratory. If the sample is going to be analyzed, make sure to do so as soon as possible. Blood gas analysis (see **Figure 13–8**) involves measurement of the partial pressure of oxygen (pO_2), partial pressure of carbon dioxide (pCO_2), and pH.

Venous Access Devices

A **cannula** is a hollow tube that is inserted and left in a vein. It is referred to as a *venous access device*. The most commonly used type for obtaining blood samples is called a **heparin lock**. This is a special winged needle set left in a patient's vein for between 48 and 72 h. In specific circumstances, heparin locks are used when obtaining blood is difficult or the patient needs multiple draws over a short time. However, these locks are primarily used to administer certain medications. The

Table 13–3 Commonly Monitored Medications

Type of Medication	Examples	Indications
Antibiotics	Amikacin, gentamicin, tobramycin, vancomycin	Infections
Anticonvulsants	Phenobarbital, phenytoin	Abnormal discharge of central nervous system electrical impulses, treatment of seizure activity
Antidepressants	Thorazine (chlorpromazine)	Elevation of mood, treatment of depression
Blood thinners	Heparin, warfarin	Heart conditions, coagulation disorders
Cardiac glycosides	Lanoxin (digoxin)	To increase strength of heart contraction, slow heart rate, treat heart failure (such as congestive heart failure)
Mood stabilizers	Lithium	Stabilization of mood swings, treatment of manic-depressive psychosis
Xanthine derivatives	Theophylline	Opening of airway passages, treatment of asthma and bronchitis

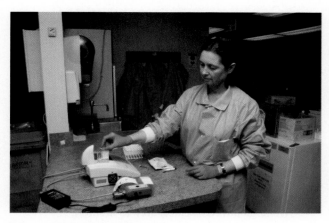

Figure 13–8 Blood gas analysis.

cannula must be periodically flushed with heparin or normal saline to keep clots from forming. If heparin is chosen, the first 5 mL must be discarded before any specimens are collected. Only specially trained personnel should do this—phlebotomists usually are not sufficiently trained.

Other venous access devices include **shunts** and **central venous therapy lines**. Arterial venous shunts are devices that are inserted into the forearm to allow hemodialysis to occur. The shunt is connected to a machine that filters the blood, as is often done for patients with severe kidney disease. Central venous therapy involves introducing a cannula into a vein other than a peripheral vein. Phlebotomists usually do not perform these functions. *Vascular access devices* are defined as those that allow frequent access to a patient's veins without using IV needles or other large catheters. An example is a "chemo port," which is used to infuse chemotherapy.

Summary

Blood specimens may be taken at specific times to ensure accuracy. They can be affected by intake of alcohol, food, medications, and tobacco as well as exercise, posture, stress, and time of day. Bleeding time tests assess platelet function. Phlebotomists must have special training to obtain blood for donations. Patients may donate blood for their own future needs. Blood alcohol testing requires written consent from patients. Forensic specimens may be used as evidence in court. Toxicology specimens detect drugs, medications, and poisons. Therapeutic drug monitoring ensures correct amounts of drugs to provide the desired effects. Alternative methods of blood collection include arterial venous shunt, heparin lock, arterial punctures, and central venous therapy lines.

CRITICAL THINKING

An emergency physician ordered a blood alcohol test for a 27-year-old patient who was brought into the emergency room after a car accident. The accompanying police officer had indicated suspicion of alcohol use.

1. What are the most important procedures that the phlebotomist must follow in collecting blood from this patient?
2. What form of consent must be obtained from the patient and why?

WEBSITES

http://www.buzzle.com/articles/forensic-toxicology.html

http://www.emedicinehealth.com/venous_access_devices/article_em.htm

http://www.givelife2.org/donor/faq.asp

http://www.mclno.org/webresources/pathman/BT_web/Bleeding_time.htm

http://www.nhlbi.nih.gov/health/dci/Diseases/bt/bt_whatis.html

http://www.nlm.nih.gov/medlineplus/ency/article/003430.htm

http://www.nlm.nih.gov/medlineplus/ency/article/003466.htm

http://www.ou.edu/oupd/bac.htm

http://www.redcrossblood.org/

http://www.who.int/violence_injury_prevention/resources/publications/en/guidelines_chap5.pdf

REVIEW QUESTIONS

Multiple Choice

1. The testing of glucose levels helps to diagnose
   A. diurnal variation
   B. hemophilia
   C. pregnancy
   D. diabetes mellitus
2. Blood donors are placed into which position prior to venipuncture?
   A. standing
   B. prone
   C. inverted
   D. reclined
3. Two conditions that utilize therapeutic phlebotomy include
   A. hemophilia and diabetes
   B. alcoholism and drug addiction
   C. polycythemia and hemochromatosis
   D. glycolysis and lipemia
4. A lipemic specimen is an indication that the patient is
   A. drinking milk
   B. not fasting
   C. drinking coffee
   D. chewing tobacco
5. Fasting specimens are preferred for which of the following tests?
   A. hemoglobin
   B. creatinine
   C. triglycerides
   D. thyroid function
6. Which of the following causes would give plasma or serum a milky appearance?
   A. hyperlipidemia
   B. protein disorder
   C. vegetarian diet
   D. cancer

7. For fasting blood sugar, patients must fast for
   A. 2 to 3 h
   B. 4 to 5 h
   C. 6 to 7 h
   D. 8 to 12 h

8. The needle gauge for collecting blood from an adult donor is
   A. 16
   B. 19
   C. 21
   D. 25

9. The venipuncture site for blood alcohol testing must be cleaned with
   A. iodine
   B. hydrogen peroxide
   C. an alcohol prep pad
   D. methyl alcohol

10. Which statement is false in the collection of forensic specimens?
    A. Collect the specimen as soon as possible
    B. Avoid contamination
    C. Discard the chain-of-custody form
    D. Make sure the specimen is tamper-proof

11. Therapeutic drug monitoring must be collected when
    A. patients fast
    B. medicines are at their highest blood levels
    C. elderly patients are at risk of internal bleeding
    D. individuals are using illegal drugs

12. How many times during the classic oral glucose tolerance test must blood glucose be checked over the 3-h period?
    A. two
    B. three
    C. four
    D. five

13. Which color-stoppered tube should be used to collect fasting blood glucose?
    A. gray
    B. red
    C. black
    D. yellow

14. Hemoglobin A1c is measured to monitor
    A. hemolytic disease of the newborn
    B. diabetes
    C. anemia
    D. transfusion reactions

15. Hypoglycemia is found with
    A. hyperthyroidism
    B. pregnancy
    C. pancreatitis
    D. insulinoma

CHAPTER 14

Specialized Phlebotomy

OUTLINE

Introduction
Pediatric Phlebotomy
Special Neonatal Blood Collection and Screening
Blood Spot Collection
Geriatric Phlebotomy
    Venipuncture Procedures
Blood Cultures
Arterial Blood Gases
Phlebotomy for Anticoagulated Patients
Phlebotomy for Obese Patients
Phlebotomy for Psychiatric Patients
Summary
Critical Thinking
Websites
Review Questions

OBJECTIVES

After studying this chapter, readers should be able to:

1. In which condition would capillary puncture be preferred over venipuncture?
2. What are the most common methods of neonatal and infant blood collection?
3. Describe the methods used to draw blood from the capillaries of geriatric patients.
4. List the types of patients most commonly requiring capillary puncture.
5. Explain the indications of blood cultures.
6. Describe the most common conditions that require arterial blood gas testing.
7. Discuss why blood collection may be difficult for anticoagulated patients.
8. Explain how phlebotomists should deal with blood collection from obese patients.
9. Explain the Allen test.
10. Discuss the collection of blood from psychiatric patients.

KEY TERMS

Bacteremia: A general term that indicates the presence of bacteria in the blood; it is also called *septicemia*.

Globules: Spherical masses of lipid tissue under the skin.

Jaundice: Disease characterized by yellowish color of the skin, sclera, mucous membranes, and body fluids.

Microhematocrit tube: A common, heparin-coated capillary tube used for determining the percentage of packed red blood cells in microhematocrit tests.

Introduction

Phlebotomists are required to be skillful to collect blood specimens from children and elderly patients. They must be specialized and trained for collecting blood specimens for blood cultures and arterial blood gases. Dealing with these types of blood specimen collections poses unique challenges for phlebotomists. Only specially trained and skilled phlebotomists should collect blood samples from neonates, infants, and children because of the risk of complications that may occur during or after these procedures. Capillary puncture is usually performed on the heel of the foot for neonates and infants. For children over the age of 1 year or adults, a finger is used for capillary puncture. In adults, the distal segment of the middle finger is usually used. Collected specimens must be handled properly to maintain their quality for accurate test results. The recommendations for pediatric and geriatric phlebotomy in this chapter conform to the standards of the Clinical and Laboratory Standards Institute (CLSI). Blood cultures that are collected before antimicrobial therapy require special tubes or bottles that contain a nutrient medium that promotes the growth of microorganisms present in blood. Arterial blood gases are obtained by arterial puncture and require special training; usually, the individuals performing this procedure must be certified by their healthcare facility.

Pediatric Phlebotomy

Phlebotomy for infants and children requires special knowledge and abilities. Younger patients are not fully able to understand what types of tests have to be administered, and they are usually afraid of the experience. The phlebotomist must be prepared to handle a variety of difficulties concerning infants and children. Another consideration is that the blood vessels of children are smaller and more difficult to visualize and palpate.

For neonates and infants under the age of 1 year, skin puncture is done for blood collection. The heel of the foot is the puncture site of choice, with the capillaries providing the collected blood. The depth of heel puncture must be carefully controlled to avoid injuring the calcaneus bone, which can cause osteomyelitis. For children older than 1 year, collection of blood for routine capillary puncture is obtained from the fingers.

In children younger than 2 years of age, use only the superficial veins. Use a butterfly collection set and a 23-gauge needle. The flexible tubing that this utilizes allows the child to move slightly during blood collection. The butterfly set will show a flash of blood in the tubing when the needle enters the vein. Often, young children can remain on their parent's lap as the procedure is performed (see **Figure 14–1**). Another method of restraint is the *papoose*, a specially designed board

with attached canvas flaps. Cooperative children may undergo phlebotomy while lying on an examination table or sitting in a phlebotomy chair. A child phlebotomy station is especially designed for this purpose.

Skill is required to perform blood collection from a child as painlessly and nontraumatically as possible. If the child is not extremely young, involve him or her in the process. Ask the child to hold the gauze pad or adhesive bandage and tell you exactly when he or she feels pain—this will help to focus attention on the minimal amount of pain actually caused and away from the needle itself. Sometimes the use of a doll or stuffed animal can help you to demonstrate to the child exactly how the procedure is done before you begin. It is crucial to ensure that all supplies are gathered before the actual procedure. From children, only the minimum amount of blood needed for the required tests is drawn—a quantity much less than that from an adult.

Blood is collected drop by drop into Microtainers through a funnel-like device. Capillary tubes are another way to collect blood from dermal punctures. They are made of glass or plastic and fill by normal capillary action, after the puncture is made by a *lancet*. These narrow tubes do not utilize suction. If the capillary tube is coated with the anticoagulant heparin, a red band will be seen at the top. A common ammonium heparin-coated capillary tube is the **microhematocrit tube**, used for manually determining the percentage of packed red blood cells in the microhematocrit test. Some microhematocrit tubes are plain, meaning that they have no additives. Microtubes should not be overfilled because there is not enough anticoagulant for the increased volume of blood. Therefore, overfilling may cause the formation of microclots. Blood from a capillary puncture can also be used to test neonates for certain metabolic disorders such as phenylketonuria (PKU). Capillary puncture blood is a mixture of arterial, venous, and capillary blood. It does not contain serous fluid.

Special Neonatal Blood Collection and Screening

When bilirubin is overproduced, it is due to accelerated red blood cell hemolysis. This is associated with *hemolytic disease of the newborn* (HDN). High levels of bilirubin may result in **jaundice**, which causes the skin to become yellow. In premature infants, temporary abnormal liver function often causes impaired bilirubin excretion. Bilirubin is dangerous in infants because it can accumulate to toxic levels, causing permanent brain damage and even death. Jaundiced infants are often placed under special ultraviolet (UV) lights to lower bilirubin levels because bilirubin breaks down in the presence of light. UV lights must be turned off prior to collecting any blood samples because a darkened Microtainer is not adequate to protect the sample from these lights during capillary collection.

When bilirubin specimens are collected, accuracy is crucial—this usually requires collection by heel puncture. The procedure must be performed quickly to minimize exposure to light. The same minimal light exposure must be maintained during transportation and handling. To reduce light exposure, amber-colored microcollection containers are often used. Microcollection containers are sometimes called

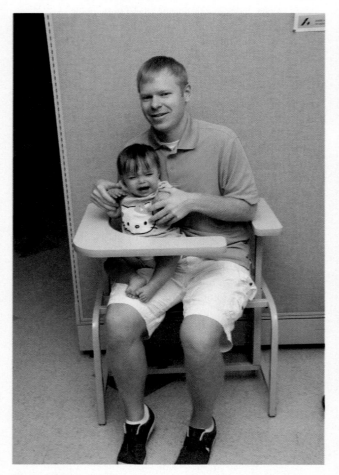

Figure 14–1 A child being restrained while sitting on a parent's lap as phlebotomy is being performed.

bullets. Hemolysis of specimens must be avoided because this can falsely decrease bilirubin levels. Specimens should be collected as closely as possible to when they are requested because the rate of increase in bilirubin levels depends on accurate timing.

The routine testing of newborns for certain genetic, metabolic, hormonal, and functional disorders is referred to as *newborn/neonatal testing*. These tests help to detect, on a timely basis, potential disorders that may lead to mental and physical impairments such as phenylketonuria, galactosemia, and hypothyroidism. Certain states in the United States also test for infectious agents such as toxoplasma and human immunodeficiency virus (HIV). The March of Dimes recommends that all newborns be tested for 30 specific disorders, including hearing loss. Newborn/neonatal tests are usually done when the infant is between 24 and 72 h old.

Blood Spot Collection

Blood spot testing for screening is performed within 72 h after birth. All newborn screening tests are usually performed on just a few drops of blood, obtained via heel puncture. The blood drops are absorbed onto circles that are printed on a specific filter paper usually asked for on the requisition form. The blood-filled circles are called *blood spots*.

After the infant's heel has been punctured and the first drop of blood wiped away, the filter paper is brought close to the heel, and a large drop of free-flowing blood is applied to the center of the first printed circle. The paper must never touch the surface of the heel in order to avoid smearing, blotting, stopping of blood flow, or incomplete penetration of blood through the paper. The paper's position must be maintained as blood continues to flow and completely fill the circle on both sides of the paper.

The same process is continued until all circles are completely filled. Each circle must be completely filled, or the required tests cannot be performed. The circles must be filled from one side of the paper only; each large drop spreads throughout. If multiple drops are used or the circles are filled from both sides of the paper, the blood may become layered, making the results inaccurate.

The collected specimens should be air-dried while the collection paper is in an elevated, horizontal position kept away from heat or sunlight. The papers should not be hung or stacked. Hanging them can cause blood to move toward the lower part of the paper, making results inaccurate. Stacking them can cross-contaminate between specimens. Once fully dried, the requisition containing the samples is placed in a special envelope and sent to a state public health (or other approved) laboratory for tests. Once complete, results are sent to the physician or other healthcare provider.

Geriatric Phlebotomy

The geriatric (elderly) population comprises about 15% of the population of the United States and uses 31% of all healthcare services. Within 25 years, this population will be equivalent to 20% of the total U.S. population. Skin puncture may be more difficult in these patients because of the effects of such conditions as arthritis or Parkinson's disease. Often, the elderly patient requires point-of-care testing and other healthcare services in the home, rehabilitation center, nursing home, or other long-term care facility.

Geriatric patients should always be treated with the utmost respect and courtesy. Their privacy must always be respected. Aging causes a variety of physical and emotional problems that may affect venipuncture procedures. Because of hearing problems, it is important to ensure that the patient has heard and understood instructions. Patients should always be addressed with respectful terms such as *Mr., Mrs., Ms.,* or *Miss.* Because of vision problems, it is also important to ensure that the patient can get to blood collection seats. Memory loss may mean that a patient has forgotten to take a medication that was required to be taken prior to a blood collection procedure.

Geriatric patients may experience edema caused by the accumulation of excessive fluid in the tissues. These areas should be avoided for venipuncture. Because of edema, it is difficult to palpate the vein. The skin does not bounce back, and a "finger" impression may be observed in the palpated area. The specimen can also become diluted by tissue fluid.

Venipuncture Procedures

With geriatric patients, thinner skin tissue makes venipuncture more difficult. The skin must be held more tautly so that the patient's vein does not "roll." The patient's arm should not be tapped with too much force to locate the vein because this can easily cause bruising. Heated compresses may be helpful. Because the muscles are smaller in elderly patients, the angle of penetration of the needle may need to be shallower. Elderly patients often complain of feeling cold, which may be due to increased susceptibility to accidental hypothermia (a subnormal drop in body temperature). Often, the venipuncture site will need to be warmed prior to the procedure. The elderly also often have increased sensitivities and allergies, which must be determined prior to any venipuncture procedure.

When the phlebotomist goes to the home of an elderly patient to perform venipuncture, it is important to follow these steps:

- Bring extra supplies and equipment (including biohazard containers for disposable items, temperature-controlled specimen transport containers, hand sanitizer, other disinfecting supplies and equipment).
- Positively identify the patient. If this is not possible, develop and follow the healthcare organization procedures carefully.
- Ensure that the patient is comfortable, preferably in a reclining position in case of fainting.
- Locate a bathroom so that hand washing can be completed quickly.
- Because many elderly patients take medications that prolong bleeding, wait for the puncture site to stop bleeding.
- Make sure not to leave any trash or used supplies in the living area after the procedure.
- Label specimens and place them in leakproof containers with biohazard signs.
- Verify the appropriate temperatures for specimen transport.
- If the patient lives in a high-crime area, take security precautions, including bringing a mobile phone, and

have the area mapped in advance to avoid becoming lost on the way to or from the home.

■ Carefully document any delays concerning the return of specimens to the laboratory.

Common tests ordered for geriatric patients are listed in **Table 14–1.**

Blood Cultures

Physicians order blood cultures when they suspect that a patient has **bacteremia** or *septicemia* or has a high fever of unknown origin. Blood cultures can determine the presence of infection, its extent, and the antibiotics to which the bacterium is most susceptible. Blood cultures can also provide information about the effectiveness of antibiotic therapy and the patient's response to it. They are are often timed procedures. Specimens are collected at the height of a fever, when microorganisms are likely to be most plentiful.

When used to monitor antimicrobial therapy, blood cultures are drawn in special collection bottles containing a resin that inactivates them and allows the bacteria to grow. These are called *antibiotic removal device* (ARD) *bottles.* The resin separates the antimicrobial agent from the blood, and specimens must be submitted to the laboratory as soon as possible. Blood should not be exposed to the device for more than 2 h.

Blood cultures drawn before antimicrobial therapy are collected in containers with a nutrient medium that promotes the growth of microorganisms. One type is an *anaerobic* bottle designed for organisms that grow best without oxygen. The second type is *aerobic*, designed for organisms that grow best when oxygen is present. If a syringe is used to collect blood, the anaerobic bottle is filled first. If a butterfly collection kit is used, the aerobic bottle is filled first. This is done so that any air in the tubing is released into the oxygen-containing bottle.

There are also specially designed collection bottles that eliminate the need for either syringe or butterfly collections. These bottles have long necks that fit into evacuated tube holders, allowing for the collection of other blood specimens via evacuated tubes without additional venipuncture.

Up to 10 mL of blood is usually collected (from adults) for the optimal recovery of microorganisms. From infants and children, only 1 to 5 mL is collected. The amount collected must be correct because too little blood causes inhibition of the growth of microorganisms. Too much blood can cause a risk to the patient of hospital-induced anemia and a lack of optimal growth of the microorganisms.

Blood cultures are often ordered in sets, which occurs in two ways. Both sets can be collected at the same time from different sites, or they can be collected from the same site, but 30 min apart. Laboratory protocol should be followed if the timing method is not noted on the order. Correct bottle labeling is essential.

Antisepsis of the patient's skin is critical in collecting blood cultures in order to avoid contamination of the specimen with surface microorganisms, which can produce a false-positive blood culture. Every found microorganism must be reported, and the physician must interpret whether each microorganism is clinically significant. **Figures 14–2** (**A** through **F**) show the steps involved in performing blood cultures.

Arterial Blood Gases

Arterial blood gases (ABGs) are performed to determine a patient's status of oxygenation, ventilation, and *acid-base balance.* Arterial blood is used because its composition is relatively consistent throughout the body. Venous blood is avoided for these tests because it fluctuates with the metabolic needs of whichever tissues surround the chosen vein. Extremely skilled phlebotomists are the only professionals who should attempt arterial blood gas collection. Usually, these professionals are certified by their healthcare institutions because this form of blood collection may cause serious injury. Criteria for this skill include theory training, observations of others performing the technique, and actual performance of the procedures while being supervised.

■ **Table 14–1 Phlebotomy for Geriatric Patients**

Blood Test	Clinical Indications
Acid phosphatase	Prostatic cancer, metastatic bone cancer, hyperparathyroidism
Arterial blood gases (ABGs)	Asthma, chronic obstructive pulmonary disease (COPD), cystic fibrosis, drug overdose, heart failure, kidney failure, severe infections, sleep disorders, uncontrolled diabetes
Blood urea nitrogen (BUN), creatinine	Diagnose kidney disorders
C-reactive protein (CRP)	Active rheumatic fever
Bicarbonate	COPD, hypoventilation, pulmonary edema
Glucose	Detect and monitor diabetes mellitus
Hemoglobin M	Drug or chemical toxicity
Prothrombin time (PT), partial thromboplastin time (PTT)	Monitor blood-thinning medications, coagulation problems
Serum protein electrophoresis (SPEP), immunoprotein electrophoresis (IPEP)	Multiple myeloma
Uric acid	Gout and kidney stones
Venereal disease research laboratory (VDRL)	Diagnose or rule out syphilis

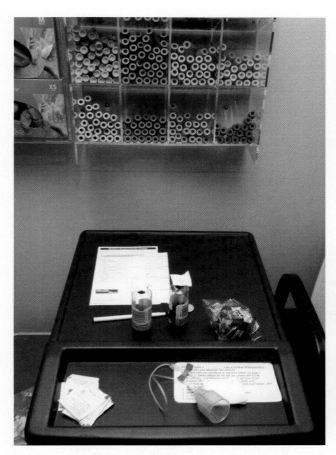

Figure 14–2A Assembling the equipment.

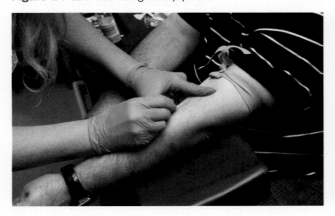

Figure 14–2B Locating the vein while tourniquet is in place.

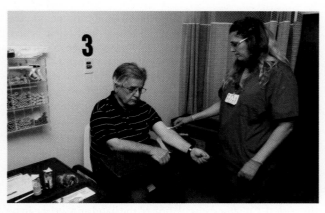

Figure 14–2C Cleansing the arm for one minute.

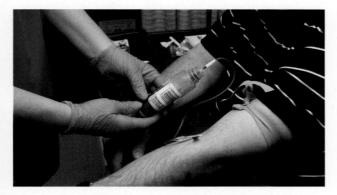

Figure 14–2D Drawing blood through the butterfly set into the container.

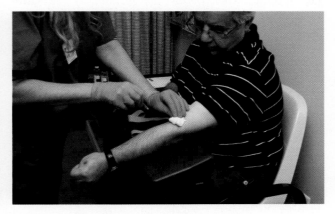

Figure 14–2E Removing the butterfly set and applying gauze.

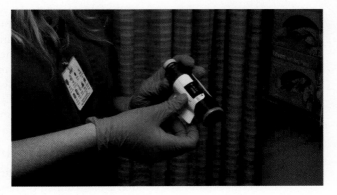

Figure 14–2F Labeling the container.

The main sites chosen for arterial puncture include the radial artery (preferred), brachial artery, and ulnar artery. The radial artery is most commonly selected because it usually has the best collateral circulation (see **Figure 14–3**). Site selection depends on the size and accessibility of the artery, stability of surrounding tissues, and *collateral circulation*. The chosen site should not be near a wound, should not be inflamed, and should not have an AV shunt or fistula.

Collateral circulation is defined as blood supplied to an area by more than one artery. For example, the hand and wrist are normally supplied with blood from the radial and ulnar arteries. If the radial artery were damaged during arterial puncture, the ulnar artery would continue to supply blood to the region. Collateral circulation of the hand and wrist can be determined by a Doppler ultrasonic flow indicator, or by performing the *Allen test*. This test is a method of determining collateral circulation prior to performing arterial puncture. The Allen test is performed in five steps:

1. The patient is asked to make a tight fist.
2. The phlebotomist applies pressure to the patient's wrist by using the middle and index fingers of both hands to compress and occlude both the radial and ulnar arteries simultaneously.
3. Pressure is maintained as the patient is asked to slowly open the hand, which should appear to be drained of color.
4. The patient's hand should be lowered and the pressure released on the ulnar artery.
5. The hand should flush pink within 15 s.

The laboratory technician performs the arterial blood gas test using a *rapid arterial blood gas analyzer* (see **Figure 14–4**). This machine aspirates the blood from the syringe

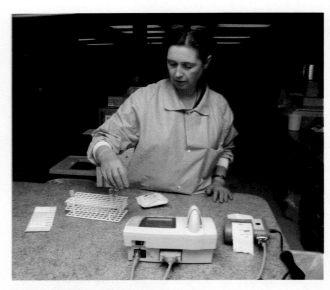

Figure 14–4 Arterial blood gas testing.

and measures the pH and the partial pressures of oxygen and carbon dioxide. The bicarbonate concentration is also calculated. Results are usually available for interpretation within five minutes. There are two types of tests commonly performed: the alpha-stat and the pH-stat tests. The alpha-stat test is preferred. In this test, the arterial carbon dioxide tension and the pH are maintained at 5.3 kPa (40mmHg) and 7.40 when measured at 37°C. When a patient is cooled down, the pH-value will increase and the pCO2-value and the pO2-value will decrease with lowering of the temperature if measured at the patient's temperature.

In the pH-stat test, the arterial carbon dioxide tension (paCO2) is maintained at 5.3 kPa (40 mmHg) and the pH is maintained at 7.40 when measured at the actual patient temperature. It is then necessary to add CO2 to the sample to calculate results.

The phlebotomist should record the results on the laboratory requisition form—the hand flushing pink within 15 s indicates a positive result, meaning that collateral circulation is present. If the result is positive, the arterial puncture may be performed. If negative, there is an absence of collateral circulation, and the radial artery cannot be used for arterial puncture—another site must be selected.

In this case, the brachial artery is chosen next, but it carries an increased risk of hematoma. The third choice would be the femoral artery, located in the groin area. Usually only physicians or specially trained emergency room personnel are allowed to puncture this artery. The femoral artery is seldom used for arterial puncture, but is a site of last choice. In newborns, the umbilicus may be punctured for this purpose. In adults, the dorsalis pedis may be punctured also. However, only physicians or specially trained emergency room personnel are allowed to perform these punctures.

Phlebotomy for Anticoagulated Patients

When a patient is on anticoagulation therapy, blood collection is more difficult. These patients may continue bleeding. After venipuncture, the site should have pressure applied for at

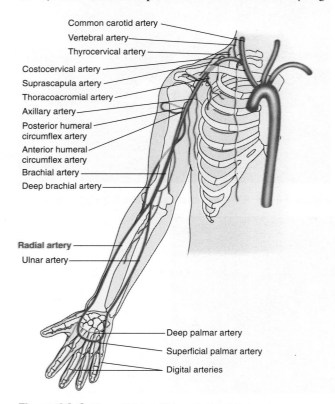

Common carotid artery
Vertebral artery
Thyrocervical artery
Costocervical artery
Suprascapula artery
Thoracoacromial artery
Axillary artery
Posterior humeral circumflex artery
Anterior humeral circumflex artery
Brachial artery
Deep brachial artery

Radial artery
Ulnar artery

Deep palmar artery
Superficial palmar artery
Digital arteries

Figure 14–3 The radial, brachial, and ulnar arteries.

least 5 min. A 2-in by 2-in pad of gauze should then be folded down the middle and folded down the middle again to make a thick 1-in square. It should be taped over the puncture site to produce a pressure dressing. It should be checked in 15 min to determine any bleeding through the gauze. If an outpatient, the patient must not be allowed to leave before waiting 15 min to determine stoppage of bleeding. Any patient carrying a purse should use the other arm so that the puncture site does not start bleeding again.

If the patient immediately bleeds through the gauze square, several layers of gauze should be placed over the site and the arm should be wrapped with an elastic bandage. A nurse should monitor the patient. Sites where bleeding has occurred should be avoided for future punctures. Each anticoagulated patient must be treated on an individual basis to determine his or her level of bleeding.

Phlebotomy for Obese Patients

Drawing blood from obese patients is usually challenging for phlebotomists. They must be skilled in working with these patients because of a variety of factors caused by excessive weight. It is more difficult to access a vein through additional layers of fatty tissue. Often, it is difficult to feel an obese patient's veins through these tissue layers. Therefore, tourniquets must be tighter to exert enough pressure to slow the venous blood flow. Phlebotomists must palpate the desired vein to make sure it is the correct one before attempting venipuncture. Obese patients often have tissue **globules** under the skin that can resemble veins upon first *palpation* (examination by touch). The cephalic vein is the most common site for venipuncture in obese patients, and it is the easiest to feel. If it is not easy to feel this vein, the veins of second choice should be those in the wrist or on the back of the hand.

Phlebotomy for Psychiatric Patients

Often, psychiatric patients do not understand the procedure that must be done, and the nurses of these patients need to be informed. Usually, the nurse will be present during the procedure to assist in any way needed. Often, psychiatric patients trust only their caregivers or relatives. These people may need to be asked to assist. Often, the patient may feel intimidated and insecure. Many psychiatric patients exhibit similar behaviors to those of young children. They can be unpredictable, and the phlebotomist should be ready for sudden movements. Some of these patients may be suicidal, and care should be taken to keep equipment away from them that could be used to harm themselves or others.

Summary

Capillary puncture of the heels is used for newborns and infants. Newborn screening for phenylketonuria, galactosemia, and hypothyroidism is required by law in all 50 states. For children and adults, the fingers are used for capillary puncture. They are also used for geriatric patients and for those who are anticoagulated or obese or have psychiatric conditions. It is important for the phlebotomist to be skilled in working with all of these different patients, each having special needs. For blood cultures, phlebotomists must be familiar with the procedures used and the purposes of these tests. Arterial blood gases are measured for patients suffering from conditions such as COPD, asthma, cystic fibrosis, and heart failure.

CRITICAL THINKING

A 12-day-old newborn presented in the pediatric office with a high fever, no appetite, vomiting, and swelling of the left heel. The patient history shows that 24 h after birth, she had a heel puncture to screen for PKU. Her pediatrician diagnosed that all of these signs and symptoms were related to the heel puncture procedure.

1. What are the most common complications of heel puncture in newborns?
2. What would be the consequences to the phlebotomist who performed this heel puncture?

WEBSITES

http://findarticles.com/p/articles/mi_m3230/is_1_34/ai_82272880/

http://www.cdhb.govt.nz/ch_labs/cap_blood_collecting.htm

http://www.mgh.org/lab/specimen.html

http://www.ncctinc.com/SpecialtyCourses/Preview/Geriatrics%20for%20Phlebotomists.pdf

http://www.phlebotomypages.com/child_venipuncture.htm

http://www.virginiahopkinstestkits.com/bloodspottestadvantage.html

http://www.webmd.com/a-to-z-guides/blood-culture

http://www.webmd.com/lung/arterial-blood-gases

REVIEW QUESTIONS

Multiple Choice

1. Before a routine capillary puncture, the site is typically cleaned with
   A. soap and warm water
   B. povidone-iodine solution
   C. ethyl alcohol
   D. isopropyl alcohol
2. Blood obtained via capillary puncture can be collected in
   A. microhematocrit tubes
   B. Microtainer tubes
   C. capillary tubes
   D. all of the above
3. The device used for dermal puncture is a
   A. butterfly
   B. lancet
   C. Vacutainer
   D. Unopette
4. Capillary puncture blood is
   A. nearly identical to a venous blood specimen
   B. mostly tissue fluid mixed with arterial blood
   C. a mix of venous, arterial, and capillary blood
   D. only tissue fluid

5. Capillary specimens contain all of the following, EXCEPT
   A. tissue fluids
   B. venous blood
   C. arterial blood
   D. serous fluids

6. Which equipment is used to collect a manual packed cell volume test?
   A. microhematocrit tube
   B. circles on filter paper
   C. glass microscope slide
   D. mixing bar and magnet

7. A microcollection container is sometimes called a
   A. lancet
   B. microtube
   C. bullet
   D. pipette

8. Which test is particularly performed via capillary puncture?
   A. PKU
   B. PTT
   C. GTT
   D. CBC

9. What is the reason to control the depth of lancet insertion during heel puncture?
   A. to avoid unnecessary bleeding
   B. to avoid puncturing an artery or a vein
   C. to avoid injuring the calcaneus bone
   D. all of the above

10. The most common and proper site for finger puncture on an adult is the
    A. proximal phalanx of the index finger
    B. distal segment of the middle finger
    C. end segment of either of the thumbs
    D. medial segment of the index finger

11. The safest area of an infant's foot for capillary puncture is
    A. the medial plantar heel
    B. the posterior curvature
    C. any area of the arch
    D. the center of the big toe

12. Which of the following arteries is most commonly selected for arterial puncture?
    A. ulnar
    B. brachial
    C. radial
    D. femoral

13. Obese patients often have which of the following types of tissues that may resemble veins upon first palpation?
    A. cartilage
    B. globules
    C. muscular
    D. collagenous fibers

14. Psychiatric patients exhibit similar behaviors to which of the following?
    A. pregnant women
    B. teenagers
    C. young children
    D. elderly people

15. Blood supply to an area by more than one artery is called
    A. capillary circulation
    B. shunting
    C. collateral circulation
    D. portal circulation

CHAPTER 15

Complications of Phlebotomy

OUTLINE

Introduction
Complications of Phlebotomy
    Hematoma
    Hemoconcentration
    Nerve Damage
    Fainting
    Seizures
    Allergic Response
    Collapsed Vein
    Excessive Bleeding
    Accidental Artery Puncture
    Uncooperative Patients
Summary
Critical Thinking
Websites
Review Questions

OBJECTIVES

After studying this chapter, readers should be able to:
1. List the possible complications of phlebotomy.
2. Define *hemoconcentration* and its possible causes.
3. Define *hematomas* and their causes.
4. Describe how nerve damage may occur during phlebotomy.
5. Explain how a phlebotomist should handle a patient who may be about to faint.
6. Describe how collapsed veins may occur.
7. Define *anaphylactic shock* and list its signs and symptoms.
8. Explain accidental artery puncture.
9. Describe how to effectively handle complications when they occur during or after blood collection.
10. Describe the common factors that may result in patients becoming uncooperative.

KEY TERMS

Anaphylactic shock: An immediate allergic reaction characterized by acute respiratory distress, hypotension, edema, and rash. Anaphylactic shock can be life-threatening.

Anticoagulants: A group of agents that prevent or delay blood coagulation (clotting).

Hematoma: An abnormal localized collection of blood within tissues or organs.

Hemoconcentration: A relative increase in the number of red blood cells resulting from a decrease in the volume of plasma.

Hemophilia: A hereditary blood disease marked by greatly prolonged blood coagulation time, with consequent failure of the blood to clot, and abnormal bleeding that is sometimes accompanied by joint swelling.

Hyperventilation: Abnormally fast, deep breathing that sometimes results in fainting.

Seizure: A sudden spasm or convulsion, especially one associated with epilepsy.

Syncope: Fainting.

Topical: Pertaining to a specific area of the body or surface area of the skin.

Introduction

It is important for phlebotomists to recognize potential complications of phlebotomy. Complications can occur at any time, in many different situations. Appropriate precautions must be taken to prevent complications of phlebotomy from occurring. When they do occur, complications must be handled quickly and professionally.

Complications of Phlebotomy

If a problem arises that keeps blood collection from occurring, the phlebotomist must systematically determine what caused the situation. The most common complications of venipuncture may include hematoma, **hemoconcentration**, nerve damage, fainting, seizures, allergic response, collapsed vein, excessive bleeding, and accidental artery puncture.

Hematoma

Blood loss into a tissue, organ, or other confined space is called a **hematoma**. Hematomas may compress nearby organs, causing pain and impairing their function. Hematomas are most common after trauma or as a side effect of anticoagulant medications. In many cases, hematomas must be surgically drained. In the case of phlebotomy, hematomas are caused by excessive probing to locate a vein, failure to insert the needle far enough into the vein, or the needle penetrating all the way through the vein (see **Figure 15–1**). When this occurs, the tissue around the puncture site will swell. A hematoma may also form if the tourniquet is not removed before the needle is removed, if inadequate pressure is applied on the puncture site, or if the elbow is bent while pressure is applied to the puncture site.

If a hematoma should form, discontinue the procedure immediately. Apply pressure to the area for 3 to 5 min, then apply an ice pack. The patient should not bend the arm at the elbow because this will cause additional bruising. It is important *not* to place the ice pack directly on the patient's skin. Instead, first put a towel or sheet over the injured area. Then apply the ice pack for 20 min and remove it for 20 min, in rotation. Notify the physician, observing the site to determine whether bleeding has stopped. An incident report must be completed and recorded in the patient's record.

Hemoconcentration

Leaving a tourniquet tied on a patient's arm for longer than the recommended time results in **hemoconcentration**. It is defined as a decrease in plasma volume with an increased concentration of cells and larger molecules (such as red blood cells and cholesterol). Hemoconcentration may also be caused by massaging, probing, or squeezing a venipuncture site; by the patient pumping his or her fist during the draw; as a result of long-term intravenous therapy; and by occluded or sclerosed veins. Hemoconcentration compromises the quality of laboratory test results, so these practices should be avoided as much as possible to avoid causing hemoconcentration.

Nerve Damage

The potential for nerve damage due to venipuncture also exists. Do not probe with the needle if the vein is missed because this may cause contact with a nerve. Contact with a nerve during a venipuncture results in a painful burning sensation. Avoiding the use of the basilic vein for venipuncture also minimizes the risks of nerve damage. Make only two attempts to draw blood from a single patient. If you are unsuccessful, ask the patient whether he or she would prefer to have another healthcare professional try or would like to return at another time. At one time or another, everyone experiences the failure of an unsuccessful blood draw, so understand that it is acceptable under these conditions.

Fainting

Another problem associated with venipuncture is **syncope** (fainting). Always be prepared for this to occur. The use of a blood collection chair, which secures the patient and keeps her or him from falling, is preferred. Keeping conversation going with the patient helps to determine how he or she is feeling. Observe the breathing rate and the appearance of the patient's face for anything abnormal. Signs of fainting include increased nervousness and **hyperventilation**, decreased blood pressure, a slow and weak pulse, pallor and mild sweating, and sometimes nausea and vomiting.

Patients may admit that they feel faint every time their blood is drawn. If a patient says this, have him or her lie down prior to drawing the blood. If the procedure is begun and the patient says that he or she is feeling faint, quickly remove the tourniquet and needle from the arm, making sure the needle is placed out of the patient's way. Talk to the patient to divert attention from the blood collection process and help him or her to stay alert and conscious. Assist the patient in lowering the head between the knees (see **Figure 15–2**), and have the patient breathe slowly and deeply.

Physically support the patient, and loosen any tight clothing he or she is wearing. Place a cold cloth on the forehead and the back of the neck. If the patient experiences nausea, give the patient an emesis basin. Alert the nurse or physician as quickly as possible. Keep monitoring the patient's vital signs. When patients actually faint, they are generally laid on their backs and monitored closely until they become conscious, then instructed to remain in the position for at least 15 to 20 min.

Seizures

Fainting may progress until the patient is fully unconscious and, in extreme cases, may include a **seizure**, which is also called a *convulsion*. Although they are rare, when seizures develop, the phlebotomist must stay calm and remove the needle and tourniquet. Apply pressure to the site without restricting the patient. Gently help to guide the patient to the floor to protect him or her from injury, and call for help. Never leave the patient unattended or put anything in the mouth. Protect the head and move potentially harmful items out of the way.

When a seizure subsides, keep the patient in the same area for at least 15 min. Have the nurse or physician check the patient before he or she is released, and make sure the patient will not operate a motor vehicle for at least 30 min. In fact, it is best that a friend or family member drive the patient home. Document the incident fully in the patient's record.

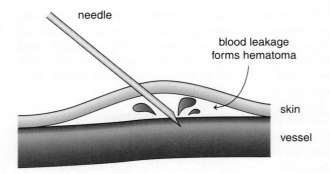

needle

blood leakage forms hematoma

skin

vessel

Figure 15–1 Improper placement of needle in the arm, causing a hematoma to form.

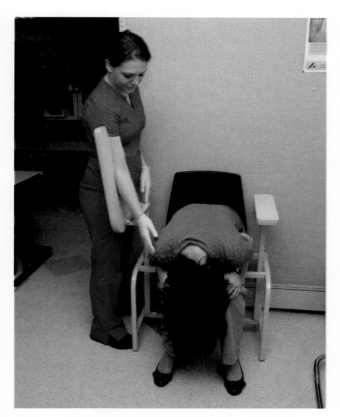

Figure 15-2 A phlebotomist assisting a patient who is feeling faint.

Allergic Response

Allergic responses may occur as a result of blood collection due to latex allergies, adhesives used on bandages, and antiseptics used in procedures. Phlebotomists should remember to take the precaution of asking each patient about these allergies. If the patient is allergic, nonlatex gloves and tourniquets, paper tape, and gauze pads may be used. Isopropyl alcohol or povidone-iodine can be used alternatively for the same antiseptic purpose in case the patient is allergic to one of them.

If the patient states that he or she does not have any of these allergies and an allergic response occurs, complete the procedure as quickly as possible. If the reaction is extreme, wash the affected area with a nonallergenic soap and running water. Report the reaction to the nurse or physician immediately. Most allergic responses are mild and cause an itchy rash or redness of surrounding tissue. The patient should avoid scratching to prevent infection. The physician may prescribe **topical** ointments to treat the condition. Severe allergic responses may require treatment with a systemic medication.

In very severe cases, allergic responses can lead to **anaphylactic shock**. This requires immediate treatment to avoid unconsciousness and potential death, which occurs because of edema that causes the airway to become blocked. The phlebotomist must be aware of the signs and symptoms of anaphylactic shock to intervene in time. These include acute respiratory distress, edema, hives, hypotension, pale and cool skin, convulsions, tachycardia, and cyanosis. The nurse and physician should be notified immediately if these symptoms develop.

Collapsed Vein

A collapsed vein most commonly occurs in elderly or otherwise frail patients. Their veins may be too fragile to tolerate the force of the vacuum in an evacuated tube. A vein may collapse because of the use of too large an evacuated tube, or if too much force is used in drawing back the plunger of a syringe. Also, an extremely tight tourniquet or one that is positioned too near the venipuncture site may cause a vein to collapse. If the patient states that his or her veins have collapsed before, this should alert the phlebotomist to use another collection method, such as a butterfly infusion set, a smaller syringe, or smaller evacuated tubes such as those used for pediatric patients. It is important to pull the blood slowly into the tube regardless of the chosen method.

Excessive Bleeding

Sometimes a patient who is taking **anticoagulants** or who has **hemophilia** will continue to bleed after venipuncture. If bleeding continues after a few minutes, apply direct pressure over the site and raise the affected arm above the patient's heart level. Pressure must be maintained until the bleeding stops. If it continues for another 5 min, notify the nurse or physician. Never leave the patient unattended if this situation develops. Another bleeding condition that may occur is *petechiae* (small hemorrhagic spots on the skin); it may occur if the tourniquet is left in place for more than 1 min. Petechiae can also be an indication of a coagulation problem.

Accidental Artery Puncture

If an artery is accidentally punctured, the phlebotomist must immediately remove the tourniquet and withdraw the needle from the patient's arm. Direct pressure must be applied for at least 5 min or until the bleeding has stopped. If an artery has been punctured instead of a vein, it is easy to tell. The blood will be spurting into the tube and have a bright red color. Accidental artery puncture may cause infection, numbness, and hematoma.

Uncooperative Patients

Uncooperative patients include small children, extremely ill patients who are tired of having blood drawn, and patients who are under the effects of drugs or alcohol or who otherwise cannot understand that what is occurring is for their benefit. As a last resort, the phlebotomist may have to restrain or request assistance in restraining an uncooperative patient. Usually, the only patients put into restraints are children, not adults. Immobilization before venipuncture is done for the patient's safety. The phlebotomist must use interpersonal skills in these situations in an attempt to calm and encourage the patient that the procedure is absolutely required and must proceed.

The patient should be told that his or her feelings are understood, as is any anxiety being felt. The procedure should be explained step by step. If, after every attempt has been made to calm the patient, he or she is still uncooperative, then the nurse and/or physician must be notified. Patients do have the right to refuse any procedure. If this ultimately occurs, the refusal should be thoroughly documented on the requisition form and/or the patient's chart, and the nurse should be notified. If possible, a person whom the patient trusts should be asked to encourage the patient to cooperate. The phlebotomist should not give up on the patient and should never take the patient's refusal to cooperate personally.

Summary

Phlebotomists regularly encounter complications to phlebotomy. Each situation must be recognized and dealt with properly. Professionalism must be maintained. The following of emergency procedures should be "second nature" because there may be no time to stop and check the policies and procedures manual for the correct steps to take. Common complications to phlebotomy include hematoma, hemoconcentration, nerve damage, fainting, seizures, allergic responses, collapsed veins, excessive bleeding, and accidental artery puncture. Uncooperative patients may include small children, extremely ill patients, and those under the effects of alcohol or drugs.

CRITICAL THINKING

While a phlebotomist was drawing blood from a 25-year-old patient, he noticed that the patient was sweating and not responding to his questions. He recognized that the patient appeared to be about to faint. He immediately removed the needle from the patient's arm and left the room to notify the physician.

1. What are the common signs and symptoms of fainting?
2. What should the phlebotomist do when a patient feels faint?
3. What mistake did this phlebotomist make?

WEBSITES

http://www.gomcl.com/PLHDOCS/PLH407.pdf

http://www.medicinenet.com/hematoma/article.htm

http://www.medicine.uiowa.edu/path_handbook/Appendix/ TechServ/phleb_policies.html

http://www.medscape.com/viewarticle/509098

http://www.righthealth.com/topic/Complications_In_Phleb otomy?p=l&as=goog&ac=519&kgl=7765694

http://www.saferinjecting.info/sihowveinscollap.html

http://www.webmd.com/brain/nerve-pain-and-nerve-damage-symptoms-and-causes

REVIEW QUESTIONS

Multiple Choice

1. When a hematoma occurs during a venipuncture, the phlebotomist should NOT do which of the following?
    A. withdraw the needle
    B. apply an ice pack
    C. apply direct pressure over the site
    D. continue drawing blood

2. Which of the following statements is false about nerve damage?
    A. It may result in a painful burning sensation.
    B. Avoiding the use of the cephalic vein for venipuncture minimizes the risks of nerve damage.
    C. Only two attempts should be made to draw blood from a single patient in order to avoid nerve damage.
    D. Avoiding the use of the basilic vein for venipuncture minimizes the risks of nerve damage.

3. Hemoconcentration compromises the
    A. certification of the phlebotomist
    B. certification of the laboratory technologist
    C. quality of laboratory test results
    D. confidentiality of the patient

4. All of the following are the signs and symptoms of fainting, EXCEPT
    A. hypertension
    B. weak pulse
    C. pallor
    D. nausea and vomiting

5. The term *hyperventilation* means
    A. abnormally increased muscle tone
    B. an abnormal increase in fluid volume
    C. abnormally high levels of uric acid
    D. abnormally fast breathing

6. If fainting progresses and the patient becomes fully unconscious, which of the following may occur?
    A. fever
    B. seizures
    C. heart attack
    D. stroke

7. An immediate allergic reaction that is characterized by acute respiratory distress, hypotension, edema, and rash is called
    A. urticaria
    B. distributive shock
    C. neurogenic shock
    D. anaphylactic shock

8. If a patient is allergic to isopropyl alcohol, which of the following antiseptics may be used instead?
    A. povidone-iodine
    B. wood alcohol
    C. sodium hypochlorite
    D. potassium chloride

9. All of the following factors may cause collapsed veins, EXCEPT
    A. tying a tourniquet extremely tightly
    B. using a larger evacuated tube
    C. using a butterfly infusion set
    D. using a smaller evacuated tube

10. Which of the following hereditary blood disorders may increase blood coagulation time?
    A. hemolytic anemia
    B. hemophilia

    C. sickle-cell anemia

    D. lymphoma

11. Which of the following is important to do for preventing collapsed veins?

    A. Use force when drawing back the plunger of a syringe.

    B. Pull the blood slowly into the tube regardless of the chosen method.

    C. Use a small needle.

    D. Make sure the tourniquet is tight.

12. Small hemorrhagic spots on the skin are called

    A. cyanoses

    B. varicoses

    C. aneurysms

    D. petechiae

13. Accidental artery puncture may cause all of the following complications, EXCEPT

    A. numbness

    B. hematoma

    C. hyperlipidemia

    D. infection

14. Which of the following patients are usually uncooperative to the collection of blood specimens?

    A. obese patients

    B. pregnant women

    C. elderly patients

    D. small children

15. Which of the following is the most appropriate for the phlebotomist to do if an artery is accidentally punctured?

    A. Continue collecting blood from the arm of the patient by moving the needle in the arm.

    B. Immediately remove the tourniquet and withdraw the needle from the patient's arm.

    C. Ask the patient if everything is all right.

    D. Call the nurse to assess the hole in the arm of the patient.

CHAPTER 16

Urinalysis and Other Specimens

OUTLINE

Introduction
Anatomy of the Urinary System
Urine Formation
Collecting the Urine Specimen
Transporting the Urine Specimen
Urine Characteristics
Pregnancy Testing
Urine Toxicology
Sputum Specimens
Cerebrospinal Fluid Specimens
Amniotic Fluid Specimens
Semen Specimens
Fecal Specimens
Summary
Critical Thinking
Websites
Review Questions

OBJECTIVES

After studying this chapter, readers should be able to:

1. Describe the steps involved in a standard urinalysis.
2. Explain pregnancy testing.
3. Describe the process of urine formation.
4. Differentiate between 24-h urine specimens and clean-catch midstream urine specimens.
5. Perform a urinalysis using a chemical reagent strip.
6. Describe how urine is tested for the presence of drugs.
7. Explain the purpose of sputum specimen collection.
8. Describe the role of the phlebotomist in collecting cerebrospinal fluid specimens.
9. Explain the reasons for semen collection and examination.
10. Describe the guaiac test.

KEY TERMS

Bilirubin: The yellow breakdown product of normal heme catabolism.

Bilirubinemia: The presence of bilirubin in the blood.

Breathalyzer: A device for estimating blood alcohol content from a breath sample.

Chemical reagent strip: A plastic strip to which chemically treated reagent pads are attached—it allows for the testing of various components of urine.

Culture and sensitivity: A microbiology procedure involving the culturing of a specimen on artificial media to detect bacterial or fungal growth, followed by screening for antibiotic sensitivity.

Filtrate: The fluid remaining after a liquid is passed through a membranous filter.

Guaiac: A type of tree resin that chemically reacts to small amounts of blood.

Human chorionic gonadotropin: A hormone that normally increases in pregnancy, is secreted from the placenta, and prevents spontaneous abortion.

Icterus: Jaundice.

Ketones: The waste products of fat metabolism.

Myoglobinuria: The presence of myoglobin, an oxygen-storing pigment of muscle tissue, in the urine.

Oliguria: An abnormally small amount of urine produced, particularly if fluid consumption significantly exceeds urine output; oliguria is often a sign of kidney disease, obstruction of the urinary tract, or dehydration.

Phenyl ketones: Metabolites of phenylalanine that, when present in urine, signify phenylketonuria, an inborn metabolic disorder.

Pheochromocytoma: A vascular tumor of the chromaffin tissue of the adrenal medulla or sympathetic paraganglia, causing persistent or intermittent hypertension.

Polyuria: Excessive elimination of urine; polyuria is often a symptom of undiagnosed or poorly controlled diabetes mellitus.

KEY TERMS CONTINUED

Refractometer: An instrument for measuring the refractive index of a substance; used primarily for measuring the refractivity of solutions such as urine.

Renal thresholds: Levels above which substances cannot be reabsorbed by the renal tubules and therefore are excreted in the urine.

Renin: An enzyme released by the kidneys that raises blood pressure by activating angiotensin.

Spinal tap: The puncture of the subarachnoid space of the lumbar area of the spine with a needle to examine and

culture cerebrospinal fluid, or to inject a drug or dye for other purposes, such as myelography; also called a *lumbar puncture.*

Suprapubic: Pertaining to a location above the symphysis pubis (the slightly movable interpubic joint of the pelvis).

Urinometer: Any device for determining the specific gravity of urine.

Urochrome: A pigment that causes the yellow color in urine.

Introduction

For many diseases, a routine *urinalysis* is used because it can be quickly and easily performed for the diagnosis and treatment of disease. Usually, urinalysis is not an invasive procedure. A routine urinalysis can reveal bladder, kidney, systemic metabolic, endocrine, and liver diseases as well as obstructions in the urinary system. All patients requiring physical examinations or entering a hospital for treatment undergo urinalysis. The urinary system has three major functions: excretion of organic wastes from body fluids, elimination of these wastes into the environment, and homeostatic regulation of the volume and solute concentration of blood plasma. Other forms of testing include pregnancy testing, urine toxicology to detect poisonous substances as well as drugs or alcohol, sputum collection, cerebrospinal fluid collection, amniotic fluid collection, semen collection, and fecal collection.

Anatomy of the Urinary System

Phlebotomists must have a basic knowledge of the urinary system and urine formation. The urinary system consists of two kidneys, two ureters, one bladder, and one urethra (see **Figure 16–1**).

The functional unit of the kidney is the nephron. Each kidney has more than 1 million nephrons. Each nephron consists of a glomerulus, which acts in filtering (see **Figure 16–2**), and a *renal tubule*, through which the **filtrate** passes. As the filtrate passes through, various changes occur. Certain solutes are reabsorbed, and others are secreted into the kidney for eventual excretion. Almost all of the water that passes through the glomeruli is reabsorbed.

The glomerulus consists of a capillary network surrounded by a membranous *Bowman capsule*. Blood is carried by the afferent arteriole from the renal artery into the glomerulus, where it divides to form a capillary network. The capillaries reunite to form the efferent arteriole, through which blood flows out of the glomerulus.

The nephron's *proximal convoluted tubule* and *distal convoluted tubule* are part of a loop known as the *loop of Henle*. Filtrate from several nephrons is drained into a collecting tubule. A number of these tubules join to form a collecting duct. Then these ducts join to form the papillary ducts, emptying into the calyces near the tips of the papillae. Filtrate

drains into the renal pelvis and is now called *urine*. It passes from the renal pelvis down the ureter and into the bladder, and it remains there until it is voided through the urethra.

Aside from urine formation, the kidneys help to maintain homeostasis. They accomplish this by regulating the composition, pH, and volume of the extracellular fluid, which involves removing metabolic wastes from the blood and diluting them with water and electrolytes. The kidneys also secrete the hormone *erythropoietin*, which helps to control red blood cell production. The kidneys help to activate vitamin D and maintain blood volume and pressure via secretion of the enzyme called **renin**.

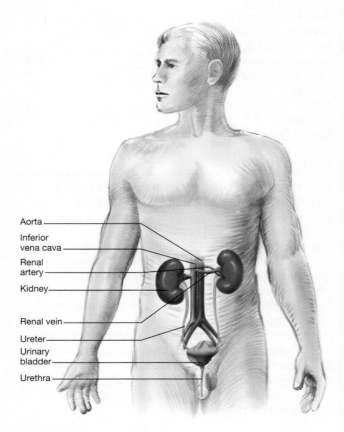

Aorta

Inferior vena cava

Renal artery

Kidney

Renal vein

Ureter

Urinary bladder

Urethra

Figure 16–1 The urinary system.

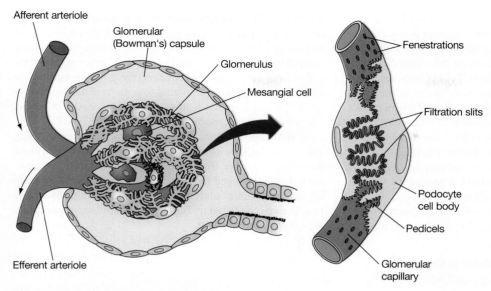

Figure 16–2 Structure of the renal corpuscle.

Urine Formation

Urine formation begins as the kidneys excrete or retain substances based on the body's needs and **renal thresholds**. About 1,200 mL of blood flows through the kidneys every minute, entering the glomerulus through the afferent arteriole. The capillaries surrounding the *proximal tubules* partially or completely reabsorb filtrate components such as glucose, amino acids, and water. The *collecting tubules* and *loop of Henle* concentrate the urine.

Every day, the kidneys convert approximately 180,000 mL of filtered plasma into a final urine volume of 750 to 2,000 mL. This amount is about 1% of the filtered plasma volume. Urine is mostly made up of water, with solutes that include urea, chloride, potassium, sodium, phosphate, sulfate, creatinine, and uric acid.

Collecting the Urine Specimen

Today, urine is the most commonly analyzed nonblood specimen in the clinical laboratory. It is analyzed to detect both extrinsic conditions caused by an imbalance in homeostasis and intrinsic pathologic conditions.

Urine collection requires between 12 and 50 mL per specimen. Each collected specimen must be properly labeled (on the container, not the cap) with the patient's name and date and the time of collection. Females should not undergo urine tests while they are menstruating. For all patients, any medications being taken must be recorded on both the laboratory requisition form and the patient's chart.

If the patient is required to collect a urine specimen at home, he or she must be fully instructed on the proper methods. The patient should urinate in an appropriate container with a wide opening, and nothing should be added to the container. However, if the patient has been provided with a container containing a preservative, she or he must not throw away the preservative. After collection, the container must be covered with a lid and refrigerated.

The most common type of urine sample is a single, *random specimen*, which can be taken at any time. When a random specimen is collected in a physician's office, a urine specimen container is provided, and the patient utilizes a restroom to provide the specimen, which should be left on the sink. The technician should transport the specimen to the laboratory immediately or refrigerate it.

A *clean-catch midstream specimen* refers to a urine specimen that is collected after the genital area is cleaned. It is often ordered to diagnose urinary tract infections or to evaluate how effective a drug is. Its purpose is to collect a urine specimen that is free from contamination. Written instructions are given to the patient to make sure he or she fully understands how to complete the procedure without contamination of the specimen. If a technician assists a patient with a clean-catch midstream specimen collection, antiseptic towelettes must be used to clean either the perineal area (in females) or the penis (in males). Any soap residue that can affect the pH of the specimen must be rinsed away. The patient must understand that he or she must void urine first into the toilet, and then into the container, and any remaining urine must be voided into the toilet again. Collection must be done in a sterile container. A clean-catch midstream specimen is required for culture and sensitivity tests.

A *timed specimen* is collected over a predetermined time period to obtain additional information about the patient's health status. The patient should discard the first specimen. Then all urine should be collected for a specified time period. The timed specimen test typically requires serial urine specimens collected at specific times for glucose tolerance tests. The urine should not come into contact with stool or toilet paper. The specimen must be kept refrigerated until it is brought to the doctor's office or laboratory.

A *24-h specimen* is collected to measure urine output in a 24-h period. This type of specimen is tested for substances that are released sporadically into the urine. Bedpans, urinals, and toilet paper must be avoided during this type of collection because they can retain the substances for which the test is being done. The first specimen should be discarded. The patient should urinate directly into the small collection container and then pour the urine into the large container.

Between collections, the small container must be cleaned with soap and warm water. This type of specimen is used in the diagnosis of renal disease, dehydration, urinary tract obstructions, and **pheochromocytoma**. The urine creatinine clearance test is used to diagnose renal disorders. A 24-h urine specimen is required, and refrigeration of the urine is also needed.

A *first-voided morning specimen* is collected after a night's sleep. It is also called an *8-h specimen*. It contains greater concentrations of substances that collect over time than do specimens taken during the day. Either a urine specimen container or an approved clean, dry jar may be used. This type of specimen is commonly used for pregnancy testing, microscopic examination, and culturing.

Catheterization is the insertion of a sterile, narrow, flexible, plastic tube (*catheter*) through the urethra and directly into the bladder to withdraw urine. It is used to obtain a sterile urine specimen, when a patient cannot void naturally, or to measure the amount of residual urine in the bladder after normal voiding. Catheterized specimens are sometimes collected from female patients to prevent vaginal contamination of the specimen, or from infants to obtain *culture and sensitivity* (C&S) specimens. Catheterization may cause infection. Therefore, it is not routinely used.

A **suprapubic** urine specimen can be collected by using a sterile syringe, in which the needle is inserted directly into the urinary bladder, from which urine is aspirated. Suprapubic collection is used for samples needed for cytology studies or for microbial analysis. Common abbreviations related to urinalysis are listed in **Table 16–1**. Standard urine values are listed in **Table 16–2**.

Table 16–1 Abbreviations Related to Urinalysis

ADH	Antidiuretic hormone	RBCs	Red blood cells
BIL, bili, BR	Bilirubin	SPG, sp gr, sp.gr.	Specific gravity
BJP	Bence Jones proteins	U/A	Urinalysis
Ca	Calcium	UBG	Urobilinogen
CC	Clean catch (urine)	U/C	Urine culture
CCMS	Clean catch, midstream (urine)	UC	Urinary catheter
CL VOID	Clean voided specimen (urine)	UC&S	Urine culture and sensitivity
CrCl	Creatinine clearance	UcaV	Urinary calcium volume
CSU	Catheter specimen (urine)	UCRE	Urine creatinine
Cys	Cysteine	UFC	Urinary free cortisol
CYS	Cystoscopy	UK	Urine potassium
EMU	Early morning urine(s)	Una	Urinary sodium
HCG, hcg, hCG	Human chorionic gonadotropin	Uosm	Urine osmolarity
IVP	Intravenous pyelogram	UTI	Urinary tract infection
K	Potassium	UUN	Urinary urea nitrogen
pH	Hydrogen ion concentration	UV	Urinary volume
PKD	Polycystic kidney disease	Vol	Volume
PKU	Phenylketonuria	WBCs	White blood cells

Table 16–2 Standard Urine Values

Test	Value	Test	Value
Acetone	None	Ketones	Negative
Albumin, qualitative	Negative	Lead	0.021–0.038 mg/L
Albumin, quantitative	10–140 mg/L (24 h)	Odor	Distinctly aromatic
Bacteria (culture)	< 10,000 colonies/mL	pH	4.5–8; generally acidic
Blood, occult	Negative	Phenylpyruvic acid	Negative
Calcium, quantitative	100–300 mg/24 h	Protein	Negative
Color	Pale yellow to dark amber	Specific gravity, single specimen	1.005–1.030
Creatine, nonpregnant women or in men	< 6% of creatinine	Specific gravity, 24-hour specimen	1.015–1.025
Creatine, pregnant women	≤ 12% of creatinine	Turbidity	Clear
Creatinine, men	1–1.9 g/24 h	Volume, adult females	600–1,600 mL/24 h
Creatinine, women	0.8–1.7 g/24 h	Volume, adult males	800–1,800 mL/24 h
Crystals	Negative	White blood cells	0–8/high-power field

Containers used for urine specimens must be extremely clean. A medical laboratory or other facility usually supplies containers. The most commonly used containers are made of plastic, disposable, nonsterile, or coated paper containers. However, the container must be sterile if the sample is to be sent to the laboratory for a culture. These containers are packaged with an intact paper seal over the cap, and they may also have a sterile envelope into which they must be placed.

For children and infants, special polyethylene bags with adhesive may be used for urine collection. For timed specimens, containers have wide mouths and screw-cap tops. Most routine urinalysis testing, abnormal analyte testing, and pregnancy testing utilize nonsterile containers. All types of specimens must have labels containing the patient's name, date and time of collection, and type of specimen. The technician must wear gloves when handling filled specimen containers.

Transporting the Urine Specimen

Proper handling while collecting and transporting urine specimens is essential. Components of urine change if the specimen is allowed to stand at room temperature (see **Table 16–3**).

Urine specimens should be refrigerated and processed within 1 h of collection. For transporting to a referral laboratory, evacuated transport tubes are available that contain preservatives and resemble blood collection tubes.

The vacuum in these tubes allows for delivery of 7 to 8 mL of urine. A transfer straw or urine collection cup is used with an integrated sampling device. Also, the urine can be poured into the tube after the stopper is removed. A *BD Vacutainer* cherry red/yellow-stoppered tube consists of chlorhexidine, ethylparaben, and sodium propionate. These preservatives prevent bacterial overgrowth and stop changes from occurring in the urine that can affect the test results. On preserved specimens, chemical reagent strip testing can be performed,

but this must be done within 72 h. The tubes may be kept at room temperature until this time.

For urine specimens intended for culture, a different preservative must be used. Sodium formate or boric acid helps preserve the level of bacteria present in the urine at the time of collection. This method of transport should be used only for urine specimens intended for culture. These preservatives can alter the results on the chemical reagent strip. **Culture and sensitivity** tests should be performed within 72 h, and again the tubes may be held at room temperature.

For all specimens that will be transported to another site for analysis, a laboratory request form must be completed. The information on these forms should include the patient's name, the date, the type of UA ordered, the name of the requesting physician, the appropriate ICD-9-CM code for diagnosis, and a line where the physician can sign after reviewing the results. Plastic biohazard bags with zipper seals are used to contain specimens when they are sent to the laboratory. These bags have an outside pocket where the laboratory request is placed.

Urine Characteristics

When urine is tested, it is evaluated for numerous different properties and conditions. Normal urine is yellow, ranging from pale straw to dark amber. Its color depends on the concentration of water in the specimen as well as the pigment **urochrome**. A dilute specimen should be pale, while a more concentrated specimen should be darker. The color of a patient's urine can indicate various diseases, but can also be influenced by other causes, including diet and medications. **Table 16–4** lists possible causes of changes in urine color.

The turbidity of a patient's urine can also indicate various diseases. For example, cloudy urine can indicate infection, glomerular nephritis, or inflammation. Cloudiness can be caused by bacteria, cells, vaginal contaminants, yeast, or crystals. However, a vegetarian diet can also cause the urine to appear cloudy. As clear urine cools, it may become cloudy due to the formation and precipitation of crystals.

On a random specimen, the amount of urine is rarely measured. However, urine volume is measured during a timed specimen by pouring the entire collection into a large, graduated cylinder. It is not accurate enough to use the markings on the side of the collection container. After measurement and recording, a portion of a well-mixed specimen (*aliquot*) is removed for testing. The laboratory then may store or discard the remainder of the specimen.

Excessive production of urine is called **polyuria**, and it is common in patients with diabetes and various kidney disorders. **Oliguria** is insufficient production of urine, caused by dehydration, decreased fluid intake, renal disease, or shock. *Anuria*, the absence of urine production, occurs in renal failure or obstruction.

When *foam* appears in a urine specimen, identified as small bubbles that persist for a long time after the specimen has been shaken, it may indicate the presence of increased protein. When the foam is green-yellow, it can indicate **bilirubinemia**. These specimens must be handled very carefully because the color of the foam can indicate viral hepatitis.

Although the *odor* of urine, like foam, is not normally recorded, it can signify metabolic disorders. While normal

Table 16–3 Urine Changes at Room Temperature

Urine Component	Changes
Bacteria	Double in amount approximately every 20 min
Bilirubin and urobilinogen	Undergo degradation in light
Blood	May hemolyze; false-positive results may occur due to bacterial peroxidase
Casts	Lyse or dissolve in alkaline urine
Cells	Lyse or dissolve in alkaline urine
Clarity	Becomes cloudy as crystals precipitate and bacteria multiply
Color	May change if pH becomes alkaline
Crystals	Precipitate as urine cools and may dissolve if pH changes
Glucose	Decreases as it is metabolized by bacteria
Ketones	Decrease due to evaporation
Nitrite	May become positive as bacteria multiply and reduce *nitrate*
pH	Becomes alkaline as bacteria form ammonia from urea
Yeast	Multiply

Table 16–4 Abnormal Urine Color

Color	Pathologic Conditions	Other Causes
Colorless or pale straw (dilute)	Anxiety, chronic renal disease, diabetes	Diuretic therapy, excessive fluid intake (water, beer, coffee)
Milky white	Fats, pus	Amorphous phosphates, spermatozoa
Dark yellow, dark amber (concentrated)	Acute febrile disease, diarrhea or vomiting (fluid loss or dehydration)	Excessive sweating, low fluid intake
Orange-yellow, orange-red, orange-brown	Bile duct obstruction, bilirubin, diminished liver-cell function, excessive RBC destruction	Drugs (such as pyridium and rifampin), dyes

urine is described as "aromatic," changes in odor can indicate the presence of bacteria. For example, when the urine has a "fruit" odor, this is often caused by the presence of **ketones** and may indicate uncontrolled diabetes. If the urine smells like ammonia or is putrid, there may be an infection present. However, this type of odor can also be caused by allowing the urine to stand before being tested. Bacteria break down the urea in the urine, forming ammonia. Abnormal urine odor can also be caused by various foods, including asparagus or garlic. The condition known as *phenylketonuria* can cause a "mousy" smell, which is described as smelling like wet animal fur.

Specific gravity is the weight of a substance compared with the weight of an equal volume of distilled water. In urinalysis, it is the concentration of substances dissolved in the urine. Specific gravity of distilled water is 1.000, and the specific gravity of urine ranges from 1.005 to 1.030, based on fluid intake. An abnormal specific gravity reading is an early indicator of kidney disease or other organ diseases. However, specific gravity can be affected by the presence of glucose, protein, or x-ray contrast media. Specific gravity is measured using a **urinometer**, **refractometer**, or a **chemical reagent strip** (see **Figure 16–3 A, B,** and **C**).

The chemical reagent strip, also referred to as a *dipstick*, is the most commonly used method in modern laboratories to measure specific gravity. The pad located on the strip contains a chemical sensitive to positively charged ions such as sodium and potassium. The strip detects specific gravity between 1.005 and 1.030.

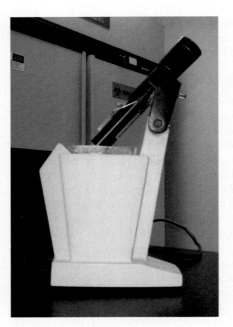

Figure 16–3B A refractometer.

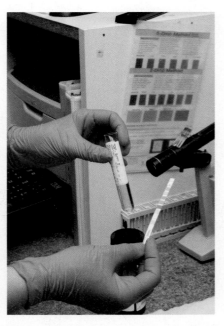

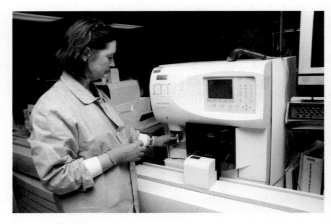

Figure 16–3A A urinometer.

Figure 16–3C A chemical reagent strip.

Chemical tests are performed on urine specimens to detect a wide variety of chemicals present. Again, the reagent strip is the most commonly used technique for this purpose. There are many different types of chemical reagent strips (used in computerized or manual urinalysis). Usually, they consist of plastic strips to which one or more pads containing chemicals are attached (see **Figures 16–4A** and **B**). They allow testing for pH, specific gravity, leukocyte esterase, vitamin C, ketones, protein, blood, glucose, bilirubin, nitrite, urobilinogen, **phenyl ketones**, and other chemicals. Today, most laboratories use computerized urinalysis for various urine tests (see **Figure 16–5**).

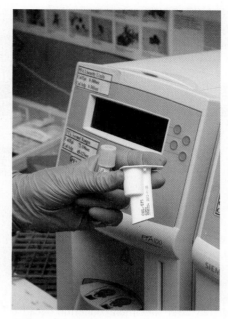

Figure 16–5 A computerized urinalysis machine.

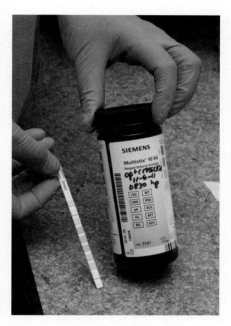

Figure 16–4A A urine reagent used for manual urinalysis.

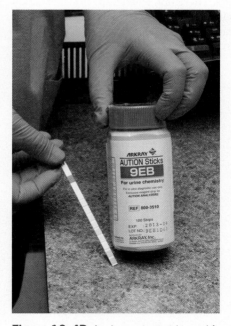

Figure 16–4B A urine reagent strip used for computer urinalysis.

Reagent strips are used once and then discarded, and instructions on proper use are included in their packaging. The container label contains a color comparison chart. Also, various reagent tablet tests are available. Both strips and tablets must be kept tightly sealed in containers located in a cool, dry area. They should only be removed from their containers immediately before testing. Any strip that has been exposed to urine should never be touched to the color comparison chart on the bottle. If both a urinalysis test and a culture and sensitivity test have been ordered, the urine must be cultured before starting the urinalysis. This is done because the introduction of the reagent strip into the urine will contaminate it.

The pH of urine is its degree of acidity or alkalinity. Neutral specimens have a pH of 7. **Figure 16–6** shows a pH scale. If the value is below 7, the urine is acidic, and if above 7, it is alkaline. Freshly voided urine may have a pH ranging from 5.5 to 8. The pH can vary based on diet, metabolic status, disease, and drug therapy. Conditions such as bacteriuria cause it to be alkaline due to bacterial conversion of urea to ammonia. Crystals can also be identified in urine based on the pH.

Under normal conditions, glucose is filtered at the glomerulus and reabsorbed in the tubules. Reagent testing normally does not detect tiny amounts of glucose present in the urine. However, when the renal tubules cannot reabsorb the filtered glucose load, detectable glycosuria occurs. Patients with diabetes may be first diagnosed by a positive glucose finding in the urine. Reagent strip glucose testing is based on *enzymatic reactions* that are specific for only glucose.

Protein in the urine in detectable amounts (*proteinuria*) is an early sign of renal disease. Protein is present normally in only tiny amounts in the urine. Proteinuria is a common finding in pregnancy, and it is also almost always present after heavy exercise. Reagent strips are highly sensitive to urinary albumin and less sensitive to hemoglobin, immunoglobulin, and mucoproteins.

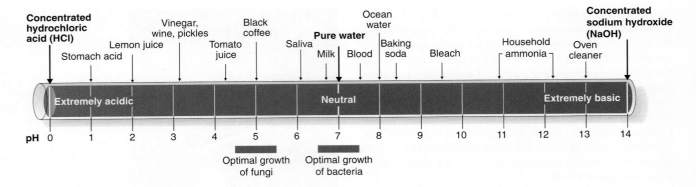

Figure 16–6 A pH scale.

Ketones are the end products of fat metabolism. Acetoacetate, acetone, and beta-hydroxybutyric acid are examples of ketones, which are also called *ketone bodies*. Ketonuria occurs due to low-carbohydrate diets, starvation, diabetes mellitus, and excessive vomiting. Urine testing for ketones must occur immediately after specimen collection because ketones evaporate at room temperature. If immediate testing is not possible, the specimen should be tightly covered and refrigerated. While the reagent strip detects only acetoacetate, another test called *Acetest* can also detect acetone.

Blood in the urine can indicate bleeding in the kidneys and infection or trauma to the urinary tract. On a reagent strip, the blood test pad reacts with hemoglobin from red blood cells. The presence of red blood cells in urine is called *hematuria*. In some rare cases, after massive muscle injury, physical trauma, or electrical injury, **myoglobinuria** may occur. When hematuria is present, the color reaction on the strip ranges from yellow to dark green, giving a speckled appearance. Causes of hematuria include irritation of the bladder, ureters, or urethra as well as cystitis or the passage of kidney stones. If a woman is menstruating, a random specimen may contain blood from vaginal contamination.

Bilirubin, a product of the breakdown of hemoglobin, is a bile pigment not normally found in urine. Hemoglobin is released from old red blood cells (RBCs) and is gradually converted to bilirubin in the liver, then converted to urobilinogen in the intestines. When bilirubin is present in urine, it may be an early sign of liver disease or related infections such as mononucleosis. Bilirubinuria can occur before jaundice (**icterus**) or other symptoms of liver disease, and it results from liver cell damage or obstruction of the common bile duct by neoplasms or stones. When it is present in high amounts, the urine is yellow-brown to green-orange. Urine samples must be protected from light until testing is completed because direct light causes decomposition of bilirubin. Urobilinogen may increase in the urine with increased RBC destruction and liver disease. Reagent strip methods cannot detect a decrease in urobilinogen. An *Ictotest* is used to detect and confirm the presence of bilirubin in the urine.

Nitrite occurs in urine due to bacteria breaking down nitrate, which is a common urine component. When nitrite is present, it may indicate a urinary tract infection (UTI). *Escherichia coli*, which causes most UTIs, reduces nitrate to nitrite. If the specimen is allowed to sit at room temperature and bacteria multiply, a false-positive result may occur. False-negative results may occur if bacteria further metabolize the nitrite they have produced so that it becomes ammonia.

Leukocytes appear in urine due to UTIs, but can also be contaminants from the vagina. On a reagent strip, the leukocyte esterase test detects both intact and lysed *polymorphonuclear leukocytes*, but does not detect *mononuclear leukocytes*. The test also does not react with the small amounts of leukocytes that exist in normal urine.

Reagent strips are reliable if used properly. **Table 16–5** shows normal urine reference ranges for reagent strips.

However, errors in the use of reagent strips can be due to excessive soaking of the strip in the specimen, which dilutes its chemicals. Holding the strip in any way other than horizontally may cause the chemicals to bleed into one another. Certain chemicals, such as ascorbic acid (vitamin C), can affect the results of certain tests. Ideally, patients should not consume large amounts of vitamin C for at least 24 h before urine testing.

Some laboratories use automated equipment to read reagent strips (see **Figure 16–7**). This equipment offers consistent timing and color interpretation, but cannot identify or compensate for highly pigmented urine, which can lead to false-positive results. Therefore, when a specimen is darkly pigmented, the technician should manually test it.

Microscopic examination of urine categorizes and counts casts, cells, crystals, and other constituents of urine sediment

Table 16–5 Normal Reagent Strip Reference Ranges

Reference	Range
Bilirubin (mg/dL)	NEG
Blood (mg/dL)	NEG
Clarity	Clear to slightly turbid
Color	Pale yellow to straw
Glucose (mg/dL)	NEG
Ketone (mg/dL)	NEG
Nitrite (mg/dL)	NEG
pH	4.6–8
Protein (mg/dL)	NEG
Specific gravity	1.001–1.035
Urobilinogen (Ehrlich units)	0.1–1
White blood cells	NEG

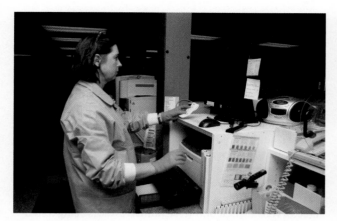

Figure 16–7 A urine analyzer with a sample printout of results.

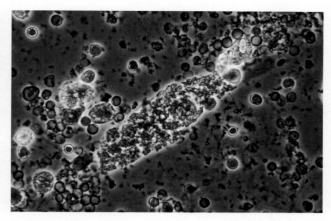

Figure 16–9 Granular casts.

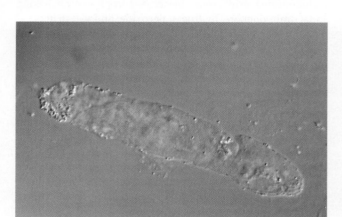

Figure 16–8 Hyaline casts.

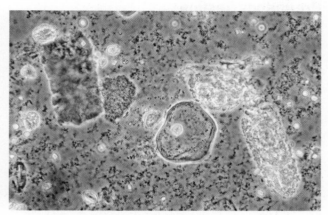

Figure 16–10 Epithelial cells in urine.

after urine is centrifuged. Urine cytology studies look for the presence of abnormal cells. This type of testing requires additional, specialized training. Microscopic observation requires a bright field, phase contrast, or polarizing microscope. *Casts* are formed as protein accumulates and precipitates in kidney tubules and is washed into the urine. Casts are cylindric, with flat or rounded ends. Certain types of casts are associated with renal conditions, but may also be related to strenuous exercise. Because casts dissolve in alkaline urine as it stands, examination of fresh specimens is required. Examples of *hyaline casts* and *granular casts* are shown in **Figures 16–8** and **16–9**.

Epithelial cells, RBCs, and white blood cells (WBCs) may be found in the urine. Epithelial cells (see **Figure 16–10**) are derived from the lining of the genitourinary tract. RBCs may enter the urinary tract at any point, due to inflammation or injury. WBCs in the urine are associated with inflammation or contamination of the specimen.

Crystals are common in urine specimens, especially after cooling occurs. Abnormal crystals may be caused by metabolic conditions or may be of iatrogenic origin, related to medications or other treatments. After crystals are identified due to pH changes, their color, shape, and refractivity are observed with a polarized or phase microscope, or a supravital stain. Various types of crystals in the urine are shown in **Figure 16–11**.

Other miscellaneous findings in the urine may occur. *Oval fat bodies* are related to nephrotic syndrome. *Yeast* may indicate vaginal contamination or infection of the urine with candidiasis, and it is common in the urine of diabetic patients (see **Figure 16–12**).

Bacilli (rod-shaped bacteria) or cocci (spheric bacteria) may indicate a UTI. Spermatozoa may also be present in the urine. Parasites may include *Trichomonas vaginalis*. Mucous threads in increased numbers may be seen with inflammation and in specimens contaminated with vaginal secretions.

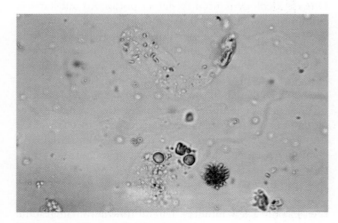

Figure 16–11 Crystals of various types.

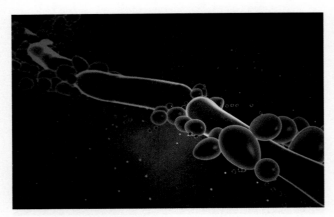

Figure 16–12 Yeast in the urine.

Pregnancy Testing

All pregnancy tests detect the presence of **human chorionic gonadotropin** (hCG) in the urine. This hormone is produced by the placenta of a pregnant female. Once a fertilized egg is implanted in the uterus, hCG levels double every few days, rapidly rising for about 7 weeks, then declining. The most common type of test for pregnancy is the *lateral flow immunoassay test*, and many forms of this test are now available over the counter. They can detect the presence of hCG as early as 1 week after implantation, or 4 to 5 days before a missed menstrual period. They can usually be performed in less than 5 min, and a simple color change usually signifies pregnancy.

Pregnancy tests should optimally be performed on the first morning-voided specimen. A first morning-voided specimen is normally the most concentrated. The pregnancy test cartridge contains a membrane with an absorbent pad that overlaps a strip of fiberglass paper. This paper has been impregnated with a freeze-dried conjugate of gold particles and antibodies to hCG. When the urine specimen dissolves the freeze-dried conjugate, the hCG antigen attaches to the antibodies in the colloidal solution, and the gold particles accumulate, forming a pink line. Another line, called the "C" (control) line, will change color from all samples, and it is used to indicate that the test has been carried out correctly.

Urine Toxicology

Urine toxicology is used to detect poisonous substances, certain therapeutic drugs, illegal drugs, and alcohol. Urine drug screening may be used to monitor therapeutic drug use, determine prescription drug abuse, or detect the use of illegal drugs. Urine is the specimen of choice for most routing screening procedures, with a random specimen usually being collected. In some cases, a strict chain of custody for these tests is required. Urine screening is favored over blood or serum screening because the substance for which the test is performed, or its *metabolite*, often remains in urine much longer than intoxication or impairment from the agent persists.

Rapid drug-screening devices are dipped into a urine sample, or urine is directly applied to the device. Results are seen in only a few minutes. Lateral flow chromatographic immunoassay tests are used for a variety of drugs, including amphetamines, barbiturates, benzodiazepines, cocaine, methadone, morphine, phencyclidine (PCP), marijuana, tricyclics, methamphetamines, and Ecstasy. These tests work by separating the components of substances being tested via the activity of antigens and antibodies.

In these tests, urine mixes with a labeled antibody–dye conjugate and causes a specific color banding to occur. Additional testing is usually conducted to ensure that samples have not been adulterated (intentionally manipulated in order to pass the test). Temperature detectors are used to ensure that the urine sample has been freshly voided from the bladder and has not been introduced after being carried in some sort of container hidden within the test subject's clothing. Other detectors ensure that only fresh human urine is being tested—common substances that have been used to pass these tests include animal urine, water, bleach, eyedrops, vinegar, baking soda, drain openers, hydrogen peroxide, and soft drinks.

Note that alcohol testing is performed not on urine, but on saliva. A swab that is saturated with saliva is usually used for workplace testing to detect ethanol. This is common in "drug-free workplaces." Another form of alcohol testing is the **Breathalyzer**, which is primarily used by the police in cases of *driving under the influence* (DUI). These devices determine approximate blood alcohol levels by measuring the amount of alcohol in an individual's breath. The individual is asked to exhale deeply into the device for at least 5 s, usually until the police officer signals him or her to stop. Chemicals inside the Breathalyzer cause a reaction to occur if the individual's blood alcohol level is at or above accepted state levels. **Figure 16–13** shows a common Breathalyzer.

Sputum Specimens

Sputum is mucus or phlegm ejected from the trachea and lungs via deep coughing. In some cases, sputum may also contain pus or blood. It is collected in a sterile container for microbiology specimens to test for pathogenic organisms (such as tuberculosis). Sputum can also be collected in containers that have a preservative for cytology testing. Both the patient and the phlebotomist must be careful during collection because this preservative is poisonous. Additional care must be taken when transporting these specimens. **Figure 16–14** shows how a sterile sputum specimen is collected from a patient.

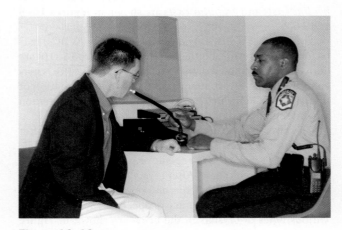

Figure 16–13 A Breathalyzer.

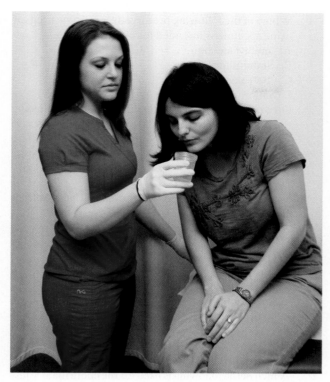

Figure 16–14 A patient about to spit into a sputum collection container.

Cerebrospinal Fluid Specimens

Cerebrospinal fluid is normally clear, and it resembles blood plasma. It circulates around the brain, in the brain cavities, and in the space surrounding the spinal cord. The **spinal tap** (lumbar puncture) procedure is performed by a physician to diagnose conditions such as meningitis, brain tumors, or multiple sclerosis. Cerebrospinal fluid is often tested for cell counts, chloride, glucose, and total protein. After this procedure, the phlebotomist may transport the specimen into the laboratory. The fluid is usually collected in three sterile containers that are numbered in the order of collection. Personal protective equipment must be worn during transporting by the phlebotomist.

Amniotic Fluid Specimens

Amniotic fluid surrounds the fetus inside the amniotic sac. A physician collects it at approximately 16 weeks of gestation to detect fetal abnormalities. It is sometimes also collected in the last trimester to determine the lung maturity of the fetus. The phlebotomist may transport amniotic fluid specimens *immediately* to the laboratory, and she or he must wear gloves while doing this. Also, the specimen must be protected from light.

Semen Specimens

Semen must be collected in clean containers that are free of any detergents or spermicides. Sometimes patients performing semen collection themselves use condoms as the collection devices—it is important to ensure that these condoms do not contain spermicides, which would alter the results. Semen is examined for various reasons, including to determine if a vasectomy was effective, to assess fertility, and as evidence

in sexual criminal cases. The patient will collect the semen himself and bring it to the ordering physician immediately. Also, specimens must not be exposed to extreme temperature or light, and they should be kept as close to body temperature (37°C or 98.6°F) as possible. The phlebotomist may assist in the transport of samples, and he or she must wear gloves while doing this—remember that the sample must be transported to the laboratory as soon as possible, which must be less than 2 h.

Fecal Specimens

Fecal (stool) specimens are frequently collected to detect parasites, enteric disease organisms (such as *Salmonella*, *Shigella*, *Clostridium difficile colitis*, or *Staphylococcus aureus*), occult blood, and colorectal cancer. Specimen containers are wide-mouthed, with tight-fitting lids. If the patient will perform the collection at home, he or she must be instructed to avoid getting any urine into the sample because this can kill microorganisms that are to be studied. The outside of the container should be cleaned thoroughly. It must be transported immediately to the laboratory and maintained at body temperature. Fecal occult blood testing requires small amounts of feces collected on special test cards on 3 separate days. A chemical called **guaiac** is used because it can detect small amounts of blood. A fecal fat analysis may require a 72-h refrigerated stool specimen.

Summary

Routine urinalysis is performed often as a screening test to detect metabolic and physiologic disorders. Urine is formed in the kidneys via the nephrons, and its filtrate passes the tubules with various changes occurring. Urine is stored in the bladder and voided through the urethra. Some urine collections must be performed following meals or fasts, may require cleansing of the external genitalia, and may require the addition of preservatives. Only urine that will be cultured must be collected in a sterile container. Timed urine specimens are collected to determine the amount of a particular analyte during a given time frame.

Physical examination of urine involves determination of color, turbidity, and specific gravity. Chemical examination involves determining levels of glucose, pH, ketones, protein, bilirubin, blood, nitrite, urobilinogen, leukocyte esterase, and specific gravity. A complete UA involves physical, chemical, and microscopic assessment, often involving reagent strips or tablets. Formed elements in the urine sediment include casts, cells, and crystals. Pregnancy tests detect hCG, a hormone produced by the placenta. Drug testing utilizes lateral flow technology, and measures must be taken to prevent adulteration of specimens.

Sputum from the trachea or lungs may be collected to test for pathogenic organisms or for cytology testing. Cerebrospinal fluid specimens are obtained by spinal tap (lumbar puncture) to diagnose meningitis, brain tumors, multiple sclerosis, and other conditions. Amniotic fluid specimens may be collected to detect fetal abnormalities. Semen specimens may be collected to determine if a vasectomy was effective, to assess fertility, and as evidence in sexual criminal cases. Fecal (stool) specimens are frequently collected to detect parasites, enteric disease organisms, occult blood, and colorectal cancer.

CRITICAL THINKING

A phlebotomist works in a large clinic. One day she received an order to collect urine from two different patients. The first was for a urine culture, and the second was for drug screening.

1. What type of sample should be collected for a urine culture?
2. What type of sample should be collected for drug screening?

WEBSITES

http://www.bd.com/vacutainer/labnotes/ Volume14Number2/

http://www.ivy-rose.co.uk/HumanBody/Urinary/Urinary_ System_Composition_Urine.php

http://www.nlm.nih.gov/medlineplus/ency/article/003578 .htm

http://www.nsbri.org/humanphysspace/focus4/ep-urine .html

http://www.medindia.net/animation/anatomy_urinary.asp

http://www.uch.edu/for-healthcare-professional/ Clinical-Laboratory/Guide/packaging-and-transporting-specimens-to-the-laboratory/

http://www.womenshealth.gov/publications/our-publications/fact-sheet/pregnancy-tests.cfm

REVIEW QUESTIONS

Multiple Choice

1. Urine is carried to the urinary bladder by
   A. blood vessels
   B. lymphatics
   C. the urethra
   D. the ureters
2. The process of filtration occurs at
   A. the distal convoluted tubule
   B. the collecting duct
   C. Bowman's capsule
   D. the loop of Henle
3. Each of the following is a characteristic of a normal urine sample, EXCEPT
   A. cloudiness
   B. amber color
   C. acidic pH
   D. ammonia odor
4. The most common type of urine collection is
   A. timed
   B. 24-h
   C. random
   D. first-voided morning
5. Specific gravity may be measured by all of the following methods, EXCEPT
   A. a microscope
   B. a refractometer
   C. a reagent strip
   D. a urinometer

6. Which of the following preservatives must be used for urine specimens intended for culture?
   A. methyl alcohol
   B. sodium formate
   C. 10% bleach
   D. chlorhexidine
7. On a urinalysis reagent strip, infection is indicated by the presence of
   A. ketones
   B. leukocytes
   C. protein
   D. bilirubin
8. Which of the following is the causative agent of candidiasis?
   A. virus
   B. protozoa
   C. yeast
   D. bacteria
9. The presence of which of the following substances in urine most likely indicates metabolism of fat?
   A. glucose
   B. ketones
   C. hemoglobin
   D. bilirubin
10. Which of the following is used for the confirmatory test to detect the presence of bilirubin in urine?
    A. Multistix
    B. Clinitest
    C. Ictotest
    D. Acetest
11. Cytology studies of urine determine the presence of
    A. illegal drugs
    B. glucose
    C. abnormal cells
    D. lead poisoning
12. Which of the following tests determines the presence of occult blood?
    A. guaiac
    B. lactose
    C. troponin
    D. cholesterol
13. Semen specimens must be collected by
    A. laboratory personnel
    B. nurses
    C. physicians
    D. patients
14. Which of the following fluids is obtained via lumbar puncture?
    A. sputum
    B. spinal
    C. amniotic
    D. gastric
15. Sputum specimens are collected in the diagnosis of
    A. strep throat
    B. lung maturity
    C. whooping cough
    D. tuberculosis

CHAPTER 17

Specimen Handling and Transport

Outline

Introduction
Handling Specimens after Venipuncture
Delivery Methods
Clinical Laboratory Specimen Processing
Reporting of Laboratory Results
Summary
Critical Thinking
Websites
Review Questions

OBJECTIVES

After studying this chapter, readers should be able to:

1. Define the term *turnaround time* in phlebotomy.
2. Describe handling and transport methods for blood after collection.
3. Explain pneumatic tube systems and their disadvantages.
4. Discuss the three basic processing steps for clinical laboratory specimens.
5. Describe a variety of general packing requirements to ship infectious substances.
6. Explain automated carriers used to transport specimens.
7. Describe *special handling*.
8. Compare verbal laboratory reports with computerized reports.
9. Describe transportation of microbiological specimens.
10. List the components of labeling of laboratory specimens.

KEY TERMS

Additive tube: A blood collection tube that contains any type of additive, most commonly an anticoagulant.

Agitation: Putting into motion by shaking or stirring.

Aldosterone: A hormone that has major effects upon blood volume and pressure.

Aliquots: Portions of a total amount of solution.

Calcitonin: A hormone that acts to reduce blood calcium, opposing the effects of parathyroid hormone.

Dry ice: The solid form of carbon dioxide; it is used as a cooling agent.

Pneumatic tube system: A system of carrying items in cylindrical containers, propelled through a network of tubes by compressed air or partial vacuum.

Thermolabile: Easily destroyed or altered by heat; also called *heat labile*.

Turnaround time: The total time needed for a blood sample to be collected, analyzed, and reported on.

Introduction

Analysis of blood specimens after venipuncture must take place as quickly as possible to ensure accuracy. The phlebotomist and other healthcare workers have continued responsibilities throughout the processes of collection, transport, analysis, and reporting. Appropriate documentation is always required. A variety of transportation methods may be utilized to carry specimens. Hazardous agents require careful monitoring during shipping. Computerization offers rapid communication of test results.

Handling Specimens after Venipuncture

The time between venipuncture and delivery to the laboratory for testing is critical. Analysis must take place as quickly as possible to ensure accuracy. Test results, upon which physicians make accurate decisions, must be totally correct. In phlebotomy, the term **turnaround time** describes the entire amount of time required for blood specimens to be ordered, collected, transported, processed, analyzed, and reported.

The following factors are important invariables in phlebotomy:

- *Patients:* age, identification, gender, pregnancy, fasting versus nonfasting, medications, diurnal variations, level of cooperation, availability, anxiety, and stress
- *Transportation and handling:* correct filling and mixing of specimens, leakage, tube breakage, and excessive shaking of specimens
- *Specimen processing and storage:* adequate centrifugation, sample registration, sample distribution, processing delays, specimen contamination, and heat or light exposure
- *Specimen quality:* hemolysis, inadequate specimen volume, and inadequate mixing with anticoagulant

The duties of the phlebotomist and healthcare workers who assist in transporting specimens continue throughout the process. The Clinical and Laboratory Standards Institute (CLSI) defines standards for specimen handling and processing. The following are the basic steps in the handling and transporting of the specimen once it arrives at the testing laboratory:

- *Mixing:* Gentle inversion of tubes should be effected so that additives are evenly distributed throughout the blood. This should be done as quickly as possible after the specimen enters the **additive tube**. If not handled gently, blood cells will be damaged, resulting in hemolysis. Inadequate mixing causes tiny clots to form. If gel separation tubes are not thoroughly mixed, incomplete clotting may occur. Remember, specimen tubes without additives do not require mixing.
- *Labeling:* Whenever possible, tube labels should be compared with patient identification bracelets, or patients can be asked to verbally verify that the label information is correct (see **Figure 17–1**). Information that should be included is the patient's first and last names, date, identification number, collection time, name of the person performing the collection, and, if required, the ordered tests, volume requirements, physician's name, etc.
- *Use of biohazard bags:* Blood specimens may be placed in biohazard bags, racks, or other safe carrying equipment. Bags must usually be leakproof to protect healthcare workers from pathogenic microorganisms (see **Figure 17–2**). If possible, evacuated tubes and microcollection tubes should be kept upright and closed. Gentle handling of all types of containers is recommended.

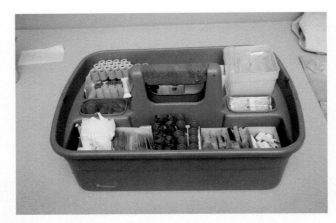

Figure 17–2 Specimen bags and a specimen rack in a phlebotomy tray.

- *Transportation:* Again, this should occur as soon as possible after collection. Significant delays may greatly affect test results. For example, glycolytic action may interfere with the analysis of glucose, **calcitonin, aldosterone**, phosphorus, and enzymes. Rough handling or **agitation** of blood specimens may affect coagulation tests.
- *Special handling:* Certain tests require cooling to slow metabolic processes. Others require transporting at body temperature to prevent agglutination or precipitation. Still others require protection from light to prevent various components from breaking down. **Table 17–1** lists special handling requirements.

  Figure 17–3 shows transportation racks for cooled specimens, a specimen in an ice slurry, and a specimen wrapped in foil for protection from light.
- *Microbiological specimens:* These include blood or throat cultures, sputum, semen, stool, and urine specimens. Quick transport is also required for these

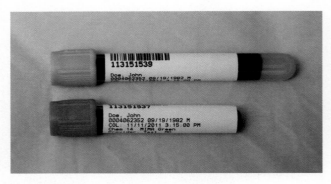

Figure 17–1 The labeling of a blood specimen.

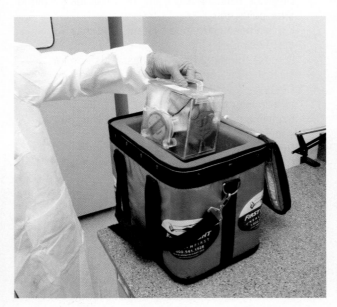

Figure 17–3 Transportation racks for cooled specimens, a specimen in an "ice slurry," and a specimen wrapped in foil for protection from light.

Table 17–1 Special Handling Requirements

Requirement	Tests
Photosensitive specimens *Photosensitive* means "sensitive to light"—these specimens will decompose after being exposed to bright light. These specimens should be protected from bright light with amber/brown biohazard bags, aluminum foil wrapping around tubes, or transport containers that do not allow light to enter.	Beta-carotene Bilirubin Folate Porphyrins Vitamin A Vitamin B$_6$
Specimens requiring chilling (thermolabile) *Thermolabile* means "sensitive to higher temperatures"; these specimens need to be chilled immediately after collection, which inhibits blood cell metabolism and stabilizes most constituents. An "ice slurry" may be used, which is a mixture of ice and water—large chunks of ice should not be used because they can freeze specimens. For *blood gases*, delivery speed is essential to prevent loss of these gases from the specimen. If analysis can occur within 30 min, plastic syringes are recommended, and specimens can be transported at room temperature. If analysis is delayed, glass syringes are recommended, which should be cooled soon after collection. Chilling can harm certain analytes, such as potassium. If a potassium test is ordered and collected in tubes with other analytes that require chilling, it should be tested within 2 h or collected in a separate tube. If it is chilled for more than 2 h, potassium leaks out of cells, causing a false elevation. Electrolyte specimens should not be chilled.	Ammonia Blood gases Catecholamines Gastrin Lactic acid Parathyroid hormone Pyruvate
Plasma-based coagulation assays Temperatures must be kept constant, and ice or cold packs should be avoided because they may activate clotting factors or disrupt platelets. Transportation should occur within 1 h after collection, although some assays (such as *prothrombin time*) can be delayed up to 24 h. Follow the laboratory guidelines for each type of specimen. Specimens should be stored with their caps shut tightly. PT can remain uncentrifuged or centrifuged at room temperature for up to 24 h. Activated partial thromboplastin time (APTT) specimens, if the patient is not on heparin therapy, can remain uncentrifuged or centrifuged at room temperature for up to 4 h after collection. If they contain unfractionated heparin, they should be kept at room temperature and centrifuged within 1 h. Anticoagulated whole blood (citrate or ethylenediaminetetraacetic acid [EDTA]) can be stored at room temperature for up to 8 days or at 2 to 8°C before DNA is extracted. Always follow manufacturers' directions for any molecular hemostasis assays.	Time delays depend on the actual test
Specimens requiring 37°C transport These specimens must be heated via a controlled heat source or heating block during transportation and handling.	Cold agglutinins Cryofibrinogen Cryoglobulins

specimens. Blood culture specimens are usually collected into culture media, minimizing possible contamination and speeding up contact with the media itself. Incubation is required as soon as possible for accuracy.

■ *Transportation to remote sites:* Handling guidelines must still follow standard precautions. All protection equipment and clothing must be worn. Lockable containers should hold specimens during driving so that in case of an accident, they cannot spill outside the containers. These containers should be labeled with biohazard warning labels. Cold packs or heat packs should be used to ensure controllable temperatures within these containers.

Figure 17–4 shows a transport container for transportation to remote sites.

Delivery Methods

Laboratories in larger facilities are usually responsible for delivering blood specimens to the place of analysis. Urine or sputum specimens are often delivered by nursing staff members or transportation department members. Guidelines for delivery should include pickup schedules, steps to deliver STAT specimens, where specimens should be placed, electronic or manual log-in of symptoms, etc. Appropriate

documentation must always be completed. Sometimes commercial specimen couriers are used for transport. Adequate packaging and handling, especially in hot or cold temperatures, must always be maintained.

Many specimens are hand-carried. In the laboratory, a log sheet is usually used for hand-delivered specimens. In the hospital, blood collection trays or carts are usually arranged to hold specimens to be delivered in test tube racks, holders

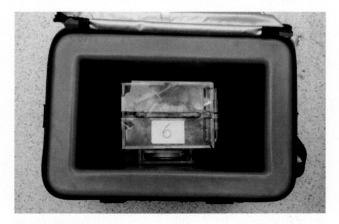

Figure 17–4 A transport container for the transportation to remote sites.

(for microscopic slides), cups, plastic holders, or leakproof ice water containers.

Pneumatic tube systems are used to transport messages, patient records, bills, letters, medications, X-rays, and laboratory test results. **Pneumatic tube systems** must be mechanically reliable, with control mechanisms, shock absorbers, and a variety of other considerations to ensure accuracy. This type of transport can damage tests, such as those used to determine levels of potassium and plasma hemoglobin, and the system must be carefully evaluated before transporting any test specimens. For the majority of substances to be analyzed, pneumatic tube systems are safe. Specimens are contained within shock-absorbent padding and biohazard bags.

Automated carriers used to transport specimens may be motorized as well as computerized. A small "container car" attached to a track network is used to route specimens to appropriate laboratory sites, nursing states, or specimen collection areas. Similar safety and mechanical factors must exist to those utilized in pneumatic tube systems.

Clinical Laboratory Specimen Processing

In the clinical laboratory, blood specimens with additives are analyzed after having been mixed gently. Specimens are placed on a tray that feeds them into an analyzer. Other specimens require greater processing than those containing additives. These other specimens are divided into smaller portions (**aliquots**) for testing on a variety of analyzers. There are three basic processing steps:

- Precentrifugation: after collection but before centrifugation
- Centrifugation: during the actual centrifuge processes
- Postcentrifugation: after centrifugation but before removal of an aliquot of plasma or serum for testing

Table 17–2 lists detailed information about the handling and processing of blood specimens that do or do not require centrifugation.

Aliquot preparation is not standardized, and therefore, errors may occur. Automated instrumentation is often used to prepare aliquots. When laboratory staff prepare them by hand, it is important to use measurable steps, review the steps (by more than one person), use random testing of aliquots against original tubes, and use repetition to reinforce training on procedures.

Hazardous agents require cautious monitoring during shipping. There are nine hazard classes of substances that can cause harm when transported by air. Class 6 of these hazardous substances includes infectious substances and requires specific packaging and handling. They include diagnostic specimens that may contain human or animal materials that are being shipped for diagnostic or investigative purposes.

When hazardous agents are shipped, adequate training of employees must be undertaken. Properly absorbent materials must be used, all labeling must be sufficient, and carriers should be properly contacted in advance of shipping. There should be a receipt confirmation of prompt delivery, sharing of all shipping details with carriers, and follow-up of any problems immediately after they occur.

Aircraft used to ship infectious substances have a variety of general packing requirements. These include double packaging, watertight seals, absorbent material, individual wrapping of tubes, specific thicknesses of protective materials, correct marking designating the material as infectious substances, proper shipping paperwork, adequate temperature control, protection of infectious substances from **dry ice** or other temperature-regulating substances, and prompt verification of proper shipping when infectious substances arrive at their destination.

Shipping requirements for diagnostic specimens are slightly less rigid, but similar. For any type of shipment, serious legal ramifications and fines apply if regulations and guidelines are not followed. Upon arrival at a healthcare facility, packages must be thoroughly inspected for maintenance of storage criteria. Many commercial shipping companies provide sophisticated and reliable tracking methods, able to monitor shipping status at each stopping point along the way.

Reporting of Laboratory Results

Permanent reports should be maintained in the laboratory about laboratory results. Each report must contain adequate patient and testing information. This applies regardless of whether results are stored on paper or in electronic format. Written reports should include patient identification, location, physician, date and time of collection, specimen source and description, labeled precautions, adequate shipment or mailing packaging, format consistency, clear instructions or orders, record keeping in logical places in the patient chart, sequential order of multiple results, listing of reference ranges and normal/abnormal values, assurances of accuracy, and administrative/record keeping value. Quality control is vital.

Today, verbal or telephone reports of laboratory results have greatly declined. They are more prone to error than written or computerized reports. If they are used, verbal reports should be accompanied by documentation of patient name and identification number, name of the person who receives the report, date, time, information given, and name of the person issuing the report.

Computerized reports offer rapid communication of test results. In hospitals, computer terminals are usually located throughout the facility. Once tests are verified, results can be displayed immediately wherever there is a computer. Attached printers can generate hard copies of test results. Patient privacy and confidentiality must always be maintained.

Summary

Phlebotomists and other healthcare workers have many different responsibilities during blood collection, transport, analysis, and reporting. Analysis must take place as quickly as possible to make sure that test results are accurate. The Clinical Laboratory Standards Institute defines standards for specimen handling and processing. The three basic steps of specimen processing include precentrifugation, centrifugation, and postcentrifugation. The basic steps of handling and transporting specimens include mixing, labeling, use of biohazard bags, transportation, special handling, quick

Table 17–2 Handling and Processing Blood Specimens

No Centrifugation	Precentrifugation	Centrifugation	Postcentrifugation
Instead of centrifugation, some specimens may require no additional processing except for gentle mixing. Usually hematology specimens are placed on automatic mixing trays or placed directly into analyzers.	Serum or plasma should be removed from cells as soon as possible and not exceed 2 h from the time of collection.	Serum specimens should be allowed to clot before centrifugation. Incomplete clotting can leave fibrin residue in the serum, interfering with analysis.	Unless otherwise instructed, if not tested completely within 48 h, separated serum/plasma should be frozen at or below −20°C. Do not use frost-free freezers. Aliquots are prepared when specimens must be subdivided for different tests. Make sure there is proper storage for each analyte being tested.
Tubes with additives should be gently inverted 5 to 10 times to mix the specimen with the additive—first at the patient's side before transportation and again prior to analysis.	Anticoagulated plasma specimens can be centrifuged immediately. Those without anticoagulant additives (serum specimens) should be clotted before centrifugation (usually 30–60 min at room temperature).	Tubes should be centrifuged with stoppers or caps in place to prevent exposure and evaporation. They should be balanced in the centrifuge to avoid breakage. Follow all laboratory instructions.	Serum/plasma should not be repeatedly frozen and thawed. It may be left in contact with a gel, barrier, or separator device. Tubes should be inspected after centrifugation to check for complete barriers between serum/plasma and cells.
It is preferred that CBC, differentials, reticulocyte counts, and nucleated red blood cell (NRBC) counts be performed as soon as possible.	Clotting time is affected (delayed) by anticoagulant therapy. Chilling the specimen delays clotting. Clotting may be accelerated by glass or silica particles, thrombin, snake venom/thrombin, reducing clotting times 15–30 min.	The centrifuge should have a secure top and should not be opened until the cycle is completed. It should be temperature-controlled to protect heat-sensitive analytes.	Tubes should be stored upright with secure closures. Serum/plasma and whole blood should be kept covered at all times. Excessive agitation causes hemolysis and affects the quality of test results.
Some hematology parameters may be reliable for 3–4 days if specific instrumentation is used. Add a comment about the age of the specimen used.	Light-protective containers should be used for photosensitive analytes.	Specimens should not be centrifuged more than once. Specimens containing separation devices should never be recentrifuged.	Lipemic specimens should be handled according to laboratory rules. Plunger-type filters should be used to separate serum/plasma from clots only if they can fully prevent particulate matter from passing into the filtered serum/plasma. For potassium, ACTH, cortisol, catecholamines, and lactic acid, removal of sera from the cells should occur in a shorter time.
Blood smears should be made from EDTA specimens within 1 h to minimize changes in cellular morphology.	Although you may "rim the tube" with a wooden applicator stick to release blood clots attached to the tube surfaces, this is not recommended and may cause hemolysis.	Gel and nongel devices enable a barrier to form between serum/plasma and blood clot/cells during centrifugation. They vary in viscosity and specific gravity. Follow manufacturers' instructions.	Some studies show that certain analytes (albumin, bilirubin, calcium, etc.) may not be affected even if serum is not removed for 48 h or longer. However, some analytes are affected significantly after just 2 h if serum/plasma is not removed. Analyte stability is also affected by temperature.

transport for microbiological specimens, and special measures when transporting specimens to or from remote sites. Documentation must follow each specimen on its entire path from collection to reporting of results.

CRITICAL THINKING

Mike was a courier who regularly transported blood specimens between area hospitals and laboratories. On a Friday afternoon, he was called to pick up a variety of specimens from the downtown hospital and transport them to the large testing laboratory across town. He arrived at the hospital, completed the paperwork for the transportation of the specimens, and transported the specimens to the laboratory. Upon arriving at the laboratory, he received an emergency telephone call from his wife, handed the specimens to a laboratory technician, and left to go home. He did not complete any paperwork for the delivery of the specimens to the laboratory.

1. What could the potential outcomes be in this situation because the chain of custody was broken?
2. What potential legal actions could be brought?

WEBSITES

http://findarticles.com/p/articles/mi_m3230/is_1_34/ai_82272882/

http://homepages.gac.edu/~cellab/appds/appd-f.html

http://www.arcat.com/divs/sec/sec14580.shtml

http://www.bd.com/vacutainer/faqs/

http://www.bd.com/vacutainer/labnotes/Volume15Number1/

http://www.cdc.gov/std/syphilis/manual-1998/CHAPT3.pdf

http://www.clsi.org/source/orders/free/H21-a5.pdf

http://www.crime-scene-investigator.net/blood.html

http://www.doh.state.fl.us/disease_ctrl/std/prevent/MODULE_2_V2.1.pdf

http://www.geisingermedicallabs.com/catalog/blood_specimens.shtml

http://www.mgh.org/lab/specimen.html

REVIEW QUESTIONS

Multiple Choice

1. A blood collection tube that contains an anticoagulant is referred to as
   A. a pneumatic tube
   B. an additive tube
   C. a disposal tube
   D. none of the above
2. The entire amount of time required for blood specimens to be ordered, collected, transported, processed, analyzed, and reported is called the
   A. total time
   B. prothrombin time
   C. specimen time
   D. turnaround time
3. If gel separation tubes are not thoroughly mixed, which of the following may occur?
   A. hemolysis
   B. clotting
   C. incomplete clotting
   D. all of the above
4. Significant delays in transportation of blood collection may greatly affect test results for
   A. glucose
   B. aldosterone hormone
   C. enzymes
   D. all of the above
5. Agitation of blood specimens may affect which of the following tests?
   A. coagulation
   B. blood gases
   C. cryofibrinogen
   D. bilirubin
6. To transport blood collections to state laboratories, they must be carried in lockable containers with
   A. cold packs
   B. heat packs
   C. ice slurries
   D. A or B
7. Which of the following is usually used for hand-delivered specimens?
   A. pneumatic tube
   B. a log sheet
   C. an analyzer
   D. an invoice
8. A hormone that reduces blood calcium is referred to as
   A. thyroid hormone
   B. aldosterone
   C. insulin
   D. calcitonin
9. Written reports should include all of the following, EXCEPT
   A. date and time of collection
   B. invoice and billing information for the insurance company
   C. labeled precautions
   D. listing of reference ranges
10. What is the advantage of computerized reports?
    A. They cannot be viewed without a password.
    B. They may contain protected health information.
    C. They offer rapid communication.
    D. All of the above.
11. How long after collection should anticoagulated plasma specimens be centrifuged?
    A. immediately
    B. 1 h
    C. 5 h
    D. 24 h
12. If gel separation tubes are not thoroughly mixed, which of the following may occur?
    A. inadequate specimen volume
    B. incomplete clotting
    C. inadequate hemolysis

D. incomplete separation of blood components

13. *Thermolabile* means
    A. sensitive to lower temperatures
    B. a mixture of ice and water
    C. sensitive to higher temperatures
    D. room temperature

14. All of the following tests require chilling, EXCEPT
    A. blood gases
    B. lactic acid

C. vitamin A
D. ammonia

15. Aircraft used to ship infectious substances require all of the following steps, EXCEPT
    A. double packaging
    B. unabsorbent material
    C. watertight seals
    D. individual wrapping of tubes

CHAPTER 18

Compliance

OUTLINE

Introduction
The Need for Compliance in Phlebotomy
Compliance Regulations
The Laboratory Compliance Plan
Effects of Compliance
Legal Actions and Phlebotomy
Lawsuit Prevention
Summary
Critical Thinking
Websites
Review Questions

OBJECTIVES

After studying this chapter, readers should be able to:

1. Define *compliance*.
2. List the most important laws that regulate compliance.
3. Describe the Clinical Laboratory Improvement Act.
4. Explain the Civil Monetary Penalties laws.
5. Describe the laboratory compliance plan.
6. Explain the effects of compliance related to phlebotomists and legal concerns.
7. List complications of phlebotomy that may affect patients.
8. Describe the most widespread effect of HIPAA for phlebotomists.
9. Discuss the Stark law.
10. Explain the Anti-Kickback law.

KEY TERMS

Basilic vein: A large superficial vein of the arm that originates on the dorsal (ulnar) side of the hand, traveling up the forearm and upper arm; it is usually visible through the skin.
Compliance: Conforming to a rule, law, standard, specification, or policy.
Courier: A company or person who delivers mail, packages, or messages.
Fainting: Syncope; a sudden, usually temporary loss of consciousness due to insufficient oxygen in the brain.
Indices: Collections of information or data.
Invasive: Penetrating or breaking the skin, or entering a body cavity.
Kickback: An exchange that is illegal or unethical, such as money for a service that should not be charged for.
Standing orders: Medication orders from physicians for patients who need continual drug regimens; these are commonly utilized in long-term care facilities so that new prescriptions or orders do not have to be continually written when needed.

Introduction

The formal monitoring of how an organization follows laws and regulations is referred to as **compliance**. It helps to prevent abuse, fraud, and waste in the clinical laboratory. Quality customer service benefits greatly from compliance. *Fraud and abuse laws* have been put into force to monitor the activities of laboratories, making sure that correct testing and fair billing are being done. Inspections may be conducted by the Office of the Inspector General (OIG), and laboratories should have a compliance plan in force. It should address situations of poor conduct in the laboratory. A chief compliance officer should be selected at the laboratory to develop the compliance plan and make sure it is followed. A compliance committee, consisting of people from differing areas of the laboratory, should be formed to support the efforts of the compliance officer.

The Need for Compliance in Phlebotomy

Compliance keeps patients, insurance carriers, and healthcare programs such as Medicare and Medicaid from being overcharged. Tests that are termed *medical necessities* should be the only ones completed and charged for. There have been many cases of charging for unneeded tests that collectively amount to millions of dollars' worth of fraud. As a result, the American Medical Association has established the following panels that should be collected for determining general information about a patient's health status:

- *Basic metabolic panel:* potassium, sodium, chloride, carbon dioxide, blood urea nitrogen, glucose, and creatinine
- *Complete blood cell count* (CBC): white blood cell count and differential white cell count, red blood cell count, hematocrit, hemoglobin, red blood cell **indices** (mean corpuscular volume, mean corpuscular hemoglobin, mean corpuscular hemoglobin concentration), and the platelet count
- *Comprehensive metabolic panel:* blood urea nitrogen, glucose, creatinine, sodium, chloride, potassium, calcium, carbon dioxide, albumin, total protein, alkaline phosphatase, aspartate aminotransferase, and total bilirubin
- *Electrolyte panel (lytes):* potassium, sodium, carbon dioxide, chloride
- *Hepatic function panel:* albumin, total and direct bilirubin, alkaline phosphatase, aspartate aminotransferase (also called serum glutamic oxaloacetic transaminase), alanine aminotransferase (also called serum glutamic pyruvic transaminase)

Compliance Regulations

Usually, fraud and abuse laws result in monetary penalties for noncompliance, often two to three times the amount that was illegally billed. Certain laws have a "set" penalty of $15,000 per laboratory test or service that was billed. For more serious cases, imprisonment and criminal penalties may also be incurred, and offending companies can be excluded from future participation in programs such as Medicare or Medicaid. The most important laws that regulate compliance are listed as follows.

- **Anti-Kickback Law (1972):** This law prohibits willful payment or offer of payment, directly or indirectly, for inducing, referring, or soliciting services (including laboratory testing) paid for by a federal health program. Payment can be anything of value or service (for example, computer or laboratory equipment or free testing in the future). Payment can be made to a physician or his or her employee or relative, and it is still considered to be a kickback. If the service provided to the physician can be reasonably deemed to be directly related to the services provided, it is legal. If it provides more value than that, it is not. Penalties include imprisonment up to 5 years and/or fines up to $25,000. Future exclusion from Medicare and Medicaid may be possible. Examples include the following:
  - A phlebotomist provided by a laboratory to accomplish tasks in the physician's office not related to phlebotomy and normally done by the office staff
  - Providing computers and fax machines not exclusively used by the laboratory
  - Testing as a professional courtesy

Most lab managers and pharmacy administrators are required to have knowledge of the Anti-Kickback, False Claims, Civil Monetary, and Stark laws, while phlebotomists and other healthcare professionals must have knowledge of the Health Insurance Portability and Accountability Act (HIPAA).

- **False Claims Act (1986):** This act prohibits knowingly presenting a false claim to the government. The term *knowingly* means with reckless disregard for the truth. There does not need to be specific intent to defraud another party. Penalties include *treble damages* (three times the amount of sustained damages to the government), mandatory penalties of $5,000 to $10,000 per claim, and possible future exclusion from Medicare and Medicaid. Examples include the following:
  - Billing services not medically necessary for treatment or diagnosis of a Medicare patient
  - Billing for services that were never performed
  - Filing duplicate claims for the same service
  - Inserting diagnosis codes that were not provided by a physician
  - Misrepresenting the services performed to increase reimbursement (this is known as *upcoding*)
- **Clinical Laboratory Improvement Act (1988):** This act, known as CLIA, covers quality control and assurance, patient test management, and testing of personnel and proficiency. It assists in regulating laboratories for proven competency of their phlebotomists.
- **Stark law (1989):** This law keeps physicians from referring specimens to laboratories in which immediate family members or even the physicians themselves have a financial interest. Penalties include fines up to $15,000 per service, or twice the amount originally billed, and future exclusion from Medicare and Medicaid is possible. Examples include the following:
  - A laboratory submitting a claim to Medicare or Medicaid for a service provided to a patient whose physician has a financial interest
  - A physician referring a Medicare patient to a laboratory with which he or she has a financial relationship
- **Civil Monetary Penalties laws (1990, etc.):** These laws consist of a variety of legislation and improvements applying to claims for services that are not provided as claimed. These are similar to claims made under the False Claims Act. Penalties include fines up to twice the billed amount and up to $10,000 per service, with future exclusion from Medicare and Medicaid also possible.
- **Health Insurance Portability and Accountability Act (1996):** This act was originally designed to protect health insurance coverage for workers and their families when they were changing or losing jobs.
  - Title 1 of this act disallowed limiting or refusing coverage because of preexisting conditions and helped people to buy health insurance when they lost an employer's plan and had no other coverage.
  - Title II of this act established national standards for providers, health plans, and employers to standardize electronic data.

- The most widespread effect of this act was the requirement for healthcare providers to protect the security and confidentiality of health information, encouraging the use of electronic transfer of protected health information (PHI). PHI consists of medical information as well as personal information about a patient. HIPAA affects phlebotomists by giving them access to only information necessary for the patient's treatment and care. Phlebotomists must be very careful in sharing this information. PHI cannot be shared or looked at by employees unless there is a specific need. Computer systems have been redesigned to allow only limited access to certain files. Test results can be released only to the person ordering the test, to an authorized representative, or as required by law.

- **Various state laws:** These differ throughout the country, but usually prohibit payment of referral fees and also referral of laboratory tests to laboratories in which physicians have financial interest. State laws are not limited to only Medicare and Medicaid, but apply to insurance companies and all other payers, with varying penalties.

The Laboratory Compliance Plan

According to the Office of the Inspector General (OIG), part of the Department of Health and Human Services (HHS), seven elements should be included in a laboratory compliance plan:

1. Written standards of conduct with written policies and procedures promoting the laboratory's commitment to compliance—these should address areas of potential fraud
2. Designation of a Chief Compliance Officer and Corporate Compliance Committee
3. Compliance process maintenance to receive anonymous complaints without any fear of retaliation
4. Regular effective training programs for all affected employees
5. Auditing and other evaluations to monitor compliance and reduce identified problems
6. Investigating and remediating systematic problems, and policies developed to address them
7. A system that responds to improper or illegal activities and disciplinary action against violators

The policies and procedures of the laboratory should include the following:

- *Standards of employee conduct:* These detail the policies concerning fraud, abuse, and waste as well as adherence to government regulations.
- *Standing order reliance:* Discouragement (but not denial) of **standing orders** requires semiannual or annual reviewing and updating of these orders.
- *Medical necessity:* Order only tests appropriate for patient treatment.
- *Billing:* Correct identification of claimed services and tests to federal health programs; under the Health Care Financing Administration (HCFA), the Current Procedural Terminology (CPT) or International Classification of Diseases (ICD-9-CM) codes are used to identify these.
- *Health and Human Services fraud alert compliance:* Applicable alerts issued by the OIG about legal and enforcement issues should be reviewed by the Chief Compliance Officer to ensure laboratory compliance.
- *Physician Prices:* No inducements to gain a physician's business regarding prices charged are allowed.
- *Record Retention:* Records must be maintained for any state or federal government scrutiny if required.
- *Marketing:* All laboratory marketing should be honest, fully informative, nondeceptive, and straightforward.
- *Compliance and performance plans:* All employees must be evaluated with adherence to compliance being part of their duties; this requires periodic training in new compliance policies and procedures.

Effects of Compliance

Laboratory compliance plans and the policies and procedures are best kept in three-ring binders for easy updating. The following effects of compliance relate to phlebotomists and potential legal outcomes:

- *Client equipment and supplies:* Laboratory-supplied equipment and supplies are to be used solely for collecting and preparing samples for testing; computers and fax machines are to be used only for laboratory work; smaller items such as rubber gloves should be monitored for theft or unauthorized use.
- *Courier services:* Laboratories use paid **courier** services to pick up specimens from physicians' offices; these couriers should not transport anything from the physician to the laboratory that is not a laboratory specimen without charging the physician the fair market value for the service.
- *Design of requisitions:* Laboratory requisition forms should have standardized lists of the most commonly ordered tests; these encourage physicians to order only medically necessary tests for each patient. Forms should include only Medicare-approved profiles—if a physician requests a customized profile, Medicare may deny payment for some of the tests. Requisitions should include the patient's diagnosis to determine medical necessity; fraud may result in civil penalties.
- *Hazardous or infectious wastes:* The laboratory can only dispose of its own hazardous wastes and sharps containers, and none generated by the physician's office; sharps containers can contain only needles used for collections by the laboratory. Hazardous wastes cannot include bloody dressings (which are from the physician's office), but they can include old blood tubes (which are generated by the lab).
- *Phlebotomy:* Although a phlebotomist from a laboratory may provide specimen collection in a physician's office, he or she cannot be placed there as a cost savings for the physician. The following bullet points illustrate what the phlebotomist *can* and *cannot* do in this situation:
  - *Allowed duties:* obtaining specimens from patients when they are sent to the laboratory providing the

phlebotomist; preparing these specimens to be shipped to the lab; entering billing or other information on lab patients into a lab computer system; or performing other functions related to the lab specimen collection or testing

- *Nonallowed duties:* taking vital signs, performing other nursing functions not related to specimen collection, filing reports, answering phones, performing other functions normally handled by the physician's staff, entering billing information or performing tests for the physician's office, reviewing patient charts to see diagnosis information, or performing duties not related to the lab or specimen collection

- *Questionable requests:* If a physician's handwriting is hard to read, or a requested test is not marked on a requisition form, the patient cannot be asked what test was ordered or help to decipher the physician's handwriting—the phlebotomist must contact the physician directly. If no diagnosis is given, the phlebotomist cannot ask the patient what is wrong with him or her in order to determine the diagnosis; a diagnosis cannot be determined from an ordered test—it must come from the physician. If an ordered test is not included in the lab's list of tests, the phlebotomist cannot assume that another similar test will suffice—the physician must be contacted. All communications must be documented.

- *Release of information:* The phlebotomist can release test results to only the person who ordered the tests, authorized persons, or the individual responsible for utilizing patient results—the patient cannot receive his or her own results unless permitted by the physician. Results from a specialist cannot be sent to a patient's family physician unless the specialist allows this; results can be released to another physician only if emergency treatment by this additional physician is required. Most labs have release forms that patients can sign to have results released to them, and usually positive picture identification is required. Phlebotomists must understand what they can and cannot do legally.

Legal Actions and Phlebotomy

Phlebotomy is an **invasive** procedure that can result in complications due to patient reactions or improper procedures being followed. The following occurrences all have the potential to result in legal actions:

- *Accidental arterial puncture:* This may cause hemorrhage, hematoma, numbness, and infection. The veins of choice are the median cubital vein or the cephalic vein.

- **Fainting:** A sudden drop in blood pressure may cause a patient to faint.

- *Hematoma:* Bruising happens to many patients after blood collection, and it is best to carefully check the puncture site after the draw.

- *Mislabeling or nonlabeling of specimens:* Mislabeled tubes can cause the wrong test results to go to the patient, potentially causing over- or undermedication. This can cause many different outcomes, even death.

- *Nerve damage:* Accidental arterial puncture or going too deep for a venipuncture can cause nerve damage.

Lawsuit Prevention

To prevent lawsuits, the following established procedures should be followed:

- Avoid draws from the **basilic vein**—this reduces the chance of accidental arterial puncture and nerve damage.

- Insert needle at a 15° angle.

- Avoid deep probing venipunctures to prevent most nerve damage.

- Observe the patient after the draw for bleeding and light-headedness.

- Label all tubes beside the patient to avoid mislabeled and unlabeled specimens.

If legal action is brought, the phlebotomist's well-documented training helps to prove that the patient received the standard of care. The Center for Phlebotomy Education (CPE) follows the guidelines of the Clinical and Laboratory Standards Institute (CLSI) and offers extremely current information regarding phlebotomy procedures. It is important for certification applicants and practicing phlebotomists to adhere to these current standards and guidelines to ensure accurate patient assessment, diagnosing, and appropriate procedures.

Summary

Compliance is the term used to describe the formal monitoring of how organizations follow laws and regulations. It helps to prevent abuse, fraud, and waste. Compliance keeps patients, insurers, and healthcare programs from being overcharged. Fraud and abuse laws usually result in monetary penalties. Laws that address the issue of compliance include the Anti-Kickback law, the False Claims Act, and HIPAA. Laboratories should select a chief compliance officer as well as a corporate compliance committee to make sure that compliance is maintained. Because phlebotomy is an invasive procedure that can cause patient complications, compliance helps to reduce legal actions that could otherwise result. Lawsuits can be prevented by closely complying with all state and federal regulations.

CRITICAL THINKING

Amanda began working as a phlebotomist in a large hospital 2 weeks ago. She drew blood from a patient, who fainted during the procedure. Amanda left the patient to tell a nurse what happened, but the nurse was busy and Amanda had to wait for several minutes. The patient was alone during this entire time.

1. What did Amanda do wrong?
2. If the patient was harmed, what possible legal outcomes might result?

WEBSITES

http://labmed.ascpjournals.org/content/36/7/430.full.pdf

http://library.med.utah.edu/WebPath/TUTORIAL/PHLEB/PHLEB.html

http://oig.hhs.gov/fraud/docs/complianceguidance/cpcl.html

http://www.brighthub.com/science/medical/articles/24735.aspx

https://www.cms.gov/clia/

http://www.labcompliance.com/

http://www.labtestsonline.org/understanding/analytes/ama/test.html

http://www.medialabinc.net/hipaa-privacy.aspx

http://www.medialabinc.net/phlebotomy.aspx

http://www.medscape.com/viewarticle/509098

REVIEW QUESTIONS

Multiple Choice

1. For compliance, what is the amount of the "set" penalty commonly assessed per laboratory test or service that was billed fraudulently?
   A. $500
   B. $2,000
   C. $5,000
   D. $15,000

2. Which of the following laws keeps physicians from referring specimens to laboratories in which immediate family members have a financial interest?
   A. False Claims Act
   B. Stark law
   C. Civil Monetary Penalties laws
   D. Clinical Laboratory Improvement Act

3. Which of the following laws covers quality control and quality assurance?
   A. False Claims Act
   B. Stark law
   C. Civil Monetary Penalties laws
   D. Clinical Laboratory Improvement Act

4. Which of the following laws established national standards for providers to standardize electronic data?
   A. CLIA
   B. FCA
   C. HIPAA
   D. CMPL

5. The Office of the Inspector General is a part of the Department of
   A. Health and Human Services
   B. Justice
   C. Labor
   D. Police

6. Most accidental arterial punctures occur when attempting to draw from the
   A. cephalic vein
   B. median cubital vein
   C. basilic vein
   D. dorsal metacarpal veins

7. Which of the following is NOT a patient complication associated with arterial puncture?
   A. infection
   B. venostasis
   C. numbness
   D. hematoma

8. The formal monitoring of how an organization follows laws and regulations is known as
   A. enforcement
   B. competency
   C. policies and procedures
   D. compliance

9. A compliance committee consists of people from different areas of
   A. the hospital
   B. the laboratory
   C. law enforcement
   D. the community

10. Which of the following may be used to identify billing in federal health programs?
    A. CPT
    B. ICD-9-CM
    C. HCFA
    D. All of the above

11. The American Medical Association has established all of the following panels that should be collected for determining general information about a patient's health status, EXCEPT
    A. complete blood cell count
    B. hepatic function panel
    C. electroencephalogram
    D. electrolyte panel

12. Penalties for the Anti-Kickback law violation include imprisonment up to 5 years and/or fines up to
    A. $5,000
    B. $10,000
    C. $15,000
    D. $25,000

13. Which of the following acts prohibits knowingly billing services not medically necessary for treatment or diagnosis of a Medicare patient?
    A. Clinical Laboratory Improvement Act
    B. False Claims Act
    C. Stark law
    D. Civil Monetary Penalties laws

14. The phlebotomist can release test results to the
    A. patient
    B. lawyer of the patient
    C. parents of the patient
    D. person who ordered the test

15. To prevent lawsuits, all of the following established procedures should be undertaken, EXCEPT
    A. avoiding draws from the cephalic vein
    B. inserting the needle at a 15° angle
    C. avoiding deep probing venipuncture to prevent most nerve damage
    D. observing the patient after the draw for bleeding

CHAPTER 19

Computer Technology

OUTLINE

Introduction
Computers in the Clinical Laboratory
 Computer Hardware
 Computer Software
 Data Storage
Pneumatic Tube Systems
Bar Codes
Radio-Frequency Identification
Computer Communications
Computer Security
Summary
Critical Thinking
Websites
Review Questions

OBJECTIVES

After studying this chapter, readers should be able to:

1. List several ways that the computer can be effective in a clinical laboratory.
2. List common uses of computers in the clinical laboratory.
3. Explain the basic components of a computer.
4. Compare computer hardware with computer software.
5. Discuss bar codes and their use in the medical laboratory.
6. Explain the concept of computer networking.
7. Discuss the importance of computer security.
8. Define *radio-frequency identification*.

KEY TERMS

Bar codes: Optical machine-readable representations of data; they are "read" by scanners known as *bar code readers*.

Central processing unit: CPU; the portion of a computer that carries out instructions and is the main functioning component.

Data: Information that is processed via a computer.

Hardware: The actual programmable part of a computer system and the components that execute activities.

Health Insurance Portability and Accountability Act (HIPAA): The Kassebaum-Kennedy Act, passed in 1996; it was designed to improve the portability and continuity of health insurance coverage; to combat waste, fraud, and abuse in health insurance and healthcare delivery; to promote the use of medical saving accounts; to improve access to long-term care services and coverage; and to simplify the administration of health insurance as well as to serve other purposes.

Input: Any data entered into a computer or data processing system.

Networked: Interconnected so that various computers and other data processing devices can communicate over varying ranges of distance.

Output: Transmitted information from a computer or data processing system.

Passwords: Secret words or strings of characters used by individuals to gain access to computers or data processing systems.

Personal digital assistants: Palmtop computers that function as information managers; they commonly integrate with computers, data processing systems, and the Internet to share information.

Random-access memory: RAM; a form of computer data storage wherein information can be accessed at random.

Read-only memory: ROM; a form of computer data storage wherein information is not able to be modified but may be accessed.

Software: Computer programs and related data.

Terminal: An electronic hardware device used for entering and displaying computer data.

Universal serial bus: A specification to establish communication between computers and other devices.

Introduction

In today's world, computer skills are essential for most careers, including those of phlebotomists. Today's computers are faster and more accurate than ever before. It is essential to understand the fundamentals of computers in order to perform all the duties required in the field of phlebotomy. The computer is also effective in the medical laboratory. It performs repetitive tasks, reduces errors, increases production, recalls information, saves time, decreases paperwork, and allows for more productive use of workers' time.

Computer networks link groups of computers. They are often local, or they can cover a city or large geographic area. Some are limited to a few buildings. Networks often share resources such as printers. Computer security is critical in today's world, especially because confidential patient information is stored on computers in medical laboratories.

Computers in the Clinical Laboratory

In the clinical laboratory, computers help to collect data, tabulate, decrease errors in transcription, eliminate duplication of work, and offer a wide variety of other improvements to efficiency. They can be used for medical records management, billing, bookkeeping, inventory, scheduling, and quality control. Point-of-care systems offer computerization integrated from the bedside to many different types of workplaces, including the laboratory. Certain test results can be completely computerized, reducing the chance for human error. Automated clinical analyzing equipment integrates samples and specimens in a system that offers extremely accurate and detailed results. Computers are used in preexamination, examination, and postexamination processes (see **Figure 19–1**).

Because manual systems require human intervention at every phase of testing, semiautomated and fully automated systems are becoming the preferred methods. Semiautomated systems require little to no human intervention, and they can automatically handle sample processing, mixing of reagents with the sample, checking quality, and loading specimen tubes. Fully automated systems offer automatic performance of every stage of testing, with human intervention occurring only when an instrument error occurs or results are alerted to the operator because they fall outside the acceptable limits.

Computers in the laboratory may be handheld, laptop, desktop, **personal digital assistants** (PDAs), tablet, or mainframe, and they may be **networked** easily with many other locations. Common uses of computers in the clinical laboratory include the following:

- Entering lists of test requisitions
- Generating labels, schedules, and specimen collection lists
- Printing lists
- Updating records of laboratory specimens that have been accessed
- Reporting and storing test results
- Sending test results to nursing stations and other locations
- Sending charges for procedures to the accounting office
- Managing inventory
- Record keeping

There are a variety of laboratory equipment that can be integrated with computers to streamline their functions. Common examples of computerized equipment found in a blood bank are as follows:

- Blood bank refrigerators—microcontrolled units that maintain extremely accurate, constant temperatures (see **Figure 19–2**). These refrigerators are usually kept at 1 to 6°C. All various blood groups are kept in blood bank refrigerators (see **Figure 19–3**).
- Blood bank scales—designed for precise weighing of blood and blood components; they can measure the volume of blood components while allowing consideration of specific gravity (see **Figure 19–4**).
- Plasma freezers—also used for related blood components, vaccines, microorganism studies, and other testing; fully microcontrolled with alarms that alert the

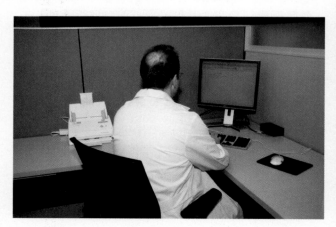

Figure 19–1 A phlebotomist working with a computer.

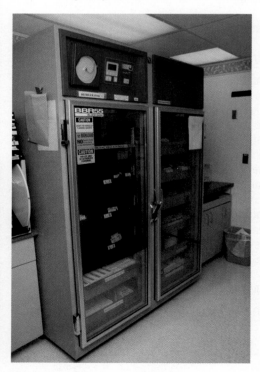

Figure 19–2 Blood bank refrigerators.

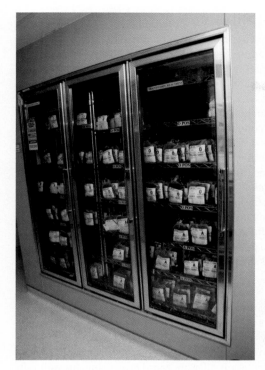

Figure 19–3 All various blood groups are kept in blood refrigerators.

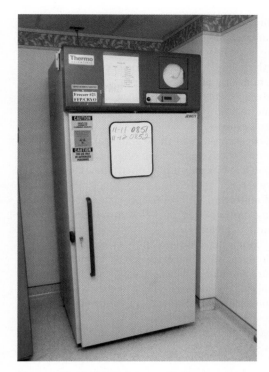

Figure 19–5 Plasma freezer with alarm system.

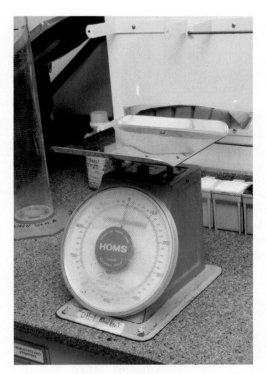

Figure 19–4 Blood bank scale.

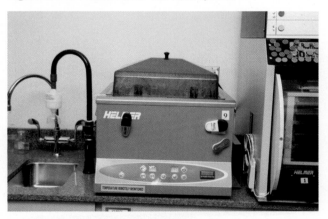

Figure 19–6 Constant temperature bath.

movable to allow agitation. The process usually takes between 10 and 18 min.

- Constant-temperature baths—for research work at preset temperatures; these microcontrolled units have circulating pumps to ensure uniform temperature, which is commonly 36.5°C (see **Figure 19–6**).
- Plasma extractors—allow microcontrolled extraction to separate blood components from the blood bag; these are also sometimes called *plasma expressors*.
- Platelet incubators—these microcontrolled units keep platelets at a constant temperature and motion.
- Bacteriological incubators—for life-cycle testing, shelf-life studies, and general incubation; temperatures can be changed widely via microcontrollers.
- Cooling incubators—to conduct life-cycle testing, shelf-life studies, general incubation, and refrigerated storage; temperatures can be changed widely via microcontrollers.

technician to any temperature variances—they offer very quick freezing capability and are commonly kept at −27.5°C (see **Figure 19–5**).

- Plasma thawing baths—offer microcontrolled quick thawing of plasma with safety and accuracy to maintain viability; frozen bags of plasma are placed inside these devices, which have automated "baskets" that are

- Stability test chambers—to conduct stability and shelf-life studies, biological studies, and many other types of testing (see **Figure 19–7**).
- Growth chambers—allow complete control of temperature, humidity, and light in order to test microorganisms, tissues, etc.; commonly used for tissue cultures, enzyme reaction studies, fermentation analysis, and many other tests.
- Blood bag tube sealers—these units seal blood bag pilot tubes via radio frequencies in only a few seconds; the bag seals can be easily pulled open when required (see **Figure 19–8**).
- Blood collection monitors—provide smooth, gentle rocking motions to thoroughly mix collected blood with anticoagulant.
- Microcontrolled donor couches—microcontrolled positioning and other extra features, such as blood pressure and blood collection monitors.
- Orbital shakers—allow for microcontrolled shaking of specimens under controlled temperatures; these shakers are available in a variety of housing configurations for specific testing needs—they are also referred to as *shaker incubators*.

Computer Hardware

Computer **hardware** consists of the actual programmable part of a computer system and the components that execute activities (see **Figure 19–9**). The **central processing unit** (CPU) is the main controller of a computer, and it is a type of microprocessor. Other forms of hardware are called *peripherals*. They include the monitor (display), keyboard, modem, printer, bar code reader, scanner, external hard drive, other handheld devices, cables, fax machine, **universal serial bus** (USB), and other equipment. A computer together with its display screen (monitor), keyboard, and mouse is commonly called a **terminal**. To **input** data is to enter them into a computer via some piece of computer hardware. Examples of input devices include keyboards and scanners. Computer **output** is defined as the information that is processed or the data that are generated. Examples of output devices include printers and speakers.

Computer Software

Computer **software** consists of the instructions for the hardware that are written in a computer programming language. Software systems include hospital information systems and laboratory information systems. Software applications include presentation software, word processing, firewall software, statistical software, antivirus protection, and Internet provider software.

Types of computer software that are used in medical laboratories may include word processing (for writing correspondence, reports, etc.), database management (for patient records and other information), scheduling, and spreadsheets (which can organize data and perform calculations, commonly used for accounting and billing).

Data Storage

Storage devices include memory and different types of external computer drives (see **Figure 19–10**). Computer **data** are stored in a variety of ways. Large amounts of information and data can be retained. Computer memory "bytes" are individual units of data that have been assigned a unique location. Forms of data storage include hard disks, magnetic tapes, compact discs, CD-ROMs (with "read-only" memory), USBs (commonly called flash, jump, or thumb drives), DVDs (digital video discs), and DVD-ROMs. Inside a computer,

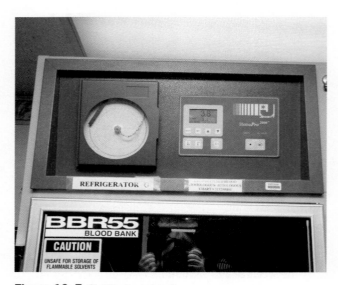

Figure 19–7 Stability test chambers.

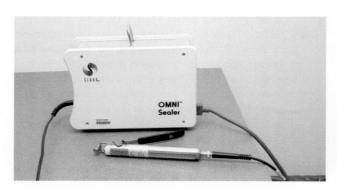

Figure 19–8 Blood bag tube sealers.

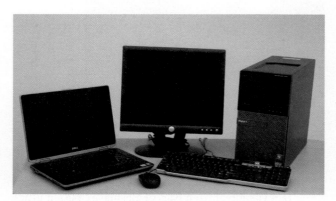

Figure 19–9 Types of hardware devices.

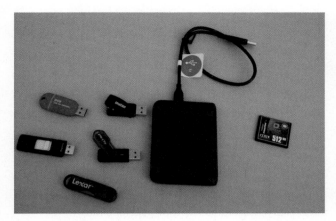

Figure 19–10 Storage devices.

information is stored in memory until the central processing unit can complete its processing functions.

Memory is of two types: **random-access memory** (RAM) and **read-only memory** (ROM). Random-access memory stores data temporarily, and these data can be lost if they are not saved to a permanent form of storage before a computer program is closed. Read-only memory is permanent memory that cannot be altered. When data are put into read-only memory by a manufacturer, they can instruct a computer to carry out user-requested operations. ROM has characteristics of both hardware and software.

Pneumatic Tube Systems

Pneumatic tube systems, also known as *air-tube systems*, allow many types of materials to be transported quickly and securely throughout a healthcare facility. These systems are used in different areas of health care and are able to transport samples to laboratories for quick analysis, especially during critical procedures such as surgeries or emergencies. Blood tests may be completed quickly, and the results sent back through the tubes to the requesting physician. Pneumatic tubes are commonly also used in pharmacies, hospitals, and non-healthcare facilities, such as banks. These systems are computerized to easily control routing of each container to the proper location within the facility. The containers (capsules) that carry items are made out of lightweight yet very solid *polycarbonate*, and they can be used for years without significant wear or breakage. **Figure 19–11** show a laboratory technician working with a pneumatic tube capsule from another location in the hospital.

Bar Codes

Bar codes reduce transcription errors and speed up the processing of samples. Scanning devices are used to "read" them. Bar codes consist of dark and light bands related to numbers and letters (see **Figure 19–12**). When the bands are sequenced, they correspond to names, tests, and codes. Bar codes are very accurate and quick to use, keeping human error out of the processing of integrating information. In phlebotomy, bar codes are used to represent the following:

- Date of birth
- Names
- Identification numbers

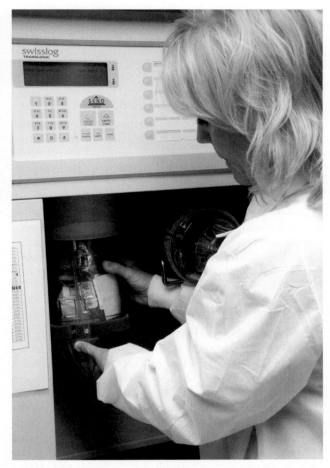

Figure 19–11 A pneumatic tube container (capsule) being put into a pneumatic tube system.

- Specimen access or log numbers
- Test codes
- Expiration dates for inventory
- Product codes for pieces of equipment
- Billing codes
- Sample identification numbers

Radio-Frequency Identification

Radio-frequency identification (RFID) is also used as an identification system for records, equipment, supplies, specimens, and patients. An RFID tag is a silicon chip that transmits data to a wireless receiver. It does not require the reading of the

Figure 19–12 Example of a bar code.

chip with any type of scanner. Many different items can be tracked at the same time using these tags. Different frequencies are used based on the distance that the tags will be from the receiver. Those requiring longer distances are usually more costly.

Computer Communications

Computer communications include the use of electronic mail (email) and the Internet. Communication software is utilized for sending messages and retrieving many different forms of data via these sources. Email allows messages to be sent quickly through a computer network, which can link unlimited amounts of computers in a company or facility as well as anywhere in the world. Information sent via this method moves very quickly, no matter how long the distance between computers. The Internet is a global computer network that allows large sources of medical information to be accessed. Information is updated frequently, so it is possible to get very recent information every time you search the Internet.

Computer Security

The **Health Insurance Portability and Accountability Act (HIPAA)** protects patient records and requires that measures be installed to make sure that this occurs. Most healthcare workers are now issued *security passwords* that give them access to computer systems. Their use of these systems can then be tracked and monitored. Various levels of security exist so that only certain individuals have access to the highest levels of information. **Passwords** should never be shared between coworkers or displayed where others can see them. HIPAA also protects electronic and facsimile (fax) transmissions of laboratory information. Each healthcare facility must develop clear policies and procedures concerning the handling of all forms of patient information.

Summary

Computers in the clinical laboratory help to organize many different types of data, including medical records, billing, inventory, scheduling, and quality control. Semiautomated and fully automated systems are becoming more popular because of their ease of integration with computer systems. Phlebotomists are required to establish computer skills to utilize these important components of laboratory work. Computers may now interface with equipment including refrigerators, freezers, scales, temperature baths, incubators, test chambers, blood collection monitors, and orbital shakers.

One important area of computer use is the storage and protection of patient health information to ensure confidentiality. Computer hardware requires computer software to operate and allow users to input information and retrieve it. The use of bar codes helps to reduce errors and increase the speed of specimen processing. Another form of the identification of information is radio-frequency identification, utilizing silicon chips that transmit data to wireless receivers.

CRITICAL THINKING

A laboratory technician is required to enter information into a computer system. The information concerns a patient's recent blood collection specimens, which have revealed a life-threatening blood disorder. The technician cannot access the patient's information for some reason and asks her supervisor for help.

1. What may be required in order for the patient's computer information to be accessed?
2. Why are barriers such as this utilized by computer systems, and what act dictated such barriers?

WEBSITES

http://electronics.howstuffworks.com/gadgets/travel/pda.htm

http://www.barcode-labels.com/pagemed.htm

http://www.bls.gov/oco/ocos096.htm

http://www.ehow.com/about_5402387_different-storage-devices-computers.html

http://www.hhs.gov/ocr/privacy/

http://www.intel.com/technology/usb/

http://www.istl.org/02-fall/internet.html

http://www.rfid.org/

http://www.unclefed.com/AuthorsRow/Daily/fwdrecord-system.html

http://www.usewisdom.com/computer/passwords.html

REVIEW QUESTIONS

Multiple Choice

1. The central processing unit (CPU) is a type of
   A. modem
   B. software
   C. microprocessor
   D. motherboard
2. Spreadsheets are most commonly used for which of the following tasks?
   A. word processing
   B. accounting and billing
   C. electronic mailing
   D. appointment scheduling
3. What legislation protects the confidentiality of patient information that is stored or transmitted electronically?
   A. OSHA
   B. HCFA
   C. FDA
   D. HIPAA
4. The actual programmable part of a computer system that executes activities is known as
   A. hardware
   B. central processing unit
   C. random-access memory
   D. read-only memory
5. In the clinical laboratory, computers help to
   A. decrease errors in transcription
   B. eliminate duplication of work
   C. tabulate
   D. do all of the above

6. A computer with its screen, keyboard, and mouse is frequently called
   A. a universal serial bus
   B. a terminal
   C. an output
   D. an input

7. Software applications include
   A. firewall software
   B. word processing
   C. antivirus protection
   D. all of the above

8. In phlebotomy, which of the following devices is used to represent expiration dates for inventory and billing codes?
   A. bar codes
   B. radio-frequency identification
   C. universal serial bus
   D. computer output

9. A specification to establish communication between computers and other devices is called
   A. computer output
   B. radio frequency
   C. bar codes
   D. universal serial bus

10. Computer programs and related data are referred to as
    A. hardware
    B. software
    C. users
    D. networks

11. Which of the following is an advantage of bar codes?
    A. They are designed for precise weighing of blood.
    B. They increase the size of the computer screen.
    C. They reduce transcription errors.
    D. They are the main controllers of a computer.

12. Which of the following allows messages to be sent quickly through a computer network?
    A. email
    B. snail mail
    C. downloading
    D. uploading

13. In the clinical laboratory, computers help to do which of the following?
    A. completely automate the blood collection process
    B. reduce electrical costs
    C. provide easier access to protected health information
    D. tabulate and eliminate duplication of work

14. Computer networks do which of the following?
    A. connect bar codes with bar codes
    B. link groups of computers
    C. completely automate the use of clean rooms
    D. use artificial intelligence to make diagnoses

15. Cooling incubators are designed to conduct
    A. life-cycle testing
    B. shelf-life studies
    C. general incubation
    D. all of the above

Units of Measurement and Conversion Tables

Units of Measurement

Type of Conversion	Units
Blood volume	Total blood volume = weight (kg) × average blood volume per kg (defined by age)
Clearance	Liter/second (L/s)
Density	Kilogram/liter (kg/L)
Dilutions	Final concentration = Original concentration × dilution 1 × dilution 2, and so on
Hematology (math)	Mean corpuscular volume (MCV) = average volume of red blood cells (RBCs); expressed in cubic microns μm^3 or femtoliters (fL) MCV = (Hct × 10) ÷ RBC count (in million) Hct = hematocrit value
	Mean corpuscular hemoglobin (MCH) = average weight of hemoglobin in RBC; expressed in picograms (pg) MCH = (hgb in grams × 10) ÷ RBC count (in millions) Hgb = hemoglobin value
	Mean corpuscular hemoglobin concentration = hemoglobin concentration of average RBC MCHC = (hgb in grams ÷ Hct) × 100%
	RBC distribution width (RDW) = numerical expression of variation of RBC size, dispersion of RBC volumes about the mean RDW = SD (standard deviation) of RBC size ÷ MCV
Mass	Kilogram/liter (kg/L)

Metric Conversions:
  Length
  Weight or mass
 	
  Volume
	1 inch (in) = 2.54 centimeters (cm); 39.37 inches = 1 meter (m)
	1 ounce (oz) = 28.35 g; 1 pound (lb) = 453.6 g;
	1 kilogram (kg) = 2.205 lb
	1 fluid ounce (fl oz) = 29.57 milliliters (mL)
	1 cubic centimeter (cc) = 1 mL
	1 ounce = 30 mL or 30 cc
	1 liter (L) = 1.057 quarts (qt)
	1 gallon (gal) = 3.78 liters

Pressure	Pascal (Pa) = $(kg/m)s^2$
Specific gravity (Sp g)	Sp g = (weight of solid or liquid) ÷ (weight of equal volume of H_2O at 4°C)

Temperature:
  Celsius or Centigrade
  Kelvin
  Fahrenheit
	°C = K − 273.15; °C = °F − 32 × 0.555
	°K = °C + 273.15 or 5/9(°F) + 255.35
	°F = (°C × 1.8) + 32

Volume	deciliter (dL) = 1/10 of a liter 10 dL = 1L centiliter (cL) = 1/100 of a liter 100 cL = 10dL = 1L milliliter (mL) = 1/1000 of a liter 1000 mL = 100 cL = 10 dL = 1L

Common Laboratory Tests

The following table lists common laboratory tests that phlebotomists should be familiar with. It is important to remember that different facilities use different tubes for specific tests, so there is some variance with these general examples.

For this table, the following ingredients are contained in these tube top colors:

Plasma, sodium citrate = LIGHT BLUE

Plasma, heparin = GREEN

EDTA = PINK or LAVENDER

Serum and/or clot activator/gel = RED or GOLD

Sodium citrate = BLACK

Plasma, sodium fluoride = GRAY

ACD = YELLOW

Test Name & Abbreviation	Specimen Type & Tube Color	Reference Interval in Conventional Units	Conversion Factor to Multiply By	Reference Interval in Systeme International Units
ABO group & RH typing	Whole blood (pink)	Reported as A, B, O, or AB as well as Rh positive/negative		
Acid phosphatase	Serum (speckled/red) or plasma (green)	0.0–0.6 units/L	1	0.0–0.6 units/L
Activated partial thromboplastin time (APTT or PTT; also, see Partial thromboplastin time)	Plasma (light blue)	Variable due to testing methods. APTT normally ranges from 30 to 40 s. If the patient is under anticoagulant treatment, the therapeutic level is 2 to 2.5 times the normal value. PTT normally ranges from 60 to 70 s, and it is normal for PTT to be longer in comparison with APTT.		
Adrenocorticotropic hormone (ACTH)	Plasma (lavender) Critical frozen	Less than 120 pg/mL	0.22	Less than 26 pmol/L
Albumin	Serum (speckled) or plasma	3.8–5 g/dL	10	38–50 g/L
Alcohol (ethanol)	Serum (red) or plasma (gray or lavender)	Less than 100 mg/dL	0.2171	Less than 21.7 mmol/L
Aldosterone	Serum (speckled) or plasma (green) Collect at 8 a.m. Patient should be on normal diet 2 weeks prior to test. Patient should be recumbent for at least 30 min prior to blood collection.	7–30 ng/dL	0.0277	0.19–0.83 nmol/L
Antibody identification	Whole blood (pink)	Reporting varies depending on antibodies tested		
Antibody to hepatitis A virus (anti-HAV), B core antigen (Anti-HBc), BE antigen, B surface antigen (Anti-HBs)	Serum (red, speckled, gold) or plasma (lavender)	Negative or positive	n/a	Negative or positive

Test Name & Abbreviation	Specimen Type & Tube Color	Reference Interval in Conventional Units	Conversion Factor to Multiply By	Reference Interval in Systeme International Units
Bilirubin, conjugated	Serum (speckled) Protect blood from light	Less than 0.3 mg/dL	17.1	Less than 5 μmol/L
Bilirubin, total	Serum (speckled) Protect blood from light	0.1–1.2 mg/dL	17.1	2–21 μmol/L
Blood cell count, CBC survey (WBC, RBC, Hgb, Hct, MCV, MCH, MCHC)	Plasma (lavender)	SEE BELOW FOR INDIVIDUAL TESTS.		
Blood cell count, differential	Blood smear	Neutrophils 40 to 60%; lymphocytes 20 to 40%; monocytes 2 to 8%; eosinophils 1 to 4%; basophils 0.5 to 1%; bands 0 to 3%	n/a	SAME
Blood cell count, eosinophil	Plasma (lavender)	Less than 350 cells/ microliter	1	Less than 350 cells/ microliter
Blood cell count, erythrocyte (RBC)	Plasma (lavender)	M: 4.6 to 6.2 million/mm^3 F: 4.2 to 5.4 million/mm^3	1	M: 4.6–6.2 $\times$ 10^{12}/L F: 4.2–5.4 10^{12}/L
Blood cell count, leukocyte (WBC)	Plasma (lavender)	4,500 to 11,000/mm^3	1	4.5 to 11 $\times$ 10^9/L
Blood cell count, platelets	Plasma (lavender)	150,000 to 400,000/ mm^3	1	150–400 $\times$ 10^9/L
Blood cell count, reticulocyte	Plasma (lavender)	25,000 to 75,000/mm^3	1	25–75 $\times$ 10^9/L
Blood gases, arterial (ABG)	Arterial blood (heparinized syringe)	SEE INDIVIDUAL TESTS BELOW.		
Base excess (BE) pCO$_2$ pO$_2$ pH Bicarbonate	SAME SAME SAME SAME SAME	–3.3 to +2.3 mmol/L 35–45mmHg 80–100 mmHg 7.35–7.45 21–28 mmol/L	1 1 1 1 1	–3.3 to +2.3 mmol/L 35–45 mmHg 80–100 mmHg 7.35–7.45 21–28 mmol/L
Blood urea nitrogen (BUN)	Serum (speckled or red)	8–23 mg/dL	0.357	2.9–8.2 mmol/L
Calcium, ionized	Whole blood (green), serum (red) DELIVER IMMEDIATELY	4.6–5.8 mg/dL	0.25	1.15–1.27 mmol/L
Calcium, total	Serum (speckled or red)	9.2–11 mg/dL	0.25	2.3–2.7 mmol/L
Carbon dioxide (CO$_2$ venous)	Serum (speckled or red)	24–30 mmol/L	1	24–30 mmol/L
Cardiac troponins (eTnI, eTnt)	Serum (speckled)	Normally too low to be measured	n/a	Normally too low to be measured
Chemistry screen (T. protein, Alb, Ca, Glu, BUN, Creat, T. bil, Alk p'tase, AST ALT, potassium, creatinine, chloride, sodium, CO$_2$)	Serum (speckled or red) or plasma (green)	SEE INDIVIDUAL TESTS BELOW.		
Chloride	Serum (speckled or red)	95–103 mEq/L	1	95–103 mmol/L
Cholesterol (total)	Serum (speckled) (FASTING)	140–200 mg/dL	0.025	3.6–5.2 mmol/L
Chromosome analysis	Sterile plasma (green)	Chromosomal abnormalities are reported.		
Complete blood count (CBC)	Plasma (lavender)	See "blood cell count" above.		
Cortisol (am)	Serum (red) or plasma (green)	5–23 μg/dL	27.6	138–635 nmol/L
Creatinine	Serum (speckled or red) or plasma (green)	0.6–1.2 mg/dL	88.4	53–106 μmol/L
D-dimer (D-D$_{IM}$)	Plasma (blue)	Highly variable due to testing methods. Negative is normal.		
Drug screen	Serum (red)	Depends on drugs tested		

Test Name & Abbreviation	Specimen Type & Tube Color	Reference Interval in Conventional Units	Conversion Factor to Multiply By	Reference Interval in Systeme International Units
Electrolytes (Na, K, Cl, HCO$_3$)	Plasma (green) or serum (red)	Na (serum or plasma): 135–145 mEq/L K (serum): 3.5–5 mEq/L K (plasma): 3.5–4.5 mEq/L Cl (serum or plasma): 96–106 mEq/L HCO$_3$ (serum): 23–29 mEq/L HCO$_3$ (plasma): 21–27 mEq/L	1	Na (serum or plasma): 135–145 mmol/L K (serum): 3.5–5 mmol/L K (plasma): 3.5–4.5 mmol/L Cl (serum or plasma): 96–106 mmol/L HCO$_3$ (serum): 23–29 mmol/L HCO$_3$ (plasma): 23–29 mmol/L
ESR (sedimentation rate, sed rate)	Plasma (lavender)	M: 0–15 mm/h; F: 0–20 mm/h	1	M: 0–15 mm/h; F: 0–20 mm/h
Ethanol (alcohol)	Whole blood (gray) or serum (red)	Less than 100 mg/dL	0.2171	Less than 21.7 mmol/L
Factor assays	Plasma (blue) test not valid if patient is taking heparin	Depends on test methods		
Fasting blood glucose (FBG)	Plasma (gray) or whole blood (green)	70–110 mg/dL	0.0556	3–6.1 mmol/L
Ferritin	Serum (speckled or red) or plasma (green)	M: 15–200 ng/mL F: 12–150 ng/mL	1 1	M: 15–200 μg/L F: 12–150 μg/L
Fibrinogen	Plasma (blue)	200–400 mg/dL	0.01	2–4 g/L
Folate, serum	Serum (speckled or red)	More than 2.3 ng/dL	2.265	More than 5 nmol/L
Glucose (fasting)	Plasma (green) or serum (red)	70–110 mg/dL	0.0556	3–6.1 mmol/L
Haptoglobin	Blood (speckled)	60–270 mg/dL	0.01	0.6–2.7 g/L
Hematocrit (HCT)	Plasma (lavender)	M: 41.5–50.4% F: 35.9–44.6%	0.01 0.01	M: 0.415–0.504 volfraction F: 0.359–0.446 volfraction
Hematology profile (Hct, Hgb, WBC, RBC, MCV, MCH, MCHC)	Plasma (lavender)	SEE INDIVIDUAL TESTS THROUGHOUT THIS TABLE.		
Hemoglobin	Plasma (lavender)	12–18 g/dL	10	120–180 g/L
INR/PT	Plasma (blue)	Depends on methodology used		
Iron binding capacity (IBC)	Serum/plasma	250–400 μg/dL	0.179	44.8–71.6 μmol/L
Iron profile (total)	Serum (speckled or red) AVOID HEMOLYSIS	60–150 μg/dL	0.179	10.7–26.9 μmol/L
Lactate dehydrogenase (LD) and LD isoenzymes (LD-1)	Serum (speckled or red) or plasma (green)	5–200 units/L	1	5–200 units/L
Lactic acid (on ice)	Blood (gray) AVOID HEMOLYSIS	5–20 mg/dL	0.111	0.6–2.2 mmol/L
Lead, blood	Blood (royal blue or lavender)	Less than 10 μg/dL	0.048	Less than 0.48 μmol/L
Lipid profile	Serum (red) or plasma (green)	Reference intervals are variable depending on methods used.		
Lithium (therapeutic)	Serum (speckled or red)	0.5–1.4 mEq/L	1	0.5–1.4 mmol/L
Magnesium, serum	Serum (red)	1.3–2.1 mEq/L	0.5	0.65–1.05 mmol/L
Malaria prep	Blood (purple)	Reported as negative, or if positive, as malaria species		
Osmolality, serum	Blood (speckled)	280–295 mOsm/kg	1	280–295 mmol/kg
Partial thromboplastin time (PTT) (APTT)	Blood (blue) INDICATE IF PATIENT IS TAKING AN ANTICOAGULANT	Reference intervals are variable depending on methods used.		
Platelet count	Plasma (lavender)	150–400 $\times$ 10^3/mm^3	10^6	150–400 $\times$ 10^{9}L
Pregnancy test (HCG)	Serum (red)	Less than 3 mIU/mL nonpregnant female	1	Less than 3 IU/L

Test Name & Abbreviation	Specimen Type & Tube Color	Reference Interval in Conventional Units	Conversion Factor to Multiply By	Reference Interval in Systeme International Units
Prostatic specific antigen (PSA)	Serum (red)	Less than 4 ng/mL	1	Less than 4 ng/mL
Protein, total	Blood (speckled)	6–7.8 g/dL	10	60–78 g/L
Red blood cell count (RBC)	Blood (lavender)	M: 4.5–5.9 10^6/mm^3 F: 4.5–5.1 10^6/mm^3	10^6 10^6	4.5–5.9 10^{12}/L 4.5–5.1 10^{12}/L
Reticulocyte count	Plasma (lavender)	25,000 to 75,000/mm^3	1	25–75×10^9/L
Sodium, blood	Blood (green)	136–142 mEq/L	1	136–142 mmol/L
Thyroid studies (T$_3$, T$_4$, TSH)	Serum (speckled or red)	Reference ranges vary with methods used.		
Triglycerides (fasting)	Serum (speckled or red) or plasma (green)	10–90 mg/dL	0.01129	0.11–2.15 mmol/L
Troponin I (cardiac)	Serum (speckled or red) or plasma (green)	Less than 0.6 mg/mL	1	Less than 0.6 μg/L
Troponin T (cardiac)	Serum (speckled)	Less than 0.2 μg/mL	1	Less than 0.2 g/L
Urea nitrogen (BUN)	Serum (speckled)	11–23 mg/dL	0.357	8–16.4 nmol/L
Uric acid	Serum (speckled or red)	3 to 7 mg/dL	59.48	179–476 mcmol/L
White blood cell (WBC) count/differential	Plasma (lavender)	See "blood cell count, differential" above.		
Zinc	Serum (blue)	50–150 μg/dL	0.153	7.7–23 μmol/L

NAACLS Phlebotomy Competencies

NAACLS is the abbreviation for the National Accrediting Agency for Clinical Laboratory Sciences. The following table lists competencies for accredited programs in phlebotomy, signifying whether each competency is considered to be a Basic (Beginning), Intermediate, or Advanced skill.

NAACLS Competency		Skill Level
1.0	Demonstrate knowledge of the healthcare delivery system and medical terminology.	B to I
1.1	Identify the healthcare providers in hospitals and clinics, and the phlebotomist's role as a member of this healthcare team.	B to I
1.2	Describe the various hospital departments and their major functions in which the phlebotomist may interact in his or her role.	I
1.3	Describe the organizational structure of the clinical laboratory department.	I
1.4	Discuss the roles of the clinical laboratory personnel and their qualifications for these professional positions.	I
1.5	List the types of laboratory procedures performed in the various sections of the clinical laboratory department.	I to A
1.6	Describe how laboratory testing is used to assess body functions and disease.	I to A
1.7	Define medical terminology commonly used in the laboratory.	I to A
2.0	Demonstrate knowledge of infection control and safety.	I
2.1	Identify policies and procedures for maintaining laboratory safety.	A
2.2	Demonstrate accepted practices for infection control, isolation techniques, aseptic techniques, and methods for disease prevention.	I
2.2.1	Identify and discuss the modes of transmission of infection and methods for prevention.	I to A
2.2.2	Identify and properly label biohazardous specimens.	I to A
2.2.3	Discuss in detail and perform proper infection control techniques, such as hand washing, gowning, gloving, masking, and double-bagging.	B to A
2.2.4	Define and discuss the term *nosocomial infection*.	I
2.3	Comply with federal, state, and local regulations regarding safety practices.	I to A
2.3.1	Use the OSHA Standard Precautions.	I to A
2.3.2	Use prescribed procedures to handle electrical, radiation, biological, and fire hazards.	I
2.3.3	Use appropriate practices, as outlined in the OSHA Hazard Communication Standard, including the correct use of the Material Safety Data Sheet as directed.	I
2.4	Describe measures used to ensure patient safety in various patient settings, including inpatient, outpatient, and pediatrics.	I to A
3.0	Demonstrate basic understanding of the anatomy and physiology of body systems and anatomic terminology in order to relate major areas of the clinical laboratory to general pathologic conditions associated with body systems.	I to A

NAACLS Competency		Skill Level
3.1	Describe the basic functions of each of the main body systems, and demonstrate basic knowledge of the circulatory, urinary, and other body systems necessary to perform assigned specimen collection tasks.	I to A
3.2	Identify the veins of the arms, hands, legs, and feet on which phlebotomy is performed.	I to A
3.3	Explain the functions of the major constituents of blood, and differentiate between whole blood, serum, and plasma.	A
3.4	Define *hemostasis*, and explain the basic process of coagulation and fibrinolysis.	I to A
3.5	Discuss the properties of arterial blood, venous blood, and capillary blood.	I to A
4.0	Demonstrate understanding of the importance of specimen collection and specimen integrity in the delivery of patient care.	I to A
4.1	Describe the legal and ethical importance of proper patient and sample identification.	I
4.2	Describe the types of patient specimens that are analyzed in the clinical laboratory.	A
4.3	Define the phlebotomist's role in collecting and/or transporting these specimens to the laboratory.	A
4.4	List the general criteria for suitability of a specimen for analysis and reasons for specimen rejection or recollection.	A
4.5	Explain the importance of timed, fasting, and stat specimens as related to specimen integrity and patient care.	A
5.0	Demonstrate knowledge of collection equipment, various types of additives used, special precautions necessary, and substances that can interfere in clinical analysis of blood constituents.	A
5.1	Identify the various types of additives used in blood collection, and explain the reasons for their use.	A
5.2	Identify the evacuated tube color codes associated with the additives.	A
5.3	Describe substances that can interfere in clinical analysis of blood constituents and ways in which the phlebotomist can help to avoid these occurrences.	A
5.4	List and select the types of equipment needed to collect blood by venipuncture, capillary puncture, and arterial puncture.	B to A
5.5	Identify special precautions necessary during blood collections by venipuncture, capillary puncture, and arterial puncture.	B to A
6.0	Follow standard operating procedures to collect specimens.	A
6.1	Identify potential sites for venipuncture puncture, capillary puncture, and arterial puncture.	B to A
6.2	Differentiate between sterile and antiseptic techniques.	A
6.3	Describe and demonstrate the steps in the preparation of a puncture site.	B to A
6.4	List the effect of tourniquet, hand squeezing, and heating pads on capillary puncture and venipuncture.	I to A
6.5	Recognize proper needle insertion and withdrawal techniques, including direction, angle, depth, and aspiration, for arterial puncture and venipuncture.	I to A
6.6	Describe and perform correct procedure for capillary collection methods on infants and adults.	I to A
6.7	Identify alternate collection sites for arterial puncture, capillary puncture, and venipuncture. Describe the limitations and precautions of each.	I to A
6.8	Name and explain frequent causes of phlebotomy complications. Describe signs and symptoms of physical problems that may occur during blood collection.	I to A
6.9	List the steps necessary to perform an arterial, venipuncture, and/or capillary puncture in chronological order.	I to A
6.10	Follow standard operating procedures to perform a competent, effective venipuncture on a patient.	B to A
6.11	Follow standard operating procedures to perform a competent, effective capillary puncture on a patient.	I to A
7.0	Demonstrate understanding of requisitioning, specimen transport, and specimen processing.	I to A
7.1	Describe the standard operating procedure for a physician requesting a laboratory analysis for a patient. Discuss laboratory responsibility in responding to physician requests.	I to A
7.2	Instruct patients in the proper collection and preservation for various samples, including blood, sputum, and stools.	I to A
7.3	Explain methods for transporting and processing specimens for routine and special testing.	I to A
7.4	Explain methods for processing and transporting blood specimens for testing at reference laboratories.	I to A
7.5	Describe the potential clerical and technical errors that may occur during specimen processing.	A
7.6	Identify and report potential preanalytical errors that may occur during specimen collection, labeling, transporting, and processing.	A

NAACLS Competency		Skill Level
7.7	Describe and follow the criteria for specimens and test results that will be used as legal evidence, including paternity testing, chain of custody, and blood alcohol levels.	I
8.0	Demonstrate understanding of quality assurance and quality controlling phlebotomy.	B to A
8.1	Describe the system for monitoring quality assurance in the collection of blood specimens.	I to A
8.2	Identify polices and procedures used in the clinical laboratory to assure quality in the obtaining of blood specimens.	I
8.2.1	Perform quality control procedures.	B to I
8.2.2	Record quality control results.	B to I
8.2.3	Identify and report control results that do not meet predetermined criteria.	I
9.0	Communicate (verbally and nonverbally) effectively and appropriately in the workplace.	I to A
9.1	Maintain confidentiality of privileged information or individuals.	I to A
9.2	Value diversity in the workplace.	I
9.3	Interact appropriately and professionally with other individuals.	I to A
9.4	Discuss the major points of the American Hospital Association's Patient's Bill of Rights or the Patient's Bill of Rights from the institution.	I
9.5	Model professional appearance and appropriate behavior.	I
9.6	Follow written and verbal instructions in carrying out testing procedures.	I
9.7	Define the different terms used in the medicolegal aspect for phlebotomy, and discuss policies and protocol designed to avoid medicolegal problems.	I
9.8	List the causes of stress in the work environment, and discuss the coping skills used to deal with stress in the work environment.	I
9.9	Demonstrate ability to use computer information systems necessary to accomplish job functions.	I

Reference Laboratory Values

Cardiac Packet

CPK-MB/CPK Relative Index	Less than 2.5%
CPK-Total	WM: 60–320 units/L WF: 50–200 units/L BM: 130–450 units/L BF: 60–270 units/L
Glucose	70–110 mg/dL
LDH-Total	100–190 units/L
LDH-1	14–26%
Troponin 1	Negative

Cerebrospinal Fluid (CSF)

Color	Clear
Glucose	45–78 mg/dL
Lymphocytes	60–80%
Monocytes	20–50%
Neutrophils	0–4%
Pressure	70–200 mm H_2O
Protein	10–45 mg/dL
WBCs—Total	Less than 5 cells/mm³

Chem 7, Chem 12, Chem 20, Hepatic Function Panel, Renal Function Panel, Abdominal Pain Panel

ALP	30–100 units/L
ALT (SGPT)	5–40 units/L
Amylase	50–190 units/L
AST (SGOT)	5–40 units/L

Bilirubin-Total
  Direct
  Indirect
	0.1–1.25 mg/dL
	0.1–0.3 mg/dL
	0.2–1 mg/dL

BUN	8–20 mg/dL
Ca^{++}–Total Ionized	9–11 mg/dL 4.25–5.25 mg/dL

Coagulation Tests

Coagulation Factors
  I (Fibrinogen)
  II (Prothrombin)
	200–400 mg/dL
	80–120%

D-Dimer	Less than 250 mcg/L
FDPs	Less than 10 mcg/mL
Platelet Count	150,000–400,000/mm³
PT	11–15 seconds
PTT aPTT	60–80 seconds 25–40 seconds
Thrombin Time	10–13 seconds

Complete Blood Count (CBC)

Agranulocytes
   Lymphocytes
   Monocytes
	1,000–4,000/mm³
	100–700/mm³

Granulocytes
   Basophils
   Eosinophils
   Neutrophils
	25–100/mm³
	50–500/mm³
	2,500–8,000/mm³

Hct	M: 40–50% F: 35–45%
Hgb	M: 14–18 g/dL F: 12–16 g/dL
Platelets Count	150,000–400,000/mm³
RBCs Count	M: 4.5–6 million/cc F: 4–5.5 million/cc

RBC Indices
   MCH
   MCHC
   MCV
   RDW
	27–31 pg
	32–36 g/dL
	80–95 μm³
	11–15%

WBCs Count	5,000–10,000/mm³

Electrolyte Panel

Cl	91–110 mEq/L
CO_2	20–30 mEq/L
K⁺	3.5–5 mEq/L
Na⁺	135–145 mEq/L

Lipid Profile

HDL	M: Greater than 45 mg/dL F: Greater than 55 mg/dL
LDL	60–180 mg/dL
VLDL	25–50%
Total Cholesterol	Less than 200 mg/dL
Triglycerides	M: 40–60 mg/dL F: Greater than 35–135 mg/dL

Toxicology—Toxic Levels

Drug Serum Screen	
Acetaminophen	Greater than 250 mcg/mL

Alcohol
   Comatose
   Intoxicated
   Stuporous
	Greater than 0.5%
	0.1–0.4%
	0.4–0.5%

ASA	Greater than 300 mcg/mL

Barbitals
   Anticonvulsant
   Sedatives
	Greater than 40 mcg/mL
	Greater than 10 mcg/mL

Carboxyhemoglobin	Greater than 20%
Dilantin	Greater than 20 mcg/mL
Lead	Greater than 40 mcg/mL
Lithium	Greater than 2 mEq/L
Drug Urine Screen	
Amphetamine	Greater than 3 mcg/mL

Diet Suppressants
   Dextroamphetamine
   Phenmetrazine
	Greater than 15 mcg/mL
	Greater than 50 mcg/mL

Methamphetamine	Greater than 40 mcg/mL
Mercury	Greater than 100 mcg/day

Urinalysis

Albumin	10–100 mg/day
Amylase	Less than 17 units/hour
Appearance	Clear
Calcium	Less than 250 mg/day
Color	Amber
Creatinine	0.75–1.5 g/day
Glucose	Less than 500 mg/day
Osmolality	250–1,000 mOsm/L
pH	4.6–8
Potassium	25–125 mEq/day
Protein	0–8 mg/dL
Sodium	40–220 mEq/day
Specific Gravity	1.003–1.030
Urea Nitrogen	10–20 g/day
Uric Acid	250–750 mg/day
Volume	750–1,800 cc/day

ABC Laboratories
Blood Transfusion Consent
Form

Name of the specialist/doctor: _____

Name of the hospital/clinic: _____

Name of the patient: _____

Age: _____   Sex: _____

Address: _____

Contact number: _____

Blood transfusion consent terms: _____

_____

What is your blood group? _____

Are you aware of the medical reason associated with your blood transfusion?

_____

Have you met the specialist and do you understand the full clinical procedure behind this process?

_____

Are you taking the medicines and liquids as referred to you? _____

Are you ready to take the responsibilities and risks associated with this medicinal procedure?

_____

Is your family aware of your blood transfusion? _____

Patient signature: _____

Signature of the head of the department: _____

Date: _____ /_____ /_____

Military Time

Military time is also used in many parts of Europe. It is based on a 24-hour clock instead of a 12-hour clock, which is mostly used in the United States. This means that there is no "a.m." or "p.m." designation needed, and each hour has its own unique name. Four digits are used to express each hour, with the first two digits representing the hour itself, and the last two digits representing the minutes within that hour.

For example, 12:00 noon is expressed as 1200 hours, and 12:00 midnight is expressed as 2400 hours. The time 3:30 p.m. would be expressed as 1530 hours, and 3:30 a.m. would be expressed as 0330 hours. However, it is important to understand that while 2400 hours is equivalent to 12:00 midnight, as soon as this passes, the hour is called 00, with the minutes displayed after that to correspond with the actual time. Therefore, the standard time of 12:05 a.m. is equivalent to the military time of 0005 hours.

The 24-hour clock is preferred in healthcare settings to eliminate confusion of the required times for treatments, specimen collections, drug administrations, testing, surgeries, etc. All healthcare workers must understand the 24-hour clock so that they can use it correctly.

The complete list of military time equivalents to a.m. and p.m. hours is shown in the following table.

Standard Time	Military Time
12:30 a.m.	0030 hours
1:00 a.m.	0100 hours
2:00 a.m.	0200 hours
3:00 a.m.	0300 hours
4:00 a.m.	0400 hours
5:00 a.m.	0500 hours
6:00 a.m.	0600 hours
7:00 a.m.	0700 hours
8:00 a.m.	0800 hours
9:00 a.m.	0900 hours
10:00 a.m.	1000 hours
11:00 a.m.	1100 hours
12:00 p.m. (noon)	1200 hours
1:00 p.m.	1300 hours
2:00 p.m.	1400 hours
3:00 p.m.	1500 hours
4:00 p.m.	1600 hours
5:00 p.m.	1700 hours
6:00 p.m.	1800 hours
7:00 p.m.	1900 hours
8:00 p.m.	2000 hours
9:00 p.m.	2100 hours
10:00 p.m.	2200 hours
11:00 p.m.	2300 hours
12:00 a.m. (midnight)	2400 hours

Answer Key

Chapter 1

Answer Key

1. B
2. A
3. D
4. C
5. A
6. D
7. C
8. B
9. C
10. A
11. B
12. D
13. B
14. C
15. A

Chapter 2

Answer Key

1. C
2. D
3. B
4. B
5. D
6. D
7. B
8. A
9. A
10. A
11. D
12. C
13. C
14. A
15. D

Chapter 3

Answer Key

1. C
2. D
3. B
4. A
5. B
6. D
7. B
8. A
9. A
10. C
11. D
12. B
13. A
14. C
15. D

Chapter 4

Answer Key

1. C
2. B
3. B
4. A
5. C
6. A
7. B
8. C
9. B
10. B
11. D
12. A
13. C
14. B
15. C

Chapter 5

Answer Key

1. D
2. B
3. A
4. B
5. B
6. D
7. C
8. A
9. C
10. A
11. A
12. B
13. D
14. B
15. C

Chapter 6

Answer Key

1. B
2. D
3. A
4. B
5. B
6. C
7. A
8. B
9. A
10. C
11. C
12. C
13. A
14. A
15. D

Chapter 7

Answer Key

1. A
2. C
3. D
4. B
5. B
6. A
7. C
8. C
9. A
10. B
11. A
12. D
13. C
14. B
15. D

Chapter 8

Answer Key

1. C
2. A
3. D
4. C
5. B
6. A
7. C
8. D
9. A
10. C
11. B
12. C
13. A
14. A
15. C

Chapter 9

Answer Key

1. C
2. C
3. B
4. A
5. C
6. B
7. D
8. B
9. A
10. B
11. C
12. C
13. B
14. D
15. B

Chapter 10

Answer Key

1. B
2. D
3. D
4. A
5. C
6. A
7. C
8. C
9. A
10. D
11. B
12. C
13. B
14. D
15. B

Chapter 11

Answer Key

1. B
2. A
3. B
4. C
5. D
6. B
7. A
8. C
9. A
10. D
11. C
12. B
13. B
14. A
15. C

Chapter 12

Answer Key

1. D
2. C
3. B
4. B
5. B
6. C
7. D
8. B
9. D
10. C
11. B
12. D
13. B
14. C
15. C

Chapter 13

Answer Key

1. D
2. D
3. C
4. B
5. C
6. A
7. D
8. A
9. B
10. C
11. B
12. D
13. A
14. B
15. A

Chapter 14

Answer Key

1. D
2. D
3. B
4. C
5. D
6. A
7. C
8. A
9. C
10. B
11. A
12. C
13. B
14. C
15. C

Chapter 15

Answer Key

1. D
2. B
3. C
4. A
5. D
6. B
7. D
8. A
9. D
10. B
11. B
12. D
13. C
14. D
15. B

Chapter 16

Answer Key

1. D
2. C
3. A
4. C
5. A
6. B
7. B
8. C
9. B
10. C
11. C
12. A
13. D
14. B
15. D

Chapter 17

Answer Key

1. B
2. D
3. C
4. B
5. A
6. D
7. B
8. D
9. B
10. C
11. A
12. B
13. C
14. C
15. B

Chapter 18

Answer Key

1. D
2. B
3. D
4. C
5. A
6. C

7. B
8. D
9. B
10. D
11. C
12. D
13. B
14. D
15. A

Chapter 19

Answer Key

1. C
2. B
3. D
4. A
5. D
6. B
7. D
8. A
9. D
10. B
11. C
12. A
13. D
14. B
15. D

Glossary

Chapter	Term	Definition
1	Bioethics	The study of ethical and moral implications of new discoveries and advances in medicine.
1	Bloodletting	The removal of blood as a therapeutic measure.
1	Chair of custody	A "paper trail"; a chronological documentation of activities.
1	Civil law	The type of law that deals with the rights of private citizens.
1	Criminal law	The type of law that deals with crimes against society.
1	Defense mechanisms	Unconscious psychological strategies used to cope with stressors.
1	Ethics	Moral principles, qualities, or practices.
1	Hemolysis	The destruction or dissolution of red blood cells.
1	Laws	Rules of conduct established by custom, agreement, or authority.
1	Malpractice	A type of negligence wherein a professional fails to follow acceptable standards, resulting in injury to a person or group of persons.
1	Phlebotomy	Opening of a blood vessel by incision or puncture in order to obtain blood.
1	Quality assurance	A formal monitoring program that assesses the level of health care being provided by health care professionals or institutions.
1	Quality control	A process that assesses all factors involved in the health care process.
1	Stressors	Events that provoke stress.
2	Caustic	Irreversibly damaging to body tissues or corroding anything else with which it comes in contact.
2	Certified medical laboratory scientists	Degreed individuals who have been accredited as proficient in the performance of complex chemical, biological, hematological, immunologic, microscopic, and bacteriological analyses.
2	Hematology	The study of the blood and tissues that form blood.
2	Immunology	The study of the immune system and immune disorders.
2	In vitro	Literally means "in glass"; this term is used for processes, tests, or procedures that take place outside the body.
2	Pathologists	Doctors who study the cause and development of disease.
2	Sensitivity testing	Procedures that determine how sensitive specific microorganisms are to various substances, such as antibiotics.
3	Active listening	A form of listening wherein the receiver pays complete attention to the speaker's verbal and nonverbal communication and then provides feedback about what was received.
3	Confidentiality	Keeping information private and away from individuals who are not authorized to receive it.
3	Defense mechanisms	Reactions often used when people feel attacked or pressured that help them to deal with difficult events.
3	Feedback	A response from the receiver back to the sender that signifies the message has been received and understood.
3	Pitch	The frequency of sound emitted by the voice; it is used in verbal communication to indicate various types of information such as questions, statements, and continuation of ideas.
3	Stereotype	To establish a preconceived image or opinion about someone.

Chapter	Term	Definition
5	Aorta	The largest artery in the body, the aorta originates from the left ventricle of the heart and extends down to the abdomen, where it branches off.
5	Aortic arch	The second section of the aorta; it branches into the brachiocephalic trunk, left common carotid artery, and left subclavian artery.
5	Aortic valve	Located at the base of the aorta, the aortic valve has three cusps and opens to allow blood to leave the left ventricle during contraction.
5	Arteries	Elastic vessels able to carry blood away from the heart under high pressure.
5	Arterioles	Subdivisions of arteries; they are thinner and have muscles that are innervated by the sympathetic nervous system.
5	Atria	The upper chambers of the heart; they receive blood returning to the heart.
5	Atrioventricular node (AV node)	A mass of specialized tissue located in the inferior interatrial septum beneath the endocardium; it provides the only normal conduction pathway between the atrial and ventricular syncytia.
5	AV bundle	The bundle of His; a large structure that receives the cardiac impulse from the distal AV node; it enters the upper part of the interventricular septum.
5	Blood volume	The sum of formed elements and plasma volumes in the vascular system; most adults have about 5 L of blood.
5	Capillaries	The smallest-diameter blood vessels, which connect the smallest arterioles to the smallest venules.
5	Cardiac conduction system	The initiation and distribution of impulses through the myocardium that coordinates the cardiac cycle.
5	Cardiac cycle	A heartbeat; it consists of a complete series of systolic and diastolic events.
5	Cardiac output	The volume discharged from the ventricle per minute, calculated by multiplying stroke volume by heart rate, in beats per minute.
5	Cardiac veins	Those veins that branch out and drain blood from the myocardial capillaries to join the coronary sinus.
5	Carotid sinuses	Enlargements near the base of the carotid arteries that contain baroreceptors and help to control blood pressure.
5	Cerebral arterial circle	The circle of Willis; it connects the vertebral artery and internal carotid artery systems.
5	Chordae tendineae	Strong fibers originating from the papillary muscles that attach to the cusps of the tricuspid valve.
5	Coronary arteries	The first two aortic branches, which supply blood to the heart tissues.
5	Coronary sinus	An enlarged vein joining the cardiac veins; it empties into the right atrium.
5	Diastole	The relaxation of a heart structure.
5	Diastolic pressure	The lowest pressure that remains in the arteries before the next ventricular contraction.
5	Electrocardiogram (EKG)	The recording of electrical changes in the myocardium during the cardiac cycle; the EKG machine works by placing nodes on the skin that connect via wires and respond to weak electrical changes of the heart; the abbreviation EKG is more commonly used than ECG.
5	Endocardium	The inner layer of the heart wall.
5	Epicardium	The outer layer of the heart wall.
5	Functional syncytium	A mass of merging cells that function as a unit.
5	Hepatic portal system	The veins that drain the abdominal viscera, originating in the stomach, intestines, pancreas, and spleen, to carry blood through a hepatic portal vein to the liver.
5	Inferior vena cava	Along with the superior vena cava, one of the two largest veins in the body; it is formed by the joining of the common iliac veins.
5	Mitral valve	The bicuspid valve; it lies between the left atrium and left ventricle, preventing blood from flowing back into the left atrium from the ventricle.
5	Myocardium	The thick middle layer of the heart wall that is mostly made of cardiac tissue.
5	Pacemaker	The term used to refer to the sinoatrial node (SA node).

Chapter	Term	Definition
5	Papillary muscles	Those muscles that contract as the heart's ventricles contract, pulling on the chordae tendineae to prevent the cusps from swinging back into the atrium.
5	Pericardium	A membranous structure that encloses the heart and proximal ends of the large blood vessels and that consists of double layers.
5	Peripheral resistance	A force produced by friction between blood and blood vessel walls.
5	Pulmonary circuit	The venules and veins, which send deoxygenated blood to the lungs to receive oxygen and unload carbon dioxide.
5	Pulmonary valve	Lying at the base of the pulmonary trunk, this valve has three cusps and allows blood to leave the right ventricle while preventing backflow into the ventricular chamber.
5	Purkinje fibers	Consisting of branches of the AV bundle that spread and enlarge, these fibers are located near the papillary muscles; they continue to the heart's apex and cause the ventricular walls to contract in a twisting motion.
5	Septum	A solid, wall-like structure that separates the left atria and ventricle from the right atria and ventricle.
5	Sinoatrial node (SA node)	A small mass of specialized tissue just beneath the epicardium in the right atrium that initiates impulses through the myocardium to stimulate contraction of cardiac muscle fibers.
5	Stroke volume	The volume of blood discharged from the ventricle with each contraction; it is usually about 70 mL.
5	Superior vena cava	Along with the inferior vena cava, one of the two largest veins in the body; the superior vena cava is formed by the joining of the brachiocephalic veins.
5	Systemic circuit	The arteries and arterioles, which send oxygenated blood and nutrients to the body cells while removing wastes.
5	Systole	The contraction of a heart structure.
5	Systolic pressure	The maximum pressuring during ventricular contraction.
5	Thyrocervical arteries	Those that branch off to the thyroid and parathyroid glands, larynx, trachea, esophagus, pharynx, and muscles of the neck, shoulder, and back.
5	Tricuspid valve	Lying between the right atrium and ventricle, this valve allows blood to move from the right atrium into the right ventricle while preventing backflow.
5	Vasoconstriction	The contraction of blood vessels, which reduces their diameter.
5	Vasodilation	The relaxation of blood vessels, which increases their diameter.
5	Veins	Blood vessels that carry blood back to the atria; they are less elastic than arteries.
5	Ventricles	The lower chambers of the heart; they receive blood from the atria, which they pump out into the arteries.
5	Venules	Microscopic vessels that link capillaries to veins.
5	Vertebral arteries	One of the main divisions of the subclavian and common carotid arteries; the vertebral arteries run upward through the cervical vertebrae into the skull and supply blood to the vertebrae, their ligaments, and their muscles.
5	Viscosity	Thickness or stickiness; the resistance of fluid to flow. In a biologic fluid, viscosity is caused by the attraction of cells to one another.
6	Abruptio placentae	A complication of pregnancy wherein the placental lining has separated from the uterus of the mother, causing late pregnancy bleeding, fetal heart rate effects, and potential fetal or maternal death.
6	Angina pectoris	Sharp pain usually felt in the chest or arm that occurs when the heart does not receive enough oxygen to support its workload.
6	Anoxia	Absence of oxygen supply to an organ or tissue.
6	Arrhythmia	An irregular heartbeat, which can range from mild to life-threatening; also called *dysrhythmia*.
6	Arthralgia	Joint pain.
6	Atherosclerosis	A form of arteriosclerosis characterized by deposits of cholesterol and other fats on the sides of the arteries.
6	Celiac disease	An autoimmune disorder of the small intestine that causes diarrhea, failure to thrive (in children), fatigue, and other effects upon multiple body systems; it is triggered by a reaction to *wheat gluten*.

Chapter	Term	Definition
6	Dysrhythmia	Also called *arrhythmia*, meaning "irregular heartbeat."
6	Eclampsia	An acute, life-threatening complication of pregnancy wherein the mother may experience tonic-clonic seizures and coma.
6	Gastrectomy	Partial or complete surgical removal of the stomach.
6	Graves' disease	An autoimmune condition caused by overactive thyroid (hyperthyroidism), causing "bulging" eyes, bone damage, and central or peripheral nervous system symptoms.
6	Hemarthrosis	Blood accumulation or hemorrhage in a joint.
6	Hematopoietic stem cells	Stem cells that develop into all the different types of blood cells.
6	Hemochromatosis	Iron overload caused by either repeated transfusions or a genetic disorder.
6	Hemoglobin S	An inherited type of abnormal adult hemoglobin, which mostly affects African-Americans, causing sickle-cell anemia.
6	Hemophilia A	The most common form of hemophilia; it is an inherited condition primarily affecting males wherein coagulation is much more prolonged than normal.
6	Hypertrophied	Enlarged, due to an increase in cell size.
6	Hypoplasia	Lack of development of a tissue or organ.
6	Hypoplastic anemia	Aplastic anemia; actually a variety of related anemias that result from destruction of or injury to stem cells in the bone marrow or its matrix.
6	Ischemia	A temporary reduction of blood supply to an organ or tissue due to obstruction of a blood vessel.
6	Lymph	Part of the interstitial fluid, which is referred to as lymph when it enters a lymph capillary; it picks up and carries bacteria to the lymph nodes to be destroyed.
6	Lymphoblasts	Immature cells that form lymphocytes; in acute lymphoblastic leukemia, lymphoblasts proliferate uncontrollably and are found in large numbers in the peripheral blood.
6	Mastectomy	Partial or complete removal of one or both breasts.
6	Megaloblastic anemia	An anemia that results from inhibition of DNA synthesis in red blood cell production; it is characterized by megaloblasts in the bone marrow.
6	Myocardial infarction	A heart attack; sudden death of cells in the heart muscle caused by an abrupt interruption of blood flow (and lack of oxygen) to part of the heart.
6	Myxedema	A type of cutaneous and dermal edema secondary to hypothyroidism and Graves' disease.
6	NSAID	Nonsteroidal anti-inflammatory drug; common examples include aspirin and ibuprofen.
6	Pancytopenia	A combination of anemia, leukopenia (decreased white blood cells), and thrombocytopenia (decreased platelets).
6	Proliferation	Growth and reproduction of cells.
6	Reed-Sternberg cells	Cells usually derived from B lymphocytes that are much larger than surrounding cells and are found via light microscopy in cases of Hodgkin's disease and certain other disorders.
6	Respiratory acidosis	A condition in which decreased respiration increased blood carbon dioxide and decreased pH.
6	Sepsis	The presence of pathogenic bacteria in tissue.
6	Thalassemia	An inherited autosomal recessive blood disorder in which hemoglobin chains are not synthesized normally, leading to anemia.
6	Thrombus	A blood clot that forms in the cardiovascular system.
6	Ventricular asystole	The absence of contraction of the ventricles.
6	Ventricular fibrillation	Abnormal discharge of electrical nerve impulses that cause the heart to stop beating.
7	Agglutination	The clumping of red blood cells following a transfusion reaction.
7	Agranulocytes	Leukocytes without granular cytoplasm.
7	Albumins	The smallest of plasma proteins; they make up around 60% of these proteins by weight.
7	Antibodies	Agglutinins; gamma globulin proteins that respond to specific antigens.
7	Antigens	Agglutinogens; red blood cell surface molecules that react with antibodies from the plasma.

Chapter	Term	Definition
7	Basophils	Leukocytes that have fewer granules than eosinophils, which become deep blue in basic stain.
7	B cells	Lymphocytes that are responsible for humoral immunity.
7	Bilirubin	An orange pigment formed from biliverdin that has potent antioxidant activity; bilirubin is orange and excreted along with biliverdin in the bile.
7	Biliverdin	A green pigment created from decomposing heme, which is converted to bilirubin.
7	Coagulation	The formation of a blood clot.
7	Colony-stimulating factors (CSFs)	Glycoproteins that can cause the proliferation and differentiation of leukocytes.
7	Embolus	A clot that dislodges or fragments, to be carried away in the blood flow.
7	Eosinophils	Leukocytes with coarse, same-sized granules that appear dark red in acid stain.
7	Erythropoiesis	The process of developing erythrocytes (red blood cells), which mostly occurs in the red bone marrow (myeloid tissue).
7	Erythropoietin	A hormone that uses negative feedback to control the rate of red blood cell formation.
7	Fibrin	Insoluble threads of protein made from the plasma protein fibrinogen.
7	Fibrinogen	A plasma protein that is important for blood coagulation. It is the largest plasma protein.
7	Globulins	Antibodies made by the liver or lymphatic tissues that make up around 36% of the plasma proteins.
7	Granulocytes	Leukocytes with granular cytoplasm, including neutrophils, eosinophils, and basophils.
7	Hematocrit (HCT)	The volume percentage of red blood cells in a sample of whole blood.
7	Hematology	The study of blood and blood disorders.
7	Hemoglobin	The substance in red blood cells that carries oxygen.
7	Hemostasis	The stoppage of bleeding.
7	Interleukins	Hormones upon which many of the effects of leukocytes depend.
7	Leukocytes	White blood cells; they protect the body against disease and develop from hemocytoblasts in red bone marrow.
7	Leukocytosis	A condition of white blood cells exceeding 10,000 per cubic millimeter (microliter), indicating an acute infection.
7	Leukopenia	A condition of the total white blood cell count being below 5,000 per cubic millimeter (microliter); this signifies conditions such as influenza, AIDS, and others.
7	Lymphocytes	Leukocytes with large, round nuclei inside a thin cytoplasm rim.
7	Macrophages	Cells that phagocytize and destroy damaged red blood cells, mostly in the liver and spleen.
7	Mast cells	Connective tissue cells that, during allergic reactions, release histamine and heparin.
7	Megakarocytes	Red bone marrow cells that fragment to produce platelets.
7	Monocytes	Leukocytes that are the largest type of blood cells, with varied nuclei.
7	Natural killer (NK) cells	Lymphocytes responsible for immune surveillance; they are important in preventing cancer.
7	Neutrophils	Leukocytes with small granules that appear light purple in neutral stain; older neutrophils are called *segs* while younger neutrophils are called *bands*.
7	Nonprotein nitrogenous substances	Amino acids, urea, and uric acid in the plasma.
7	Plasma	The liquid portion of blood.
7	Plasma cells	Specialized B cells that form and secrete antibodies.
7	Plasma proteins	The most abundant solutes (dissolved substances) in the plasma.
7	Platelets	Thrombocytes; platelets are cytoplasm fragments of megakaryocytes that are important in blood clotting.
7	Polymorphonuclear leukocytes	White blood cells with segmented lobular nuclei, such as neutrophils.
7	Prothrombin	An alpha globulin made in the liver that is converted to thrombin.

Chapter	Term	Definition
7	Red blood cells (erythrocytes)	Those red blood cells that transport gases, including oxygen.
7	Serotonin	A substance that contracts smooth muscles in blood vessels, reducing blood loss.
7	Serum	The clear, yellowish liquid that remains after clot formation; serum is plasma minus fibrinogen and some of, but not all, its clotting factors.
7	T cells	Lymphocytes that are responsible for cell-mediated immunity.
7	Thrombin	A substance that causes fibrinogen to be cut into sections of fibrin and then joined into long threads as part of the clotting process.
7	Thrombocytes	See *platelets* above.
7	Thrombopoietin	A hormone that cause megakaryocytes to develop from hemocytoblasts, resulting in eventual platelet (thrombocyte) formation.
7	Thrombus	A clot that forms abnormally in a vessel.
7	Vasospasm	An action of muscle contraction in a small blood vessel that occurs after it is cut or broken; this action can completely close the ends of a severed vessel.
7	White blood cells	See *leukocytes* above.
8	Alanine aminotransferase (ALT)	An enzyme normally present in serum and tissues of the body, especially the tissue of the liver; it is released into the serum as a result of tissue injury and increases in persons with acute liver damage.
8	Albumin (ALB)	A water-soluble protein; determination of the levels and types of albumin in urine, blood, and other body tissues is the basis of a number of diagnostic laboratory tests.
8	Alkaline phosphatase (ALP)	An enzyme present in all tissues and in high concentrations in bones, kidneys, intestines, and plasma; it may be elevated in the serum in some diseases of the liver and bones and because of other illnesses.
8	Aspartate aminotransferase (AST)	An enzyme normally present in body serum and in certain body tissues, especially those of the liver and heart.
8	Blood profile	A complete blood count (CBC).
8	Blood urea nitrogen	The result of the breakdown of proteins in the body; a blood urea nitrogen (BUN) test is commonly used to measure kidney function.
8	Creatinine	A breakdown product of creatine phosphate in muscle; creatinine blood levels rise when kidney function is deficient.
8	Erythrocyte sedimentation rate (ESR)	The speed at which red blood cells sediment in a period of 1 h; it is a common hematology test for inflammation.
8	Graves' disease	An autoimmune disease involving an overactive thyroid, causing hyperthyroidism.
8	Hypothyroidism	Underactive thyroid; a condition where the thyroid gland lacks adequate amounts of thyroid hormones.
8	Infantile cretinism	Severely stunted physical and mental growth; untreated congenital deficiency of thyroid hormones due to maternal nutritional deficiency of iodine.
8	Insulinoma	A tumor of the insulin-secreting cells of the pancreas; the majority are benign.
8	Lipoproteins	Biochemicals that contain both lipids and proteins; they function to transport fats such as cholesterol throughout the body via the bloodstream.
8	Multiple myeloma	A malignant neoplasm of the bone marrow that is composed of plasma cells and disrupts normal bone marrow functions; it causes abnormal proteins in the plasma and urine as well as anemia, weight loss, and kidney failure.
8	Salicylates	Salts, anions, or esters (such as aspirin) derived from salicylic acid.
8	Syphilis	A sexually transmitted infection caused by the spirochete *Treponema pallidum* and characterized by distinct stages of effects over a period of years.
8	Systemic lupus erythematosus	A chronic inflammatory disease affecting many body systems; it is an example of a collagen disease.
8	Treponemal antigen test	Any of various tests detecting specific antitreponemal antibodies in serum in the diagnosis of the *Treponema pallidum* infection of syphilis.

Chapter	Term	Definition
8	Tularemia	An infectious disease of animals caused by the bacillus *Francisella tularensis*, which may be transmitted by insect vectors or direct contact.
9	Algae	Unicellular or multicellular photosynthetic eukaryotes lacking roots, stems, leaves, conducting vessels, and complex sex organs.
9	Aperture	The hole in the stage of a microscope through which light is transmitted.
9	Arthropod	An invertebrate animal with an exoskeleton, such as insects, arachnids, and crustaceans.
9	Asexual reproduction	The formation of new individual organisms from the cells of a single parent organism.
9	Bacilli	A generic term that describes the morphology of any rod-shaped bacterium.
9	Bacteria	A large group of prokaryotic, single-celled microorganisms.
9	Cocci	Any bacteria that have circular shapes.
9	Condenser	The microscope structure used to collect and focus light onto the specimen.
9	Diplococci	Cocci bacteria arranged in two-celled pairs.
9	Eukaryotes	Organisms whose cells contain complex structures enclosed within membranes.
9	Fermentation	A metabolic process whereby electrons released from nutrients are ultimately transferred to molecules obtained from the breakdown of the same nutrients.
9	Microbiology	The study of microorganisms.
9	Microscopes	Pieces of equipment used to see objects that are too small to be viewed by the naked eye.
9	Mycology	The study of fungi.
9	Pathogenic	Able to cause disease or infection.
9	Periplasm	A metabolic region between the cell membrane and outer membrane of gram-negative cells.
9	Physiochemical	Relating to both physiology and chemistry.
9	Prokaryotes	A group of organisms that lack a cell nucleus and any other membrane-bound organelles.
9	Protozoa	Microorganisms generally classified as unicellular, eukaryotic organisms lacking cell walls.
9	Resolution	The capability of a microscope to visualize certain objects.
9	Spirilla	A variable resistor that controls electric current in a circuit.
9	Spores	Reproductive structures adapted for surviving over longer periods in unfavorable conditions.
9	Staphylococci	Gram-positive bacteria that form grapelike clusters.
9	Streptococci	Gram-positive bacteria that form chains or pairs of round structures.
9	Symptomatology	The study of the symptoms of diseases.
9	Teichoic acid	A negatively charged polysaccharide in the cell wall of gram-positive bacteria.
9	Virions	Complete viral particles, making up the infective forms of viruses.
9	Viruses	The smallest infectious agents; they can replicate only within living host cells.
9	Working distance	The distance between the front lens of a microscope and the specimen when the microscope is correctly focused.
10	Airborne precautions	Formerly called *respiratory isolation*, these additional safety precautions are applied to certain diseases such as tuberculosis.
10	Anoxia	Partial or complete absence of oxygen from inspired gases, arterial blood, or tissue.
10	Antiseptics	Substances that inhibit the growth of microorganisms in living tissue.
10	Asepsis	The state of being free of pathogenic microorganisms.
10	Aseptic techniques	Procedures that are performed under sterile conditions.
10	Blood-borne pathogen (BBP)	Any microorganism in the blood (or other body fluids) that can cause illness and disease.
10	Carcinogenic	Able to cause cancer or make it more likely to develop.
10	Cardiopulmonary resuscitation (CPR)	An emergency procedure commonly performed on patients who are in cardiac or respiratory arrest.
10	Carrier	An individual (host) with no overt disease who harbors infectious organisms.
10	Caustic	Capable of burning, corroding, or destroying living tissue.

Chapter	Term	Definition
10	Centrifuge	A piece of laboratory equipment used to "spin" substances such as blood samples in order to separate out various elements that they contain.
10	Chain of infection	The method of infection proliferation; it includes an infectious agent, a reservoir, a portal of exit, a mode of transmission, a portal of entry, and a susceptible host.
10	Communicable disease	An infectious disease that is able to be transmitted between individuals because of a replicating agent (rather than a toxin).
10	Contact precautions	Procedures that reduce risk of transmission of serious diseases through direct or indirect contact.
10	Disinfectants	Substances that can destroy microorganisms from nonliving objects.
10	Double bagging	The use of two trash bags for disposing of waste from patient rooms (usually from patients who are in isolation).
10	Droplet precautions	Procedures used to reduce transmission of diseases via droplets that are expelled during sneezing, coughing, or talking; these diseases include meningitis, pertussis, pneumonia, and rubella.
10	Fomites	Inanimate objects that may transmit infectious organisms or infectious agents (such as sinks, toilets, door knobs, linens, glasses, and phlebotomy supplies).
10	HazCom	The OSHA Hazard Communication Standard, which requires chemical manufacturers to supply Material Safety Data Sheets (MSDSs) for their chemicals.
10	Infection control programs	Guidelines that address community-acquired and health-care-associated infections, including their monitoring, reporting, required isolation procedures, education, and management.
10	Intensive care unit (ICU)	A specialized treatment area for critically ill patients, those needing additional monitoring, and those who are more susceptible to infections.
10	Isolation procedures	Methods used to protect health care workers from patients with certain infectious diseases; usually divided into category-specific and disease-specific types.
10	Material Safety Data Sheets (MSDSs)	Required paperwork about all chemicals used in a workplace listing chemical, precautionary, and emergency exposure information.
10	Mode of transmission	The method by which pathogenic agents are transmitted.
10	Nosocomial infections	Health-care-acquired infections; those acquired after being admitted into a health facility.
10	Protective (reverse) isolation	Precautionary methods designed to protect patients who may be highly susceptible to infections.
10	RACE: Rescus Alert Confine Extinguish	A system designed to help health care workers remember how to respond when a fire emergency occurs.
10	Source	The origin of an infection.
10	Standard precautions	Safeguards to reduce risk of transmission of microorganisms. These precautions are more comprehensive than universal precautions, applying to patients, body fluids, nonintact skin, and mucous membranes, and include barrier protection, hand hygiene, and proper use and disposal of needles and other sharps.
10	Susceptible host	A person who lacks resistance to an agent and is vulnerable to contracting a disease.
10	Teratogenic	Able to cause birth defects in an embryo or fetus.
10	Transmission-based precautions	A set of procedures designed to prevent the communication of infectious diseases.
10	Universal precautions	Approaches to infection control designed to prevent transmission of blood-borne diseases.
11	Additive	Any substance added intentionally or indirectly that becomes a part of the product.
11	Anticoagulants	Substances added to blood collection tubes to slow or stop coagulation of specimens.
11	Antiglycolytic agent	A substance that prevents glycolysis (the breakdown of glucose, which yields pyruvic acid and ATP); the most common antiglycolytic agent is sodium fluoride.
11	Benzalkonium chloride	A disinfectant and fungicide prepared in an aqueous solution in various strengths.
11	Blood-drawing chair	A special seat designed for phlebotomy procedures.

Chapter	Term	Definition
11	Butterfly needles	"Winged infusion sets," often used in phlebotomy for people who have either spasticity or thin "rolling" blood vessels that are difficult to access.
11	Chlorhexidine	An antimicrobial agent used as a surgical scrub, hand rinse, and topical antiseptic.
11	Clot activators	Substances added to blood collection tubes to speed coagulation of specimens.
11	Coagulation cascade	The series of steps beginning with activation of coagulation.
11	Evacuated tubes	Blood tubes that discharge or remove blood from blood vessels.
11	Gauge	The size of a needle's lumen.
11	Glycolysis	The breakdown of glucose into pyruvic acid and ATP.
11	Glycolytic inhibitor	A substance that stops the breakdown of glucose, such as bromopyruvic acid and dichloroacetic acid.
11	Hemolyze	To rupture the red blood cells.
11	Lancets	Small, extremely sharp bladed instruments used for puncturing the skin, as used in capillary puncture.
11	Microhematocrit capillary tubes	Collection tubes used to measure the hematocrit (the proportion of blood volume occupied by red blood cells) in very small quantities.
11	Micropipettes	Very small, thin pipettes used to measure samples that range from less than 1 μL up to 1 mL.
11	Multiple-sample needles	Double-pointed needles that allow the drawing of multiple blood samples.
11	Needle holder	A translucent cylinder that is used to hold double-pointed needles and evacuated tubes.
11	Povidone-iodine	An antiseptic microbicide.
11	Sodium fluoride	An inorganic chemical compound commonly used as an antiglycolytic agent.
11	Thixotropic gel	A material that appears to be a solid until subjected to a disturbance such as centrifugation, whereupon it becomes a liquid.
11	Velcro	A brand name of fabric "hook and loop" fasteners; usually made of nylon and polyester, the hook side of the fabric presses onto the loop side to make a firm bond.
11	Venoscopes	Devices for locating veins for blood collection.
12	Antecubital	Relating to the region of the arm in front of the elbow.
12	Basilic vein	One of the four superficial veins of the arm, beginning in the ulnar part of the dorsal venous network and running proximally on the posterior surface of the ulnar side of the forearm.
12	Bifurcation	The splitting of a structure into two parts.
12	Capillary puncture	Dermal puncture; the puncturing of the capillaries of usually the fingers or heels, to withdraw blood for testing.
12	Cephalic vein	One of the four superficial veins of the upper limb. It receives deoxygenated blood from the dorsal and palmar surfaces of the forearm.
12	Ethylenediamine tetraacetic acid (EDTA)	An anticoagulant used extensively for analysis of blood, such as in complete blood counts.
12	g Force	The unit of measure of gravitational force in the International System of units.
12	Heel stick	A method of blood collection in very young children; the heel of the foot is punctured and capillary blood is collected for testing.
12	Hemoconcentration	An increase in the concentration of blood cells resulting in loss of plasma or water from the bloodstream.
12	Hemolysis	The breaking open of red blood cells and the release of hemoglobin into the blood plasma.
12	Hemophiliac	A patient (usually male) with a group of hereditary bleeding disorders characterized by a deficiency of one of the factors necessary for coagulation of the blood.
12	Lateral	Farther from the middle or center.
12	Microcollection	Blood collection from a finger or heel into microcontainers; it requires smaller amounts of blood than from venipuncture.
12	Microtainer	A patented type of capillary tube that holds less than 1 mL of blood and often contains varieties of anticoagulants and additives.
12	Plantar	Related to the sole or bottom of the foot.

Chapter	Term	Definition
12	Smelling salts	Ammonium carbonate, packaged in small "capsules" which are broken to release a strong odor that revives fainting patients.
12	Thixotropic gel	A substance that changes from a gel to a liquid when stirred or shaken; after centrifugation, the gel forms a barrier over red blood cells in the tube, keeping them separate from the blood serum.
13	Analytes	Substances being chemically analyzed.
13	Assays	Tests to determine the purity or concentration of substances.
13	Cannula	A flexible tube that is inserted into a duct or cavity to deliver medication or to drain fluid.
13	Central venous therapy lines	Venous access devices involving the introduction of a cannula into a vein other than a peripheral vein.
13	Chain of custody	Chronological documentation, or paper trail, describing both the movement of evidence or other information and who has come into contact with it.
13	Cushing's syndrome	A metabolic disorder resulting from either the chronic and excessive production of cortisol by the adrenal cortex or the administration of glucocorticoids in large doses for several weeks or longer.
13	Diabetes mellitus	A condition caused by the inability to properly metabolize sugars; type 1 is characterized by the inability to form insulin, and type 2 is characterized by the inability to make enough insulin.
13	Diurnal variation	The time at which an organism's functions are active, change, or reach certain levels.
13	Gestational diabetes	A disorder characterized by an impaired ability to metabolize carbohydrates, usually caused by a deficiency of insulin or insulin resistance, occurring in pregnancy. It usually disappears after delivery of the infant, but may recur years later as type 2 diabetes mellitus.
13	Glycolysis	The metabolic process in which glucose is converted, by a series of steps, to pyruvic acid.
13	Hemochromatosis	A disorder that causes deposition of hemosiderin in the body tissues, leading to cirrhosis of the liver, heart failure, and destruction of the pancreas.
13	Hemostasis	The body's mechanism for controlling bleeding; normal hemostasis involves the proper functioning of the platelets and clotting factors.
13	Heparin lock	The most commonly used type of venous access device for administering medications over a longer period of time (also used for obtaining blood samples); it is a special winged needle set left in a patient's vein for between 48 and 72 h.
13	Insulinoma	A usually benign tumor of the insulin-secreting cells of the islets of Langerhans in the pancreas.
13	Lipemic	Related to lipemia, the presence of larger than normal amounts of fat in the blood.
13	Peak	The expected highest level of serum concentration of medications.
13	Platelet function assay	A test that measures both platelet adhesion and aggregation (primary hemostasis).
13	Polycythemia	An abnormal increase in production of red blood cells.
13	Reclined position	Lying back or down.
13	Reference values	Ranges used for various tests in determining how results relate to normal, healthy ranges.
13	Salicylates	Widely prescribed drugs derived from salicylic acid; they exert analgesic, antipyretic, and anti-inflammatory actions.
13	Shunts	Devices inserted into the forearm to allow hemodialysis to occur; shunts are connected to machines that filter the blood.
13	Therapeutic medication	A medicine needed to properly treat a condition.
13	Trough	The expected lowest level of serum concentration of medications.
14	Bacteremia	A general term that indicates the presence of bacteremia in the blood; it is also called *septicemia*.
14	Globules	Spherical masses of lipid tissue under the skin.
14	Jaundice	Disease characterized by yellowish color of the skin, sclera, mucous membranes, and body fluids.

Chapter	Term	Definition
14	Microhematocrit tube	A common, heparin-coated capillary tube used for determining the percentage of packed red blood cells in microhematocrit tests.
15	Anaphylactic shock	An immediate allergic reaction characterized by acute respiratory distress, hypotension, edema, and rash. Anaphylactic shock can be life-threatening.
15	Anticoagulants	A group of agents that prevent or delay blood coagulation (clotting).
15	Hematoma	An abnormal localized collection of blood within tissues or organs.
15	Hemoconcentration	A relative increase in the number of red blood cells resulting from a decrease in the volume of plasma.
15	Hemophilia	A hereditary blood disease marked by greatly prolonged blood coagulation time, with consequent failure of the blood to clot, and abnormal bleeding that is sometimes accompanied by joint swelling.
15	Hyperventilation	Abnormally fast, deep breathing that sometimes results in fainting.
15	Seizure	A sudden spasm or convulsion, especially one associated with epilepsy.
15	Syncope	Fainting.
15	Topical	Pertaining to a specific area of the body or surface area of the skin.
16	Bilirubin	The yellow breakdown product of normal heme catabolism.
16	Bilirubinemia	The presence of bilirubin in the blood.
16	Breathalyzer	A device for estimating blood alcohol content from a breath sample.
16	Chemical reagent strip	A plastic strip to which chemically treated reagent pads are attached—it allows for the testing of various components of urine.
16	Culture and sensitivity	A microbiology procedure involving the culturing of a specimen on artificial media to detect bacterial or fungal growth, followed by screening for antibiotic sensitivity.
16	Cystoscopy	Visual examination of the urinary bladder using fiber-optic instruments.
16	Filtrate	The fluid remaining after a liquid is passed through a membranous filter.
16	Guaiac	A type of tree resin that chemically reacts to small amounts of blood.
16	Human chorionic gonadotropin	A hormone that normally increases in pregnancy, secreted from the placenta, and prevents spontaneous abortion.
16	Icterus	Jaundice.
16	Ketones	The waste products of fat metabolism.
16	Myoglobinuria	The presence of myoglobin, an oxygen-storing pigment of muscle tissue, in the urine.
16	Oliguria	An abnormally small amount of urine produced, particularly if fluid consumption significantly exceeds urine output; oliguria is often a sign of kidney disease, obstruction of the urinary tract, or dehydration.
16	Phenyl ketones	Metabolites of phenylalanine that when present in urine, signify phenylketonuria, an inborn metabolic disorder.
16	Pheochromocytoma	A vascular tumor of the chromaffin tissue of the adrenal medulla or sympathetic paraganglia, causing persistent or intermittent hypertension.
16	Polyuria	Excessive elimination of urine; polyuria is often a symptom of undiagnosed or poorly controlled diabetes mellitus.
16	Refractometer	An instrument for measuring the refractive index of a substance; used primarily for measuring the refractivity of solutions such as urine.
16	Renal thresholds	Levels above which substances cannot be reabsorbed by the renal tubules and therefore are excreted in the urine.
16	Renin	An enzyme released by the kidneys that raises blood pressure by activating angiotensin.
16	Spinal tap	The puncture of the subarachnoid space of the lumbar area of the spine with a needle to examine and culture cerebrospinal fluid, or to inject a drug or dye for other purposes such as myelography; also called a *lumbar puncture*.
16	Suprapubic	Pertaining to a location above the symphysis pubis (the slightly movable interpubic joint of the pelvis).
16	Urinometer	Any device for determining the specific gravity of urine.
16	Urochrome	A pigment that causes the yellow color in urine.

Chapter	Term	Definition
17	Additive tube	A blood collection tube that contains any type of additive, most commonly an anticoagulant.
17	Agitation	Putting into motion by shaking or stirring.
17	Aldosterone	A hormone that has major effects upon blood volume and pressure.
17	Aliquots	Portions of a total amount of solution.
17	Calcitonin	A hormone that acts to reduce blood calcium, opposing the effects of parathyroid hormone.
17	Dry ice	The solid form of carbon dioxide; it is used as a cooling agent.
17	Pneumatic tube system	A system of carrying items in cylindrical containers, propelled through a network of tubes by compressed air or partial vacuum.
17	Thermolabile	Easily destroyed or altered by heat; also called *heat labile*.
17	Turnaround time	The total time needed for a blood sample to be collected, analyzed, and reported on.
18	Basilic vein	A large superficial vein of the arm that originates on the dorsal (ulnar) side of the hand, traveling up the forearm and upper arm; it is usually visible through the skin.
18	Brachial	Related to the anterior portion of the arm; for example, the brachial vein is accessed via the antecubital space (in front of the elbow).
18	Compliance	Conforming to a rule, law, standard, specification, or policy.
18	Courier	A company or person who delivers mail, packages, or messages.
18	Fainting	Syncope; a sudden, usually temporary loss of consciousness due to insufficient oxygen in the brain.
18	Indices	Collections of information or data.
18	Invasive	Penetrating or breaking the skin, or entering a body cavity.
18	Kickback	An exchange that is illegal or unethical, such as money for a service that should not be charged for.
18	Standing orders	Medication orders from physicians for patients who need continual drug regimens; these are commonly utilized in long-term care facilities so that new prescriptions or orders do not have to be continually written when needed.
19	Bar codes	Optical machine-readable representations of data; they are "read" by scanners known as *bar code readers*.
19	Central processing unit	CPU; the portion of a computer that carries out instructions and is the main functioning component.
19	Data	Information that is processed via a computer.
19	Hardware	The actual programmable part of a computer system and the components that execute activities.
19	Health Insurance Portability and Accountability Act (HIPAA)	The Kassebaum-Kennedy Act, passed in 1996; it was designed to improve the portability and continuity of health insurance coverage; to combat waste, fraud, and abuse in health insurance and health care delivery; to promote the use of medical saving accounts; to improve access to long-term care services and coverage; and to simplify the administration of health insurance; as well as to serve other purposes.
19	Input	Any data entered into a computer or data processing system.
19	Networked	Interconnected so that various computers and other data processing devices can communicate over varying ranges of distance.
19	Output	Transmitted information from a computer or data processing system.
19	Passwords	Secret words or strings of characters used by individuals to gain access to computers or data processing systems.
19	Personal digital assistants	Palmtop computers that function as information managers; they commonly integrate with computers, data processing systems, and the Internet to share information.
19	Random access memory	RAM; a form of computer data storage wherein information can be accessed at random.
19	Software	Computer programs and related data.
19	Terminal	An electronic hardware device used for entering and displaying computer data.
19	Universal serial bus	A specification to establish communication between computers and other devices.

Index

A

abbreviations
commonly used, 30–32*t*
related to urinalysis, 170
abdominal aorta, 45
abdominal pain panel, reference laboratory values, 211
ABO blood groups, 73–74, 74*f*, 74*t*
abruptio placentae, 53, 61
accession, 124
accidental arterial puncture, 190
accuracy, 6
acetaminophen, toxic level of, 212
Acetest, 174
acetylsalicylic acid (aspirin), toxic level of, 212
acid-base balance, 156
activating safety device, 116, 116*t*
active listening, 15, 18
acute lymphocytic leukemia, 59
acute myelogenous leukemia, 60
acute myeloid leukemia, 60
additive, 112
additive contamination, 128, 129*t*
additive tubes, 111*t*
additives, 109
adulterants, specimen tampering with, 147
advance directives, 5–6
aerobic bacteria, 86
aerobic bottle, 157*f*, 156
agglutination, 63, 73
agranulocytes
defined, 63
reference laboratory values, 212
airborne precautions, 93, 100
air-tube systems, 197
alanine aminotransferase (ALT), 77, 78
albumin (Alb)
defined, 63, 77
hepatic profile, 78

normal urine value for, 212
as plasma constituent, 69
albumin/globulin ratio (A/G ratio), 78
alcohol, toxic level of, 212
alcohol "prep pad," 111
alcohol testing
chain of custody and, 147
uncooperative patients, 163–164
aldosterone, defined, 179
algae, 83, 84
aliquot, 171, 179
alkaline phosphatase (ALP), 77, 78
Allen test, 158
allergic response, 163
allergies to latex, 99, 100*f*
ALP, reference laboratory values, 211
alpha-stat test, 158
ALT (SGPT), reference laboratory values, 211
American Association of Allied Health Professionals
(AAAHP), 3
American Certification Agency (ACA), 3
American Medical Association (AMA), 188
American Medical Technologists (AMT), 3
American Osteopathic Association (AOA), 4
American Society for Clinical Laboratory Science (ASCLS), 3
American Society for Clinical Pathology (ASCP), 3, 11
American Society of Phlebotomy Technicians (ASPT), 3
amniotic fluid embolism, 61
amniotic fluid specimens, 177
amphetamine, toxic level of, 212
amylase
normal serum value for, 211
normal urine value for, 212
anabolic steroids, 149
anaerobic bacteria, 86
anaerobic blood culture bottle, 157*f*, 156
analytes, 11, 141
analytical, 6
anaphylactic shock, 57, 161, 163

anastomoses, 40
anatomical pathology, 9
anatomy and physiology, medical terminology for,
    29–30t
anemias, 58–59, 66
aneurysms, 57, 58f
angina pectoris, 53, 54
anoxia, 53, 93
antecubital, 123
anterior intercostal arteries, 45
anterior tibial artery, 48
anterior tibial vein, 48
antibiotic removal device (ARD), 156
antibiotic therapy, Gram stain results and, 86
antibodies, 63, 102
antibodies (agglutinins), 73, 74f, 74t
anticoagulant therapy, phlebotomy during, 158–159,
    163
anticoagulants
    defined, 109, 161
    in evacuated tubes, 113–114, 114f
anticonvulsant, toxic level of, 212
antigen D, 75
antigens (agglutinogens), 63, 73, 74f, 74t, 102
antiglycolytic agent, 109, 114
anti-HIV, 80
Anti-Kickback Law (1972), 188
antinuclear antibody (ANA), 80
antiseptics, 93, 101, 111
antistreptolysin O (ASO) titer, 80
anuria, 171
aorta, 35, 39
aortic arch, 35, 45
aortic semilunar valve, 41
aortic valve, 35, 39
aperture, 83
aplastic anemia, 59
appendicitis, 69
aPTT, reference laboratory values, 211
arrhythmia, 53, 55
arterial blood gases (ABGs), 150, 156, 158
arterial punctures
    accidental, 163
    for blood gas specimens, 150
arteries, 35, 41, 44–48, 46f, 47f
arterioles, 35, 36, 41
arteriosclerosis, 57
arthralgia, 53, 59
arthropod, 83
arthropod vectors, 87
ASAP test status, 126t
ascending aorta, 41
ascending lumbar veins, 48
asepsis, 93, 100
aseptic techniques, 93, 100–101
asexual reproduction, 83, 87
aspartate aminotransferase (AST), 77, 78

assays, 141
Association of Genetic Technologists (AGT), 3
AST (SGOT), reference laboratory values, 211
atherosclerosis, 53, 54, 55f, 57, 73
athletic testing, 149
atria, 35, 38
atrioventricular node (AV node), 35
atrioventricular valve (AV valve), 38
atypical pneumonia, 80
auricles, 38
autologous blood donations, 146–147
AV bundle (bundle of His), 35, 40
axillary artery, 45
axillary vein, 48, 127
azygos vein, 48

B

B cells, 63, 69
bacilli, 83, 84–87
bacteremia
    blood culture collection for, 157f, 111, 111f, 156
    defined, 153
bacteria, 83, 84–87
bacterial cell wall, 84–85, 85f
bacteriophage, 87
Bacteroides fragilis, 86
bagged urine specimens, 171
bandages, 118
bands (white blood cells), 68
bar codes, 124, 193, 197, 197f
barber poles, 2
barbitals, toxic level of, 212
barrier precautions, 110
basal state specimens, 145
basic metabolic panel (BMP), 11, 188
basilar artery, 45
basilic vein, 48, 123, 127, 162, 187, 190
basophils
    defined, 63
    function of, 68
    reference laboratory values, 212
BD Vacutainer urine collection tube, 171
benzalkonium chloride, 109, 111
bevel, 115
bifurcation, 123, 134
bilirubin
    defined, 63, 167
    in RBC life cycle, 66
    reference laboratory values, 211
    in urinalysis
bilirubin (BILI), 78
bilirubin specimens, 154–155
bilirubinemia, 167, 171
bilirubinuria, 174
biliverdin, 63, 66

bilobed, 68
binocular microscopes, 88
bioassays, 88
bioethics, 1, 3
biohazard symbol, 103, 103*f*
biologic agents, 102
biologic hazards, 102
bleeding time test, 145
blind patients, caring for, 17
blood
    composition of, 64, 65*f*, 71*f*
    plasma, 69–70
    platelets, 69
    red blood cells (RBCs), 65–66, 66*f*, 67*f*, 68*f*
    white blood cells (WBCs), 64, 66–69
blood alcohol testing, 147
blood bank
    common tests performed in, 10
    laboratory equipment in, 194–196, 194*f*, 195*f*, 196*f*
blood circulation, 44–48
blood clotting, 71, 72–73, 73*f*
blood collection tubes, for common laboratory tests, 203–206
blood cultures, 111, 111*f*, 156
blood differential, 10
blood donation, 146–147
"blood doping," 149
blood films, 139
blood gas analysis, 150, 151*f*
blood gases, 69
blood glucose, 70, 70*t*
blood groups, 73–74, 74*f*, 74*t*
blood pressure, 43–44, 44*f*
blood profile, 77, 78
blood spot collection, 155
blood transfusions
    hypersensitivity reaction, 60
    misidentification error, 126–127
    role of blood groups in, 73–75, 75*t*
    sample consent form, 213
blood types, 73–75
blood urea nitrogen
    defined, 77
    in renal profile, 78
blood urea nitrogen (BUN), reference laboratory values, 211
blood vessels, 41–43, 43*t*
blood volume, 35, 44
blood-borne pathogen (BBP), 93, 100
Blood-borne Pathogens (BBP) Standard, 102–103, 103, 104
blood-drawing chairs, 109, 118–119, 119*f*
bloodletting, 1, 2, 2*f*
body language. *see* nonverbal communication
bone marrow hypoplasia, 59
Bowman capsule, 168
brachial artery, 45, 158, 158*f*

brachial vein, 48
brachiocephalic trunk, 45
brachiocephalic veins, 48
Braille system, 17
"breaking the seal," 132
Breathalyzer, 167, 176, 176*f*
"buffy coat," 71
bullets, 117, 154–155
burden of proof, 5
burning sensation, 162
burnout, 20
butterfly collection systems, 116–117, 116*f*
butterfly needles, 109, 110

C

calcitonin, 179
calcium (Ca++)
    normal urine value for, 212
    reference laboratory values, 211
calibration, 6
Candida albicans, 87
cannula, 115, 141
capillaries, 35
capillary collections
    finger sticks, 134, 137, 137*f*, 138*f*
    heel-sticks, 134–137, 135–136*f*, 137*t*
capillary punctures, 78, 123
capsid layer, 87
capsomeres, 87
carbohydrate metabolism, 79
carbonic anhydrase (CAH), 65
carboxyhemoglobin, toxic level of, 212
carcinogenic, 93
carcinogenic chemicals, 96
cardiac arrest, 56
cardiac arrhythmias, 55
cardiac conduction system, 35, 40
cardiac cycle, 35, 40
cardiac output, 35, 43
cardiac profile, 79–80
cardiac veins, 35, 40
cardiogenic shock, 57
cardiomyopathy, 56
cardiopulmonary arrest, 56
cardiopulmonary resuscitation (CPR), 56, 93, 106
cardiopulmonary system, reference laboratory values, 211
cardiovascular system
    aortic branches, 45*t*
    arteries, 46*f*, 47*f*
    blood pressure, 44*f*
    blood vessel characteristics, 43*t*
    carotid branches, 48*t*
    circulatory system, 37*f*, 41–51
    heart, 37–41

cardiovascular system *(Cont.)*
    medical terminology for, 26, 26–28*t*, 26*t*, 30, 30–31*t*
    overview, 36–37
    veins, 49*f*, 50*f*
carditis, 56
carotid sinuses, 35, 45
carrier, 94
carryover, 128
casts, in urine, 175, 175*f*
catheterized urine specimens, 170
caustic, defined, 9, 94
caustic chemicals, 96
celiac disease
    defined, 53
    iron deficiency anemia and, 58
cell-mediated immunity, 69, 102
Celsius conversion formula, 201
Center for Phlebotomy Education (CPE), 190
Centers for Disease Control and Prevention (CDC), 94, 100, 102
Centers for Medicare and Medicaid Services (CMS), 4
central processing unit (CPU), 193, 196
central venous therapy lines, 141, 151
centrifugal force, 118
centrifuges, 94, 95, 96*f*, 118, 118*f*, 119*f*
cephalic vein, 48, 123, 127
cerebral arterial circle, 36, 45
cerebral thrombosis, 73
cerebrospinal fluid (CSF), reference laboratory values, 211
certifications, for phlebotomists, 3
certified medical assistants, 11
certified medical laboratory scientists, 9, 11
certified medical laboratory technicians, 11
Certified Phlebotomy Technician (CPT), 3
chain of custody
    defined, 1, 141
    for drug testing, 80
    for forensic specimens, 147
    preventative law and, 5
chain of infection, 94, 101–102, 101*f*
"Chem 8" test
    analytes included, 11
    reference laboratory values, 211
chemical disposal, 98
chemical hazards, 96–99
chemical reagent strip, 167, 172, 172*f*, 173*f*, 174
chemical safety labels, 96, 98*f*
chemical spill cleanup, 98, 99*f*
chemistry laboratory, common tests performed in, 10–11, 78–80
chemistry panel, 78, 79*f*
Chief Compliance Officer, 189
Chlamydiae, 86–87
chlorhexidine, 109
chlorhexidine gluconate, 111
chordae tendineae, 36, 38

Christmas disease, 61
chronic lymphocytic leukemia, 59–60
chronic myelogenous leukemia, 60
circle of Willis, 45
citrates, 113
civil law, 1, 4–5
Civil Monetary Penalties laws (1990, etc.), 188
CK-MB, 80
classic hemophilia, 61
clean-catch midstream urine specimen, 169
Clinical and Laboratory Standards Institute (CLSI), 4, 78, 94, 102, 180–181, 190
Clinical Laboratory Improvement Act of 1988 (CLIA, '88), 4, 188
clinical laboratory scientists, 11
clinical pathology, 9
clonal proliferation, 60
clot activators, 71, 109, 112
clotting disorders, 60–61
clotting factors, 71
coagulation, 63
coagulation cascade, 109, 114
coagulation phases, 70
coagulation studies, 10
coagulation tests, reference laboratory values, 211
Coban, 118
cocci, 83, 84–87
coccobacilli, 84–87
Coflex, 118
cold agglutinins, 80
collapsed veins, 163
collateral circulation, 40, 158
collecting tubules, 169
collection priority, 124, 126*t*
College of American Pathologists (CAP), 3, 4, 94, 102
colloid osmotic pressure, 43, 69
colony-stimulating factors (CSFS), 63, 66
colors, of stoppers for evacuated tubes, 113–114, 114*f*
combining forms (medical terminology)
    cardiovascular system related, 26*t*
    defined, 26
comfort zones, 17
commensalism, 88
common carotid arteries, 45
common iliac arteries, 45–48
common iliac veins, 48
common laboratory tests, 203–206
communicable disease, 94, 100
communication, types of
    nonverbal, 17–18
    telephone and computer, 18–19, 19*f*
    verbal, 16–17
    written, 18
communication barriers, 20
communication cycle, 15–16, 16*f*
communication skills, improving, 19
Complete Blood Count (CBC), 10, 188, 212

compliance
  defined, 187
  effects of, 189–190
  formal monitoring for, 187
  laboratory plan for, 189
  legal actions in phlebotomy, 190
  need for in phlebotomy, 187–189
  preventing lawsuits, 190
  regulations, 187–188
comprehensive metabolic panel, 188
compromised host, 102
computer communication skills, patient care and, 18–19
computer requisitions, 124
computer technology
  communications, 18, 198
  data storage, 196–197, 197*f*
  hardware, 194*f*, 196, 196*f*
  security, 198
  software, 196
  uses in clinical laboratories, 194–196
condenser, 83
confidentiality
  defined, 15
  patient care and, 20
congenital lymphedema, 60
consent, sample consent form, 213
Consumer Bill of Rights and Responsibilities, 6
contact precautions, 94, 100
continuing education units (CEUs), 3
conversion tables, 201
convulsions, 162
coronary arteries, 36, 39
coronary artery disease, 54
coronary artery spasm, 54
coronary sinus, 36, 38
coronary thrombosis, 73
Corporate Compliance Committee, 189
courier services, 187, 189
CPK-MB/CPK relative index, reference laboratory values, 211
CPK-total, reference laboratory values, 211
C-reactive protein (CRP), 80
creatine kinase (CK), 77, 78, 80, 212
crimes, 5
criminal law, 1, 5
cross-contamination, 128
crystals, in urine, 175, 175*f*
cultural diversity, patient care and, 18
culture and sensitivity (C&S)
  defined, 167
  for urine specimens, 170, 171
cupping, 2
Current Procedural Terminology (CPT), 189
Cushing's syndrome, 141, 143
cusps, 38
Custody and Control Form (CCF), 147, 148*f*

D

data, defined, 193
data storage, 196–197, 197*f*
D-Dimer, reference laboratory values, 211
decontamination, 106
deep brachial artery, 45
deep vein thrombosis, 57
defense mechanisms, 1, 15, 20
deoxyhemoglobin, 65
Department of Health and Human Services (HHS), 147, 189
Department of Transportation (DOT), 139, 148–149
dermal puncture, 134
descending aorta, 45
dextroamphetamine, toxic level of, 212
diabetes mellitus, 141, 142
diagnosis, in medical microbiology, 88
diastole, 36, 41
diastolic blood pressure, 36, 41, 43
diet suppressants, toxic level of, 212
differential white blood cell count (diff), 69
Dilantin, toxic level of, 212
diplococci, 83, 84–87
dipotassium EDTA, 114
dipstick, 172
direct access testing (DAT), 124
direct transmission, 101
discrimination, patient care and, 20
disease transmission
  decontamination, 106
  disinfection, 106
  hand washing, 104–105
  prevention of, 104
  sanitation, 105–106
  sterilization, 106
disinfectants, 94, 106
disinfection, 106
disseminated intravascular coagulation, 61
distal convoluted tubule, 168
diurnal variation, 141, 144
double bagging, 94
driving under the influence (DUI), 147, 176
droplet precautions, 94, 100
drug testing
  employee testing, 147–149
  patient preparation for, 80
  reference laboratory values, 212
  sample handling, 80
  specimen tampering, 147
  uncooperative patients, 163–164
  urine tests for, 176
drug therapy, Gram stain results and, 86
dry ice, defined, 179
duty of care, 4
dysrhythmia, 53, 55

E

eclampsia, 54, 61
8-h urine specimens, 170
electrical hazards, 96
electrocardiogram (EKG), 3, 36, 40
electrolyte panel (lytes), 188, 212
electrolytes, 70
emboli, 57
embolus, 63, 73
employee testing, 147–149
endocardium, 36, 38
endothelium, 41
engineering controls
    BBP Standard for, 103
    needle safety device, 112, 112f
    sharp with engineered sharps injury protection
        (SESIP), 120–121
enteric disease, diagnosis of, 177
enunciation, patient care and, 17
Environmental Protection Agency (EPA), 94
eosinophils
    defined, 63
    function of, 68
    reference laboratory values, 212
epicardium, 36, 40
epidemiology, 88
epithelial cells, in urine, 175, 175f
Epstein-Barr virus (EBV), 80
erythroblastosis fetalis, 75
erythrocyte sedimentation rate (ESR), 77, 80
erythrocytes. see red blood cells (RBCs)
erythropoiesis, 63, 65, 65–66, 66f, 67f
erythropoietin, 63, 65, 168
Escherichia coli, 86, 100, 174
ethics
    defined, 1
    issues affecting phlebotomists, 3
    medical ethics, 5
ethylenediaminetetraacetic acid (EDTA), 78, 113, 123,
        134
etiquette
    patient care and, 17
    telephone communication skills, 18, 19f
eukaryotes, 83, 84
evacuated tubes, 109, 111–112, 111f, 112–114, 114f
evacuation plans, 95, 95f
evidence collection, 149, 149t
excessive bleeding, 163
expiration dates, 128–129
exposure control, 104
exposure control plan, 103, 104
exposure potential, 104
external iliac artery, 45
external iliac vein, 48
external jugular veins, 48

exudates, 102
eyewash stations, 103–104, 104f

F

facultative anaerobes, 86
Fahrenheit conversion formula, 201
fainting, 162, 163f, 187, 190
False Claims Act (1986), 188
family members, interacting with, 19–20
fasting blood glucose level, 143–144
fasting test status, 126t
fasting tests, 145
FDPs, reference laboratory values, 211
febrile agglutinins, 80
fecal fat test, 177
fecal occult blood test, 177
fecal specimens, 177
federal drug-testing programs, 147
felonies, 5
femoral artery, 48
femoral vein, 48
fermentation, 83, 87
fibrin, 63, 71
fibrinogen, 63, 69, 211
fibroblasts, 72
filtrate, 167, 168
finger-stick blood collection, lancets for, 117, 117t
finger-stick capillary collections, 134, 137, 137f, 138f
fire escape route, 95, 95f
fire hazards, 95–96, 95f, 96f, 97f
first impressions, 15
first-voided morning urine specimens, 170
"flash" of blood, 132, 134
fluorescent treponemal antibody absorption test, 80
fluoride/oxalates, 113
foam, 171
folic acid, 66
folic acid deficiency anemia, 58
fomites, 94, 101
forensic specimens, 149, 149t
Frank-Starling law of the heart, 44
fraud and abuse laws, 187, 188
friends of patients, interacting with, 19–20
"fruit" odor, 172
FTA-ABS, 80
full blood count, 10
functional syncytium, 36, 41
fungi, 87

G

g force, 123, 139
galactosemia, 155

Galen, 2
gamma globulins, 69
gamma glutamyl transferase (GGT), 78
gastrectomy, 54, 59
gastric veins, 48
gauge, 109, 112
gauze pads, 117–118
geriatric phlebotomy, 155–156, 156t
germs, 84
gestational diabetes, 141, 142, 143
G-hemoglobin, 144
G-Hgb, 144
globin, 66
globules, defined, 153
globulins, 63, 69
glomerulus, 168
gloves, 110
glucometers, 142, 142f
glucose
    normal serum value for, 211
    normal urine value for, 212
    pathogenic blood levels, 70t
    in plasma, 69–70
    testing for, 80
glucose tests, 142, 143t
glucose tolerance testing (GTT), 142–143, 144f
glycolysis, 109, 141, 143
glycolytic inhibitor, 110, 114
glycosuria, 173
glycosylated hemoglobin, 144
Gram stains, 85–86, 86f
gram-negative bacteria, 84–85, 85f, 86t
gram-negative intracellular bacteria, 86
gram-positive bacteria, 84–85, 85f, 86t
granular casts, 175, 175f
granulocytes, 64, 68, 212
granulocytic leukemia, 60
Graves' disease
    defined, 54, 77
    pernicious anemia and, 59
    thyroid profile and, 80
growth factors, 88
growth-response assays, 88
guaiac, defined, 167
guaiac test, 177

H

hand washing, 103, 104–105, 105f
hardware, 193, 194f
Hazard Communication Standard, 97
Hazardous Materials Shipping Regulations, 139
hazards
    biologic, 102
    chemical, 96–99

electrical, 96
fire, 95–96
fire hazards, 95–96
mechanical, 96
in medical laboratories, 12
physical, 94–98, 94–99
potential in medical laboratories, 12
wastes, 98, 103, 189
HazCom, defined, 94
HazCom standard, 97
HbA1c test, 144
HBV vaccination, 103
HDL, reference laboratory values, 212
Health Care Financing Administration (HCFA), 4, 189
Health Insurance Portability and Accountability Act
        (HIPAA), 188–189, 193, 198
hearing-impaired patients, caring for, 17
heart
    blood flow through, 38f
    conduction system of, 40–41, 40f
    described, 37–40
    functions of, 41
    heart valves, 39f
    structures of, 38–40
heart attack, 55, 79–80
heart failure, 56
heart murmur, 41
heel stick, defined, 123
heel warmer, 135
heel-stick capillary collections, 134–137, 135–136f,
        137t, 154–155
hemarthrosis, defined, 54
hematocrit (HCT)
    defined, 64
    reference laboratory values, 212
hematology
    common tests performed in, 10
    defined, 9, 64
hematoma, 161, 162, 162f, 190
hematomas, 72
hematopoietic stem cells, 54, 60
hematuria, 174
heme, 66
hemochromatosis, 2, 54, 59, 66, 142
hemoconcentration, 123, 127, 161, 162
hemocytoblasts, 69
hemoglobin, 10, 64, 65
hemoglobin (HbA1c) testing, 144
hemoglobin (Hgb), reference laboratory values, 212
hemoglobin S, defined, 54
hemoglobin S gene, 59
hemolysins, 75
hemolysis
    avoiding in samples, 78, 135
    defined, 1, 59, 123
    specimen rejections for, 139

hemolytic anemia, 59
hemolytic disease of the newborn (HDN), 74, 154
hemolyze, 110, 112
hemophilia, 61, 161, 163
hemophilia A, defined, 54
hemorrhagic anemia, 59
hemostasis
    bleeding time test for, 146
    defined, 64, 142
    process of, 70–71
heparin, 68, 113, 114
heparin lock, 142, 150
hepatic function panel, 188, 211
hepatic portal system, 36, 48
hepatic portal vein, 48
hepatic profile, 78
hepatic veins, 48
hepatitis B surface antigen (HBsAg), 80
hepatitis B virus (HBV), risk of exposure to, 102–103
hepatitis C virus (HCV), risk of exposure to, 102–103
high-complexity tests, 4
high-density lipoprotein (HDL), 78
Hippocrates, 2
histamine, 68
Hodgkin's lymphoma, 60
hub, 115
human chorionic gonadotropin (HCG), 80, 167, 176
human immunodeficiency virus (HIV), risk of exposure
        to, 102–103
humoral immunity, 69, 102
hyaline casts, 175, 175f
hypercalcemia, 41
hyperglycemia, 70, 80
hyperinsulinism, 142
hyperkalemia, 40
hypersensitivity reaction, in transfusion incompatibility,
        60
hypertension, 55–56
hypertrophied, defined, 54
hyperventilation, 161, 162, 163f
hypocalcemia, 41
hypoglycemia, 70, 143
hypokalemia, 40
hypoplasia, 54, 59
hypoplastic anemia, 54, 59
hypothyroidism, 77, 78
hypovolemic shock, 57

I

icterus, defined, 167
Ictotest, 174
immune surveillance, 69
immunology, 9, 88. see also serology laboratory
immunology laboratory, 10
in vitro, 9

indices, 187
indirect transmission, 101
industrial fermentations, 88
ineffective communication methods, 19
infantile cretinism, 77, 80
infant/pediatric phlebotomy stations, 119, 120f
infarction, 73
infection, 69, 100
infection control
    chain of infection, 101–102
    and disease processes, 88
    nosocomial infections, 100–101
    overview, 94
    pathogens and infections, 100
infection control programs, 94, 100
infectious agent, 101
infectious mononucleosis, 80
infectious wastes, 189
infective dose, 88
inferior hemiazygos veins, 48
inferior vena cava, 36, 38
inflammatory conditions, 80
information release, compliance and, 190
input, 193, 196
insulinoma, 143
intensive care unit (ICU), 94, 100
intentional torts, 4
interatrial septum, 38
interleukins, 64, 66
internal iliac artery, 48
internal iliac veins, 48
internal jugular veins, 48
internal thoracic artery, 45
International Classification for Diseases (ICD-9-M), 189
international normalization ratio (INR), 10
interpersonal skills, 19
interpersonal space, 17
interventricular septum, 38
intimate space, 17
invasive, defined, 187
invasive procedure, 190
iron deficiency anemia, 58
ischemia, defined, 54
isolation procedures, 94, 100

J

jaundice, 153, 154–155
Joint Commission, 3, 4, 124

K

Kassebaum-Kennedy Act, defined, 193
Kelvin conversion formula, 201
ketone bodies, 174

ketones, 167, 172
ketonuria, 174
kickback, defined, 187
kidney function. *see* renal profile
Kupffer cells, 48

L

laboratory equipment, types of, 194–196, 194*f*, 195*f*, 196*f*
laboratory requisition forms, 189, 190
laboratory technologists, 11
laboratory tests
   reference values, 211–212
   specimen requirements for common tests, 203–206
laboratory-trained phlebotomists, 11
lancets, 110, 117, 117*f*, 117*t*
language barriers
   patient care and, 16
   in patient identification, 124–125
laser lancet, 117
lateral, defined, 123
lateral flow immunoassay test, 176
lateral surface, 134
latex allergies, 99, 100*f*, 118, 163
latex allergy, 125
laws
   affecting phlebotomists, 4–5
   defined, 1
LDH-1, reference laboratory values, 211
LDH-total, reference laboratory values, 211
LDL, reference laboratory values, 212
lead, toxic level of, 212
leeches, 2
left atrioventricular (bicuspid or mitral) valve, 41
left subclavian vein, 48
legal issues. *see also* compliance
   affecting phlebotomists, 3, 4–5
   blood alcohol testing, 147
   chain of custody, 147
leukemias, 59–60
leukocytes, 64, 66
leukocytosis, 64, 69
leukopenia, 64, 69
lipemia, 145
lipemic, defined, 142
lipid profile, 78, 212
lipoproteins
   in bacterial cell wall, 85
   defined, 77
   lipid profile, 78
listening skills, 18
lithium, toxic level of, 212
lithium heparin, 114
liver function. *see* hepatic profile
living wills, 5–6

loop of Henle, 168, 169
low-density lipoprotein (LDL), 78
Luer lock, 115
lumbar artery, 45
lumbar puncture, 177
lumen, 115
lymph, 54, 60
lymphangitis, 60
lymphatic diseases, 60
lymphedema, 60
lymphoblasts, 54, 59
lymphocytes, 64, 69, 212
lymphomas, 60

M

macronutrients, 88
macrophages, 64, 66, 68, 102
malfeasance, 5
malpractice, defined, 1
malpractice claim, 5, 127
manual differential (diff) tests, 139
March of Dimes, 155
mast cells, 64, 68
mastectomy, 54, 60
Material Safety Data Sheets (MSDSs), 94, 97, 99*f*
mechanical hazards, 96
Med Emerg test status, 126*t*
median cubital vein, 127
medical asepsis, 104
medical code of ethics, 5
medical errors, 126–127
medical laboratories. *see also* compliance; safety
   divisions within, 10–11
   employee behavior standards, 12
   medical term abbreviations, 31–32*t*
   personnel, 11–12
   potential hazards in, 12
   result reporting, 182
   specimen processing, 182
medical laboratory assistants, 11
Medical Laboratory Scientist (MLS), 3, 11
medical malpractice, 5
medical microbiology, 88
medical necessity, 189
medical professional liability, 5
medical technologists, 11
medical technology, 3
medical terminology
   anatomy and physiology related, 29–30*t*
   cardiovascular system related, 26, 26–28*t*, 30, 30–31*t*
   combining forms, 26, 26*t*
   laboratory and phlebotomy related, 31–32*t*
   patient care and, 16
   prefixes, 23, 24*t*
   suffixes, 23, 24–25*t*

medical terminology *(Cont.)*
  term construction, 23
  word roots, 23
medically necessary tests, 187–188
Medicare and Medicaid, 187, 188
megakaryoblasts, 69
megakaryocytes, 64, 69
megaloblastic anemia, 54, 58
mercury, toxic level of, 212
metabolite, 176
methamphetamine, toxic level of, 212
metric conversion tables, 201
microbes, 84
microbiology, defined, 84
microbiology laboratory, common tests performed in,
    11
microcollection, 123, 134
microcollection tubes, 117, 118*f*
microhematocrit capillary tubes, 110, 117, 118*f*, 153,
    154
micronutrients, 88
microorganisms
  classifications of, 84–87
  functions of, 84
  growth of, 87–88
  medical microbiology and, 88
micropipettes, 110, 117
microscopes
  care of, 89
  defined, 83
  lenses, 88–89
  light source, 89
  stage, 89
  structure, 88
  use of, 89
microtainer tubes, 117, 123, 137
midstream voided urine specimen, 170
military time, 215
Milroy's disease, 60
misdemeanors, 5
misfeasance, 5
misidentification error, 126–127
mislabeling error, 126–127, 190
mitral valve, 36, 38
mitral valve prolapse, 56
mode of transmission, 94, 101–102, 106
moderate-complexity tests, 4
monocular microscopes, 88
monocytes, 64, 68, 212
mononuclear leukocytes, reagent strips and, 174
morphologic shapes (bacterial), 84–87, 84*f*
"mousy" odor, 172
multiple myeloma, 78
multiple-sample needles, 110, 115
mutualism, 88
Mycobacterium tuberculosis, 86, 102

mycology, 83, 87
Mycoplasmae, 86–87
myelocytic leukemia, 60
myocardial infarction (MI), 54, 55, 55*f*, 79–80
myocardium, 36, 38
myoglobinuria, 167, 174
myxedema
  defined, 54
  pernicious anemia and, 59

N

National Accrediting Agency for Clinical Laboratory
    Sciences (NAACLS), 3, 4, 207–209
National Center for Competency Testing (NCCT), 3
National Collegiate Athletic Association (NCAA), 149
National Committee for Clinical Laboratory Standards
    (NCCLS), 4
National Credentialing Agency for Laboratory
    Personnel (NCA), 3
National Fire Protection Association (NFPA), 95, 97, 99*f*
National Healthcareer Association (NHA), 3
National Institute on Drug Abuse (NIDA), 80
National Phlebotomy Association (NPA), 3
Nationally Certified Phlebotomy Technician (NCPT), 3
natural killer (NK) cells, 64, 69
needle gauges, 115–116, 116*t*
needle holders, 110, 112, 112*f*, 113*f*
needle phobia, 125
needle safety, 120–121, 121*f*
needles, 112, 112*f*, 113*f*, 115–116, 115*f*, 116*f*, 116*t*
needlestick injury prevention, 104
Needlestick Safety and Prevention Act, 103
negative communication, patient care and, 18
negligence torts, 4–5
neonatal screening, 154–155
nephron, 168
nerve damage, 162, 190
nerve injury, 127
networked, defined, 193
neurogenic shock, 57
neutralization of contaminants, 106
neutrophils, 64, 68
newborn/neonatal testing, 154–155
nonadditive tubes, 111*t*
nonfeasance, 5
non-Hodgkin's lymphoma, 60
nonprotein nitrogenous substances, 64, 70
nonverbal communication, patient care and, 17–18
normal flora, 84, 100
normal microbiota, 84
nosocomial infections, 94, 100–101
NPO test status, 126*t*
NSAID, defined, 54
NSAID use, 61

O

obese patients, phlebotomy for, 159
Occupational Exposure to Bloodborne Pathogens
        program, 102
Occupational Safety and Health Administration
        (OSHA), 12, 94, 97, 102, 110
Office of the Inspector General (OIG), 187, 189
oliguria, 167, 171
opportunism, 88
oral glucose tolerance test (OGTT), 143
order of draw, 128, 129t, 134
osmolality, normal urine value for, 212
osmotic pressure, 69
output, defined, 193
oval fat bodies, 175
overfilled tubes, 112–113, 113–114
oxygen-carrying capacity, 65
oxyhemoglobin, 65

P

pace, of speech, patient care and, 17
pacemaker, 36, 40
packed cell volume (PCV), 10
palpate (feel), 127
pancytopenia, 54, 59
panels, 78, 79f
papillary muscles, 36, 38
papoose board, 154
parasitism, 88
partial thromboplastin time (PTT), 10, 211
passwords, 193, 198
pathogenic, defined, 83
pathogenic microorganisms, 84, 86t
pathogenicity, 88
pathogens, 100
pathologists
    defined, 9
    described, 11
pathology, 9
patient care
    compassion and empathy in, 16
    cultural diversity and, 18
    language barriers and, 16–17
    sense-impairment and, 17
    warm welcomes and, 15
    young patients, 17, 18
Patient Care Partnership, 6
patient identification, 124, 126–127
patient preparation
    drug testing, 80
    lipid profile, 78
    for venipuncture, 124–127
Patient Self-Determination Act, 5–6

Patient's Bill of Rights, 6
peak, defined, 142
peak level, 149
pediatric patients
    bagged urine specimens, 171
    personal space and, 18
    phlebotomy for, 154, 154f
    uncooperative patients, 163–164
peptidoglycan, 84, 85f
pericardium, 36, 38
peripheral resistance, 36, 44
periplasm, 83, 84–85, 85f
pernicious anemia, 58–59
personal digital assistants (PDAs), 193, 194
personal prejudice, patient care and, 20
personal protective equipment (PPE), 97, 99f, 110–111,
        110f, 128
personal space, 17
personnel
    employee behavior standards, 12
    in medical laboratories, 11–12
petechiae, 163
pH
    normal urine value for, 212
    urine test for, 173, 174f
phagocytic properties, 68
phagocytosis, 102
phalanges, 137
phenmetrazine, toxic level of, 212
phenyl ketones, 167, 173
phenylketonuria, 172
phenylketonuria (PKU), 154–155
pheochromocytoma, 167
Philadelphia chromosome, 60
phlebitis, 57
phlebotomists
    certifications for, 3
    ethical issues affecting, 3
    expected behavior standards, 12
    first impressions and, 15
    as lab employees in physicians' offices, 189–190
    laws affecting, 4–5
    NAACLS competencies, 207–209
    necessary skills, 2–3
    responsibilities of, 3
    stressful work environments of, 20
phlebotomy. see also phlebotomy equipment;
        phlebotomy procedures
    compliance in, 187–188
    complications of, 161–164, 162f
    defined, 1
    history of, 2
    medical term abbreviations, 31–32t
    Patient Self-Determination Act, 5–6
    Patient's Bill of Rights, 6
    quality systems in, 6–7

phlebotomy *(Cont.)*
 regulation of, 4
 specimen requirements for common tests, 203–206
phlebotomy equipment, 110–121
 antiseptics, 111
 bandages, 118
 blood-drawing chairs, 118–119, 119*f*
 butterfly collection systems, 116–117, 116*f*
 centrifuges, 118, 118*f*, 119*f*
 evacuated tubes, 111–112, 111*f*, 112–114, 114*f*
 gauze pads, 117–118
 gloves, 110
 infant/pediatric phlebotomy station, 119, 120*f*
 lancets, 117, 117*f*, 117*t*
 microcollection tubes, 117, 118*f*
 micropipettes, 117
 needle holders, 112, 112*f*, 113*f*
 needles, 112*f*, 113*f*, 115–116, 115*f*, 116*f*, 116*t*
 personal protective equipment (PPE), 110–111, 110*f*
 sharps containers, 120, 120*f*
 specimen collection trays, 119–120, 120*f*
 syringes, 114–115, 115*f*, 116*f*
 tourniquets, 111
 venoscopes, 111
phlebotomy procedures, 124–139
 blood films, 139
 draw order, 129*t*
 finger-stick capillary collections, 134, 137, 137*f*, 138*f*
 heel-stick capillary collections, 134–137, 135–136*f*, 137*t*
 patient preparation, 124–127
 recollection of specimens, 139, 162
 specimen handling, 137–139
 test orders/requisitions, 124, 125*f*, 126*f*, 126*t*
 veins of the arm, 127*f*
 venipuncture preparation, 127
 venipuncture with butterfly set, 133–134
 venipuncture with evacuated tube, 128–131, 130–131*f*
 venipuncture with syringe, 132–133, 132–133*f*
Phlebotomy Technician (PBT), 3
photosynthesis, 87
phrenic artery, 45
pH-stat test, 158
physical hazards, 94–99
 chemical hazards, 96–99
 electrical hazards, 96
 fire hazards, 95–96
 mechanical hazards, 96
physical impairments, as barriers to communication, 20
physician-performed microscopy tests, 4
physiochemical, 83, 87
pitch, defined, 15
pitch, of speech, communication and, 16
plaintiff, 5
plantar, defined, 123
plantar surface, 135

plasma
 appearance of, 72
 composition of, 69–70
 defined, 64
 obtaining for testing, 71, 113–114, 114*f*, 118
plasma cells, 64, 69
plasma lipids, 70
plasma nutrients, 69
plasma proteins, 64, 69, 70*t*
plasmin, 72
plasminogen, 72
platelet function assay, defined, 142
platelet function assay (PFA), 145–146, 145–146*f*
platelet phase, 70
platelet plug, 71, 72*f*
platelets
 characteristics of, 70*t*
 defined, 64
 function of, 69
 reference laboratory values, 211, 212
pneumatic tube systems, 179, 182, 197, 197*f*
point-of-care testing (POCT), 144
policies and procedures, 189
polycythemia, 2, 59, 142, 147
polymorphonuclear leukocytes (PMNs), 64, 68, 174
polymorphs, 68
polys, 68
polyuria, 167, 171
popliteal artery, 48
popliteal vein, 48
portal of entry, 102
portal of exit, 101
positive communication, 18
postanalytical, 6
posterior cerebral arteries, 45
posterior intercostal arteries, 45
posterior intercostal veins, 48
posterior tibial artery, 48
postop test status, 126*t*
potassium, normal urine value for, 212
potassium oxalate, 114
potential hazards, in medical laboratories, 12
povidone-iodine, 110, 111
preanalytical, 6
precapillary sphincters, 42
precision, 6
prefixes
 commonly used, 24*t*
 defined, 23
pregnancy
 diagnosis of, 80, 176
 folic acid deficiency anemia in
 Rh antibodies and, 75
preop test status, 126*t*
preventive law, 5
primary atypical pneumonia, 87
probing venipunctures, 190

proficiency-testing program, 4
profiles, 11
prokaryotes, 83, 84
proliferation, 54, 60
protected health information (PHI), 189
protective (reverse) isolation, defined, 94
protein, normal urine value for, 212
proteinuria, 173
prothrombin, 64, 71, 211
prothrombin activator, 71, 72
prothrombin time (PT), 10
protime (PT), reference laboratory values, 211
protozoa, 83, 87
proximal convoluted tubule, 168
proximal tubules, 169
Public Health Act, 6
public space, 18
pulmonary arteries, 39
pulmonary circuit, 36, 37, 38, 44
pulmonary edema, 56
pulmonary embolism, 73
pulmonary valve, 36, 39
pulmonary veins, 39
pulse, 43
puncture lancets, 117
Purkinje fibers, 36, 38, 40
pus, 68
pyschiatric patients, phlebotomy for, 159

Q

QC samples (controls), 6
quackery, 2
quality assurance (QA)
    defined, 1
    in phlebotomy, 6
quality control log, 6, 7f
quality control (QC)
    defined, 1
    in phlebotomy, 6–7, 7f

R

RACE: Rescue Alert Confine Extinguish, 94, 95–96, 97f
radial artery, 45, 158, 158f
radio-frequency identification (RFID), 197–198
random urine specimens, 169
random-access memory (RAM), 193, 197
rapid arterial blood gas analyzer, 158, 158f
rapid plasma regain (RPR), 80
read-only memory (ROM), 193, 197
recapping of needles, mechanical devices for, 120
reclined position, defined, 142
recollection of specimens, 139, 162
record keeping, in medical laboratories, 12

red blood cell count
    defined, 65
    reference laboratory values, 212
red blood cells (RBCs)
    characteristics of, 70t
    defined, 64
    formation of, 67f
    function of, 65
    life cycle of, 68f
    RBC indices, formulas for, 201
    shape of, 66f
Reed-Sternberg cells, 54, 60, 60f
reference values, 142, 145
refractometer, 168, 172, 172f
Registered Phlebotomy Technician (RPT), 3
renal function panel, reference laboratory values, 211
renal profile, 78
renal thresholds, 168, 169
renal tubule, 168
renin, 168
requisitions, 79f, 124, 125f, 126f
reservoir host, 101
resident bacteria, 104
resistance, 88
resolution, 83, 89
respiration, 87
respiratory acidosis, 54, 56
respiratory isolation, 100
respondeat superior, 5
result reporting, 182
Rh blood group, 75
rheostat, 83, 89
rheumatic fever, 56
rheumatoid factor (RF), 80
Rickettsiae, 86
right atrioventricular (tricuspid) valve, 38
right subclavian vein, 48
"Right to Know Law," 97
ringworm, 87
routine test status, 126t

S

Safe Medical Devices Act of 1990, 5
safety
    latex allergies, 99, 100f
    overview, 94
    physical hazards, 94–98
safety manual, 103
safety needles, 120–121
safety showers, 103–104
safety transfer device, 133
salicylates, 142, 143
sanitation, 105–106
saphenous veins, 48
scarification, 2

security passwords, 198
sedatives, toxic level of, 212
segs, 68
seizures, 161, 162
semen specimens, 177
semilunar valves, 39
sensitivity testing, defined, 9
sepsis, defined, 54
septic shock, 57
septicemia, blood culture collection for, 157f, 111, 111f,
   156
septum, 36, 38
serologist, 10
serology laboratory, common tests performed in, 10, 80
serotonin, 64, 71
serum
   appearance of, 72
   defined, 64
   obtaining for testing, 71, 113, 118
sharp with engineered sharps injury protection (SESIP),
   120–121
sharps, 104
sharps containers, 120, 120f
sharps injury logs, 121
sharps injury prevention, 103f, 104
shock, 56–57
shunts, 142, 151
sickle-cell anemia, 59
sightless patients, caring for, 17
single-celled organisms, 84
sinoatrial node (SA node), 36, 40
social space, 17
sodium, normal urine value for, 212
sodium citrate, 113
sodium fluoride, 110, 114
sodium heparin, 114
software, 193, 196
source, 94, 106
specific gravity
   normal urine value for, 212
   urinalysis, 172, 172f
specimen collection trays, 119–120, 120f
specimen handling, 137–139, 179–181, 180f, 181t, 183t
specimen processing, 182, 183t
specimen requirements
   for chemistry tests, 78
   for common laboratory tests, 203–206
   rejection, 139
specimen tampering, 147
specimen transport, 180f, 181–182, 181f
sphygmomanometer, 43
spill cleanup, 98, 99f
spinal tap, 168, 177
Spirilla, 83, 84–87
splenic vein, 48
spores, 83, 86
sputum specimens, collection of, 176, 177f

standard of care, 190
standard precautions
   biologic hazards, 102
   blood-borne pathogens standard, 102–103
   defined, 94
   exposure control, 104
   hazardous wases, 103
   overview, 94
   safety showers/eyewash stations, 103–104, 104f
   sharps/needlestick injury prevention, 103f, 104
standards, 6
standing orders, 187, 189
Staphylococci, 84, 84–87
Stark law (1989), 188
STAT (stat) test status, 126t
state board of health, 4
stereotype
   defined, 15
   patient care and, 20
sterile, 104
sterilization, 106
stopper colors for evacuated tubes, 113–114, 114f
streptobacilli, 84
streptococcal infections, 80
Streptococci, 84, 84–87
stress, 20
stressors, defined, 1
strict liability torts, 5
stroke volume, 36, 43
subclavian vein, 127
suffixes
   commonly used, 24–25t
   defined, 23
superinfection, 84
superior hemiazygos veins, 48
superior mesenteric vein, 48
superior vena cava, 36, 38
suprapubic, defined, 168
suprapubic urine specimens, 170
surgical asepsis, 104
susceptible host, 94, 102
symbiosis, 88
symptomatology, 84, 87
syncope, 123, 125, 161, 162, 163f
syphilis, 78, 80
syringes, 114–115, 115f, 116f
systemic circuit, 36, 37, 44
systemic lupus erythematosus, 78, 80
systole, 36, 41
systolic blood pressure, 41
systolic pressure, 36, 43

T

T cells, 64, 69
teichoic acid, 84, 85f

telephone communication skills, patient care and, 18–19, 19f
temperature conversion formula, 201
teratogenic, defined, 94
teratogenic chemicals, 96
terminal (computer), 193, 196
test orders/requisitions, 79f, 124, 125f, 126f, 126t
test results, release of, 190
test status, 124, 126t
testing categories, 4
thalassemia, defined, 54
therapeutic drug monitoring
    specimen collection for, 149, 150t
    timed specimens for, 144–145
therapeutic medication, defined, 142
therapeutic phlebotomy, 2, 147
thermolabile, defined, 179
thixotropic gel, 110, 112, 123, 139
thoracic aorta, 45
thrombin, 64, 71
thrombin time, reference laboratory values, 211
thrombocytes, 64, 69
thrombophlebitis, 57
thrombopoietin, 64, 69
thrombus, 54, 55, 64, 73
thyrocervical arteries, 36, 45
thyroid antibodies, 80
thyroid profile, 80
thyroid-stimulating hormone (TSH), 80
thyroxine (T4), 80
timed specimens, 144–145, 169
timed test status, 126t
tinea (ringworm), 87
tinea barbae, 87
tinea pedis (athlete's foot), 87
tissue thromboplastin, 71
tone, of speech, patient care and, 17
topical, defined, 161
tort law, 4
total cholesterol, reference laboratory values, 212
total protein (TP), 78
Total Quality Management (TQM), 6
tourniquets, 111, 163
toxicology, reference laboratory values, 212
toxicology laboratory
    common tests performed in, 11
    specimen collection for, 149
    urine specimens for, 176
trace elements, 88
transfusion incompatibility reaction, 60
transient bacteria, 104
transmission-based precautions, 94, 100
transport globulins, 69
treatment, in medical microbiology, 88
treble damages, 188
Treponema pallidum, 80
treponemal antigen test, 78, 80

Trichomonas vaginalis, 87, 175
tricuspid valve, 36, 38
triglycerides, 78, 212
triiodothyronine (T3), 80
tripotassium EDTA, 114
troponin, 80
troponin 1, reference laboratory values, 211
trough, defined, 142
trough levels, 149
tuberculosis, risk of exposure to, 102
tularemia), 80
tularemia, defined, 78
tunica externa (tunica adventitia), 41
tunica interna, 41
tunica media, 41
turnaround time, 179
24-h urine specimens, 169–170
24-hour clock, 215
2-h postprandial blood glucose level test, 144
two-point check, 128

U

U-bag urine collection device, 77
ulnar artery, 158, 158f
ultrasonic sanitization, 105
uncooperative patients, 163–164
underfilled tubes, 112–113, 113–114
units of measurement, 201
universal donors, 74–75
universal precautions, 94, 100
universal recipients, 74
universal serial bus (USB), 193, 196
urea nitrogen, normal urine value for, 212
uric acid, normal urine value for, 212
urinalysis
    abbreviations related to, 170
    chemical analysis, 172–174, 173f
    microscopic analysis, 174–175
    overview, 168
    physical appearance, 171, 172t
    reference laboratory values, 170, 212
    specific gravity, 172, 172f
urinary system
    anatomy of, 168, 168f
    urine formation, 169
urinary tract infection (UTI), diagnosis of, 174
urine specimens
    collection of, 169–171
    transportation of, 171, 171t
urinometer, 168, 172, 172f
urochrome, defined, 168
U.S. Department of Health and Human Services (HHS), 4
U.S. Public Health Service, 100

V

Vacutainer systems, 111
Vacutainer tubes
    for common laboratory tests, 203–206
    for urine collection, 171
valves, 43
valvular heart disease, 56
varicose veins, 58
vascular access devices, 151
vascular phase, 70
vasoconstriction, 36, 41
vasodilation, 36, 41
vasomotor center, 44
vasomotor fibers, 41
vasospasm, 64, 70–71
vector, 88
"vein rolling," 111
veins, 36, 43, 48, 49f, 50f
veins of the arm, 127f
Velcro, defined, 110
venesection, 2
venipuncture
    with butterfly set, 133–134
    complications of, 161–164, 162f
    with evacuated tube, 128–131, 130–131f
    in geriatric patients, 155–156, 156t
    preparation for, 127
    with syringe, 132–133, 132–133f
venoconstriction, 44
venoscopes, 110, 111
venous access device, 150–151
ventricles, 36, 38
ventricular asystole, 54, 56
ventricular fibrillation, 54, 56
venules, 36, 43
verbal communication, 16
verbal permission, 125
vertebral arteries, 36, 45
viral envelope, 87

virions, 84, 87
virulence, 88
viruses
    defined, 84
    risk of exposure to, 102–103
    structure and function of, 87, 87f
viscosity, 36, 44
visually impaired patients, caring for, 17
vitamin B$_{12}$, 66
vitamin C, reagent strips and, 174
VLDL, reference laboratory values, 212
voided urine specimens, 170
volume, of speech, patient care and, 17

W

waived tests, 4
Washington, George, 2
WBCs count, reference laboratory values, 212
white blood cell count (WBC count), 69
white blood cells (WBCs), 64, 66–69
    characteristics of, 70t
    in urine, 175
whorls, 40, 137
winged infusion sets, defined, 109
winged needle set, 150
word roots, defined, 23
work practice controls, 103
working distance, 84, 89
written communication, patient care and, 18

Y

yeast, in urine, 175, 176f
young patients
    caring for, 17, 18
    phlebotomy for, 154, 154f

Credits

Chapter 1

1-1 Courtesy of National Library of Medicine

Chapter 5

5-3B © Phillipe Plailly/Photo Researchers, Inc.

Chapter 6

6-3 Courtesy of Leonard V. Crowley, MD, Century College, 6-4 Courtesy of National Cancer Institute

Chapter 7

7-8B © David M. Phillips/Visuals Unlimited

Chapter 9

9-1 © Michael Abbey/Visuals Unlimited; 9-3 Courtesy of Leonard V. Crowley, MD, Century College; 9-4C Courtesy of CDC

Chapter 10

10-2 © iStockphoto/Thinkstock; 10-3C (kitchen fire) © Michael Blann/Digital Vision/Thinkstock; 10-3D (Sodium chemical fire) © Andrew Lambert Photography/Photo Researchers, Inc.; 10-3E (large fire/explosion) © Scott Leman/ShutterStock, Inc.; 10-6 © Pedro Nogueira/ShutterStock, Inc.; 10-7 © Travis Klein/ShutterStock, Inc.

Chapter 11

11-12 Courtesy of Garrett Wade; 11-22 © FogStock/Thinkstock; 11-24 Courtesy of Garrett Wade

Chapter 16

16-3B Courtesy of Garrett Wade; 16-8, 16-9 © Dr. Frederick Skvara/Visuals Unlimited; 16-10 © Dr. Frederick Skvara/Visuals Unlimited/Getty Images; 16-11 © Custom Medical Stock Photo; 16-12 © MedicalRF.com/Custom Medical Stock Photo; 16-13 © Comstock/Thinkstock

Page xxii (photo of author) Courtesy of Garrett Wade

Unless otherwise indicated, all photographs and illustrations are under copyright of Jones & Bartlett Learning or have been provided by the authors.